ALLERGIES AND INFECTIOUS DISEASES

ANAPHYLAXIS

PRINCIPLES AND PRACTICE

Allergies and Infectious Diseases

Additional books in this series can be found on Nova's website under the Series tab.

Additional e-books in this series can be found on Nova's website under the e-book tab.

ALLERGIES AND INFECTIOUS DISEASES

ANAPHYLAXIS

PRINCIPLES AND PRACTICE

M. THIRUMALA KRISHNA
EDITOR

New York

For permission to use material from this book please contact us:
Telephone 631-231-7269; Fax 631-231-8175
Web Site: http://www.novapublishers.com

Library of Congress Cataloging-in-Publication Data

ISBN: 978-1-62618-688-0

Library of Congress Control Number: 2013936634

Published by Nova Science Publishers, Inc. † New York

Contents

List of Contributors		**vii**
Preface		**xi**
Chapter I	The Epidemiology of Anaphylaxis *Lucinda Brown and Katrina J. Allen*	**1**
Chapter II	Anaphylaxis: Clinical Approach and Differential Diagnosis *Lavanya Diwakar and S. Hasan Arshad*	**29**
Chapter III	Biomarkers of Anaphylaxis *Gabriel K. Wong and Aarnoud P. Huissoon*	**49**
Chapter IV	Management of Anaphylaxis *Priyanka Saxena Lall and Karen Demuth*	**69**
Chapter V	Food-Induced Anaphylaxis *Harshna Mehta and Scott H. Sicherer*	**83**
Chapter VI	Food-Dependent Exercise- Induced Anaphylaxis *Erick Prado de Oliveira and Roberto Carlos Burini*	**125**
Chapter VII	Anaphylaxis during General Anaesthesia *Silvia Caimmi, Naire Sansotta, Diego G. Peroni and Roberto Bernardini*	**135**
Chapter VIII	Non Steroidal Anti-inflammatory Drug-Induced Anaphylaxis *Mario Sánchez-Borges, Fernan Caballero Fonseca, and Arnaldo Capriles-Hulett*	**163**
Chapter IX	Hymenoptera Sting Anaphylaxis *M. Beatrice Bilo, Leonardo Antonicelli and Floriano Bonifazi*	**179**
Chapter X	Idiopathic Anaphylaxis *Anne Marie Ditto and Anjeni Keswani*	**227**
Chapter XI	Allergen Specific Immunotherapy and Systemic Reactions *Mark C. Glaum and Richard F. Lockey*	**251**

Chapter XII Primary Mast Cell Disorders and Anaphylaxis **263**
Jasper J. van Doormaal, Joanne N. G. Oude Elberink and Jan G. R. de Monchy

Index **297**

List of Contributors

Editor

Mamidipudi Thirumala Krishna MBBS, PhD, FRCP (Lond.), FRCPath (Lond.), DNB
Consultant Allergist and Immunologist
Head of Allergy, Birmingham Heartlands Hospital, Birmingham, UK
Honorary Senior Lecturer, University of Birmingham, UK
Honorary Fellow, University of Warwick, UK

Authors

Katie J. Allen MD
Professor and Paediatric Gastroenterologist and Allergist, Murdoch Childrens Research Institute, The Royal Children's Hospital, Melbourne, Victoria, Australia

Lucinda Brown RN, MPH
Murdoch Childrens Research Institute, The University of Melbourne, Department of Paediatrics, Melbourne, Victoria, Australia

Lavanya Diwakar MBBS, MSc (Health Economics), MRCP
Specialist Registrar, Immunology Department, Birmingham Heartlands Hospital, Birmingham, UK

Syed Hasan Arshad DM, FRCP
Professor of Allergy and Clinical Immunology and Honorary Consultant Physician, University of Southampton and Southampton University Hospitals NHS Trust, Southampton, UK

Aarnoud P Huissoon MB, PhD, FRCP, FRCPath Consultant Immunologist and Head of Immunology Department, Birmingham Heartlands Hospital, Birmingham, and Honorary Senior Lecturer, University of Birmingham, UK

Gabriel K. Wong MBBS, MSc, MRCP
Specialist Registrar, Immunology Department, Birmingham Heartlands Hospital, Birmingham, B9 5SS, UK

Karen A. DeMuth MD, MPH
Assistant Professor, Emory University School of Medicine, Emory Childrens Center, Atlanta, GA, US

Priyanka Saxena Lall, MD
Allergy and Immunology Fellow, Emory University School of Medicine, Emory Childrens Center, Atlanta, GA, US

Scott H. Sicherer MD
Professor of Pediatrics Division of Pediatric Allergy and Immunology, Jaffe Food Allergy Institute, Icahn School of Medicine at Mount Sinai, New York, New York, US

Harshna Mehta MD
Clinical Fellow, Allergy and Immunology Division of Pediatric Allergy and Immunology, Jaffe Food Allergy Institute Icahn School of Medicine at Mount Sinai New York, New York, US

Erick Prado de Oliveira MS
Researcher, UNESP - Medical School - Dept of Pathology,UNESP School of Medicine, Botucatu City, São Paulo State, Brazil

Roberto Carlos Burini PhD
University Professor and Researcher, UNESP - Medical School - Dept of Public Health, Botucatu City, São Paulo State, Brazil

Diego Peroni MD
Associate Professor, Department of Life and Reproduction Sciences, Pediatric Clinic Department of Pediatrics, University of Verona, Italy

Bernadini Roberto MD
Chief of the Pediatric Unit, "San Giuseppe" Hospital, Empoli, Florence, Italy

Sansotta Naire MD
Registrar, Department of Life and Reproduction Sciences, Department of Pediatrics, University of Verona, G.B. Rossi Hospital, Verona, Italy

Caimmi Silvia MD
Senior Registrar, Department of Pediatrics, University of Pavia, Policlinico San Matteo, Pavia, Italy

Mario Sánchez-Borges MD
Professor, Allergy and Clinical Immunology Department, Centro Medico-Docente La Trinidad and Clinica El Avila, Caracas, Venezuela

Fernan Caballero Fonseca MD
Professor, Allergy and Clinical Immunology Department, Centro Medico-Docente La Trinidad and Centro Medico de Caracas, Caracas, Venezuela.

Arnaldo Capriles-Hulett M.D.
Professor, Allergy and Clinical Immunology Department, Centro Medico-Docente La Trinidad and Centro Medico de Caracas, Caracas, Venezuela

M. Beatrice Bilò MD
Allergist and University Professor, Department of Allergy, Immunology and Respiratory Diseases, University Hospital Ospedali Riuniti - Ancona

Floriano Bonifazi MD
Director, Department of Allergy, Immunology and Respiratory Diseases, University Hospital Ospedali Riuniti – Ancona – Italy

Leonardo Antonicelli MD
Allergist and University Professor, Department of Allergy, Immunology and Respiratory Diseases, University Hospital Ospedali Riuniti – Ancona – Italy

Anjeni Keswani MD
Clinical Fellow Allergy and Immunology
Division of Allergy-Immunology,
Northwestern University Feinberg
School of Medicine, Chicago, IL, US

Anne M. Ditto MD, FAAAAI, FACP
Associate Professor in Medicine, Allergy and Immunology, Division of Allergy-Immunology, Northwestern University Feinberg School of Medicine, Chicago, IL, US

Richard F. Lockey M.D
Distinguished University Health Professor, Professor of Medicine, Pediatrics & Public Health & Director, Division of Allergy & Immunology, Joy McCann Culverhouse Chair in Allergy & Immunology, University of South Florida College of Medicine, Tampa, FL, US

Mark C. Glaum, MD PhD
Associate Professor of Medicine and Pediatrics, Division of Allergy and Immunology, University of South Florida College of Medicine, Tampa, FL, US

Jasper J van Doormaal MD PhD
Associate Professor of Internal Medicine, Department of Allergology, University Medical Center Groningen, University of Groningen, Groningen, The Netherlands

Joanne NG Oude Elberink MD PhD
Associate Professor of Allergology, Department of Allergology, University Medical Center Groningen and the Groningen Research Institute of Asthma & COPD, University of Groningen, Groningen, The Netherlands

Jan GR de Monchy MD PhD
Professor of Allergology, Department of Allergology, University Medical Center Groningen, University of Groningen, Groningen, The Netherlands

Preface

Anaphylaxis is a life threatening systemic reaction that almost always occurs unanticipated more so in a community setting. Even if symptoms are mild initially, the potential for progression to severe and irreversible outcome must be recognised and fatal reactions have been linked to delayed administration of epinephrine. Despite momentous advancement in our understanding of the pathogenesis of allergy and allergic diseases, the diagnosis and management of anaphylaxis remains a challenge for the allergist. Whilst the treatment of anaphylaxis in the acute setting has not changed over the years and epinephrine remains first line drug, there have been important in roads made with better diagnostic aids for the Allergist, in particular availability of superior *in vitro* allergy tests that are able to detect specific components of the allergen which offer greater specificity and help with 'risk stratification'. This has also added to the complexity of the subject. Furthermore, studies in the last decade have shed light on the spectrum of primary mast cell disorders which are associated with anaphylaxis and highlighted the importance of high baseline plasma tryptase as a useful surrogate biomarker for identifying 'high risk' patients.

The main objective of this project has been to improve patient care by offering the practising physician an evidence based 'problem oriented approach' in the diagnosis and management of patients with anaphylaxis from diverse aetiologies. Every chapter has tables and figures/algorithms in a simple format and special features of this book are 'Clinical Cases' to put the main text into clinical perspective for the reader as well as 'clinical pearls' summarising 'key take home messages'.

Anaphylaxis – Principles and Practice is a text book for specialists and Trainees/Fellows in Allergy and Clinical Immunology. This book has received invaluable contributions from a panel of international experts from UK, Italy, The Netherlands, North America, South America and Australia.

The chapter on 'Epidemiology' sets the scene and describes the burden of the problem across the globe and provides critical analysis of data relating to incidence, prevalence and mortality relating to anaphylaxis. The chapter on 'clinical features and differential diagnosis', is simple yet most informative on diverse clinical presentations and importantly provides an elegant description of conditions that masquerade as anaphylaxis. The chapter on management provides a systematic approach to treatment in the emergency room in children and adults based on recent international recommendations as well as long term management for the allergist and emphasises on allergen avoidance, provision of written emergency self-management plan including counselling of patient/care givers and training in the use of epinephrine auto-injectors. The chapter on 'Biomarkers' is another special feature of this book since there are not many recent comprehensive reviews on this topic and provides a critical evaluation of serum tryptase in diagnosis as well as describes potential role for 'novel biomarkers' in diagnosis and prognostication. The authors highlight the usefulness of serial measurements and lack of standardisation in interpretation of data.

There are separate chapters on various common aetiologies of anaphylaxis including food, Food-dependent exercise induced anaphylaxis (FDEIA), hymenoptera venom, non-steroidal anti-inflammatory drugs (NSAIDs), General Anaesthesia, allergen-immunotherapy and idiopathic anaphylaxis that provide an excellent systematic clinical approach for the reader when challenged with these conditions in routine clinical practice. These chapters have in particular embraced guidelines and recommendations from major international scientific societies and therefore give the reader 'best practice'. Finally, the chapter on primary mast cell disorders provides an useful overview of classification, clinical presentation, diagnostic criteria and management of these complex disorders and has colour slides depicting cutaneous mastocytosis. The authors are recognised international experts in this field and provide evidence from their own work and other international groups and distil the knowledge in an easily digestible format.

Finally, I would like to acknowledge the support of my wife Anuradha and daughter Kamya for their support whilst I was working on this project and sincerely thank all the authors for their time, effort and priceless contributions without which this project would not have been successful and it has been such a great pleasure, honour and privilege to work with them.

I hope you find this book easy to read and a useful reference to possess in your office. Happy Reading !!

Dr. Mamidipudi T. Krishna PhD, FRCP, FRCPath, DNB
Editor
Consultant Allergist and Immunologist, Head of Allergy,
Heart of England NHS Foundation Trust, Honorary Senior Lecturer,
University of Birmingham & Honorary Fellow, University of Warwick, UK
Email: mtkrishna@yahoo.com

Other Affiliations

Dr. M. T. Krishna is Chair of Specialist Training Committee and Training Programme Director for Immunology, W. Midlands Deanery, Birmingham, UK & member of Standards of Care Committee (SOCC) and audit lead for British Society for Allergy and Clinical Immunology (BSACI). He is lead author of BSACI guideline for Hymenoptera Venom Allergy and co-author for guidelines on beta lactam allergy and immunotherapy for allergic rhinitis.

Conflicts of Interest Declaration

Dr Krishna's department has received funding for educational activities from ALK Abello, Phadia, MEDA and Allergy Therapeutics in recent years.

Disclaimer

The content of this book is correct to the best of authors' and editors knowledge. However, medical science is ever changing. The authors and editor do not assume any liability for any injury or damage to persons or property arising from this publication.

In: Anaphylaxis: Principles and Practice
Editor: M. Thirumala Krishna ISBN: 978-1-62618-688-0

Chapter I

The Epidemiology of Anaphylaxis

***Lucinda Brown*[1,2] *and Katrina J. Allen*[1,2,3,*]**

[1]Murdoch Childrens Research Institute
[2]The University of Melbourne Department of Paediatrics
[3]Department of Allergy and Immunology,
Royal Children's Hospital, Melbourne, Australia

Abstract

There is now clear evidence that the incidence of anaphylaxis is rising in developed countries most likely as a reflection of the recently described phenomenon of rising rates of food allergy. Although anaphylaxis in children is most commonly food-induced, idiopathic and drug anaphylaxis are important triggers in adults. Risk factors linked to fatality from anaphylaxis include nut-induced anaphylaxis, co-existent asthma and adolescence and young adults. From a global perspective, the true rate of occurrence of anaphylaxis from all possible triggers in the general population is probably largely unknown because to date there have not been large population-based studies, other than the retrospective analysis of hospital admissions.

Estimates of the incidence of anaphylaxis range from 10.8 per 100,000 hospital admissions in Australia up to 36 per million in the United Kingdom whilst up to 1.03 million emergency department visits per year in the United States have been reported to be related to anaphylaxis. Until recently there had been little consensus on the definition of anaphylaxis but improved recent classifications will enable a better understanding of the epidemiology of this important condition in the future.

[*] Corresponding author: Professor Katrina J. Allen - Murdoch Childrens Research Institute. The Royal Children's Hospital, 50 Flemington Road, Parkville 3052, Victoria, Australia, email: katie.allen@rch.org.au. Phone: +613 99366585 Fax: +613 90905251.

Introduction

Anaphylaxis admissions has increased in the developing world with reports from Australia demonstrating a doubling in the last decade (Figure 1), with similar increases in the US, UK and Europe. Initially regarded as an uncommon occurrence at the turn of the 20th Century, anaphylaxis today has become an important clinical and public health challenge which can affect people of any age or gender.

A literature review by the American College of Allergy, Asthma and Immunology Working Group on Anaphylaxis highlighted significant gaps in the understanding of the epidemiology of anaphylaxis. In particular the review stated "An improved epidemiologic understanding of this disorder would aid ongoing efforts to reduce morbidity and mortality from anaphylaxis and could provide important clues for primary prevention" [1].

This chapter seeks to help readers understand the incidence of anaphylaxis and how it varies by age and region. We outline the commonest triggers for anaphylaxis as well as discuss the risk factors for mortality. Importantly we outline why this area of our understanding has been undermined by the difficulty in adequately defining the syndrome of anaphylaxis with recent guidelines and recommendations making some progress into a more systematized approach to this important area of allergy.

Definition of Anaphylaxis

Attempting to determine the population prevalence of anaphylaxis is made difficult because of varying clinical opinions about what constitutes anaphylaxis. Clearly variation in definition severely hampers our ability to accurately describe the incidence of anaphylaxis [2].

To understand the epidemiology of a condition it is necessary that clear and simple definitions of the condition to be studied exist, and here anaphylaxis presents a problem; there is a continuum of severity in allergic reactions and within this continuum there are variations in the combinations of symptoms, which contribute to this severity.

Non life-threatening anaphylaxis can present with dramatic and obvious signs and symptoms whilst fatal reactions may present with few or no signs and symptoms prior to cardiac or respiratory arrest [3]. None of the available definitions are ideal, primarily because not all anaphylactic responses are generalized and multi-systemic [4] although acute allergic reactions can be fatal, without being generalized. [3]

Despite this many of the definitions in common use around the globe include phrases such as: "as a *serious allergic reaction* that is rapid in onset and might cause death"; and "a serious, life threatening *generalized* or systemic hypersensitivity reaction". The definitions from the American Academy of Allergy, Asthma and Immunology (AAAAI) and the Australasian Society of Clinical Immunology and Allergy (ASCIA) are two of the most commonly utilized definitions globally. Both organizations have attempted to ensure that the definitions avoid generic terminology.

In 2006 the AAAAI developed a definition of anaphylaxis as one of three clinical scenarios:

1) 'the acute onset of a reaction (minutes to hours) with involvement of the skin, mucosal tissue or both and at least one of the following: a) respiratory compromise; b) or reduced blood pressure or symptoms of end-organ dysfunction;
2) two or more of the following that occur rapidly after exposure to a likely allergen for that patient – involvement of the skin/mucosal tissue, respiratory compromise, reduced blood pressure or associated symptoms and/or persistent gastrointestinal symptoms;' or
3) 'reduced blood pressure- after exposure to a known allergen [5]'.

ASCIA provides a simpler working definition of anaphylaxis as:

– 'any acute onset of hypotension or bronchospasm or upper airway obstruction where anaphylaxis is considered possible, even if typical skin features are not present'
  OR
– 'any acute onset illness with typical skin features (urticarial rash or erythema/flushing, and/or angioedema), PLUS involvement of respiratory and/or cardiovascular and/or persistent severe gastrointestinal symptoms (particularly for insect allergy)'.

A recent consensus document, developed by the World Allergy Organization in consultation with over 100 allergy and immunology specialists on over 6 continents, has defined anaphylaxis as a "serious allergic reaction that is rapid in onset and may cause death," and proposed diagnostic criteria for use in clinical care [2, 6]. Using this criteria, a diagnosis of anaphylaxis can be made if there is involvement of the respiratory or cardiovascular systems during an allergic reaction, or if a less severe reaction occurs in the setting of previously diagnosed allergy and likely exposure to the relevant allergen.

Anaphylactoid or pseudoallergic reactions, in the past have not been categorised as anaphylaxis. These types of reactions can be clinically indistinguishable from anaphylaxis but are not mediated by an antigen–IgE antibody interaction. In contrast the release of mediators results from an antigen acting directly on mast cells and basophils, or the antigen acting on other cascades such as anaphylatoxins of the complement system or prostaglandins and leukotrienes from arachidonic acid metabolism [1]. The same systemic manifestations as anaphylaxis occur during these reactions. Recently the World Allergy Organization (WAO) proposed the elimination of the term ''anaphylactoid reaction''and that all episodes clinically similar to typical IgE-mediated anaphylactic reactions be called anaphylaxis. They also recommended that 'anaphylaxis be divided into two types of reactions; immunologic and non-immunologic, the latter being synonymous with the older term, ''anaphylactoid." The WAO further recommend that the immunologic anaphylactic reactions be divided into two 'types' - those mediated by IgE mast cell/basophil mediator release and those occurring through other immunologic mechanisms (e.g., certain transfusion reactions)' [5].

From an epidemiological point of view it is important that there is consistency in the diagnosis of anaphylaxis which includes careful history taking and observation of clinical signs at the time of the event. There are a number of factors that should be included when doing an assessment of a person with anaphylaxis. These should outline a detailed history of the episode, which has included information about all exposures and events in the hours preceding the onset of symptoms; for example 'exercise, ingestion of prescription, non prescription and recreational drugs, ethanol, acute infections such as a cold, emotional stress, travel or other disruption to routine and premenstrual status in females' (Figure 2, Simons et al. 2011). The World Allergy Organization guidelines suggest that the "key to diagnosis involves pattern recognition: sudden onset of characteristic symptoms and signs within minutes to hours after exposure to a known or potential trigger often followed by a rapid progression of symptoms and signs over hours." Each anaphylactic episode can differ, not only in the same patient but also from one patient to another with regards to the symptoms, signs and the pattern that includes the onset, number and course of the signs and symptoms. As each episode begins it can be difficult to predict the rate of progression or the ultimate severity.

In some patients anaphylaxis can be difficult to diagnose, and if anaphylaxis is missed or attributed to another concomitant condition this can impact on the accuracy of prevalence estimates. For example: 'patients with impaired vision or hearing, neurologic disease, psychiatric illness such as depression; mental health disorders such as; substance abuse, autism, spectrum disorder, attention deficit hyperactivity disorder or cognitive disorders, might have diminished awareness of anaphylaxis triggers and symptoms. Diagnosis of anaphylaxis in patients with concomitant respiratory and cardiovascular conditions such as asthma, chronic obstructive pulmonary disease or chronic heart disease can be difficult as the signs and symptoms of these diseases can be attributed to deterioration of the underlying disease rather than anaphylaxis. Use of CNS-active medications such as sedatives, hypnotics, antidepressants and first generation sedating H1-antihistamines concurrently, can interfere with patient recognition of anaphylaxis triggers and symptoms and also with the ability of the patient to describe symptoms' [7].

From a global perspective, the true rate of occurrence of anaphylaxis from all possible triggers in the general population is probably largely unknown because to date there has not been a large population-based study of its incidence other than retrospective analysis of hospital admissions. These reports may be undermined by a variety of factors including under-recognition of anaphylaxis by patients, caregivers and health professionals, and under reporting in the acute setting [7]. Due to the varied diagnostic criteria for anaphylaxis, globally, the true incidence of the disease continues to remain a significant point of debate.

Prevalence and Incidence of Anaphylaxis

Knowledge of the actual incidence and prevalence of anaphylaxis in the population is a vital resource for public health policy and allocation of resources. This knowledge could aid governments and organizations in making choices about appropriate clinical resource allocations. Precise estimates are needed to ensure adequate research funding is made available to improve prevention and find a cure. This knowledge could also be a valuable aid in recognizing and defining the scope of the problem and ensuring that changes in prevalence and severity are documented [8]. The 2006 literature review by the WAO highlighted that there were gaps in relation to describing the population prevalence of people at high risk of experiencing anaphylaxis; and the inability to accurately ascertain those who are at greatest risk of adverse outcomes were also highlighted [7].

According to Pumphrey (3) the diversity between the statistical findings in population studies of the epidemiology of anaphylaxis can be attributed to 'differing inclusion criteria and imprecise use of terms such as incidence and prevalence' [3]. Pumphrey [3] in his book chapter 'an Epidemiological Approach to Reducing the Risk of Fatal Anaphylaxis' makes a very significant point, which should be considered when discussing the incidence and prevalence of anaphylaxis within the population. He states that: 'the imprecise use of the term incidence and prevalence, in some of the reports on the epidemiology of anaphylaxis may cause confusion'. The *incidence* of a condition is the *rate of appearance of new cases* and Pumphrey discusses how many studies, which have reported on the incidence of anaphylaxis, have generally reported the incidence of the reactions, not of 'new cases' [3]. Many of the studies recorded that most of the patients are not new cases even though they are presenting with an acute reaction as they have a history of previous reactions.

Prevalence occurs at a given time within a defined population. Prevalence is 'the probability *that an individual chosen at random will have the condition, and* is usually given as a percentage or cases per 100,000' [3]. When a person has an anaphylactic reaction it is because someone with an allergic predisposition has been exposed to a trigger in a way that will cause an anaphylactic reaction. Confusions can arise if definitions include those at risk of anaphylaxis rather than those who have actually experienced an episode of anaphylaxis. Comparison of the natural history and anaphylaxis incidence and prevalence between existing studies is difficult, mainly due to the discrepancies between, and deficits in, the various study designs, and definitions used for anaphylaxis [2]

Additionally the prevalence of anaphylaxis in the population has been difficult to quantify accurately because of the various methodologies utilized for data collection and because of the various sample populations that have been analysed (eg., emergency department presentations, hospital admissions, general practitioner presentations, specialist allergist presentations) [21].

According to recent reports incidence of anaphylaxis is rising in a number of countries including Australia [9], the United Kingdom [10], and the United States [11, 12]. Reports of an increasing incidence of food-induced anaphylaxis hospital admissions were recently confirmed in Australian study by Liew and colleagues [2, 9]. Similar findings were reported in the UK and France by Pumphrey and Stanworth [13] and Moneret-Vautrin and Kanny [14], and in Italy it was reported by Novembre et al [15] that half of the anaphylactic cases treated in the emergency departments were due to food allergy.

Reports from Australia suggest that the incidence of anaphylaxis based on the International Classification of Disease (ICD) codes may be as high as 1 per 1000 ICD presentations [16], yet if a study utilizes hospital admission rates to determine incidence of anaphylaxis there appears to be a much lower estimate of 10.8 per 100,000 hospital admissions, in Australia [17] and 36 per million in the UK [10]. The limitations with using ICD codes include inclusion of only admitted cases, diagnostic coding inaccuracies and reliance on a database from a single hospital, which may not be representative of national data. The United States reflect similar increases in hospital admissions due to allergy related anaphylaxis. One study found that in the period from 1993-2004 there were a total of 12.4 million allergy-related ED visits, which represents 1.0% (95% confidence interval, 0.93%-

1.10%) of all ED visits or 1.03 million ED visits per year [18]. Neugut et al estimated in their investigation into the epidemiology of anaphylaxis in the United States, that anaphylaxis affects between 1.21% to 15.04% of the US population, and 3.29 million to 40.9 million individuals at risk of anaphylaxis. [19]. The known rates or cases of anaphylaxis were: 0.0004% for food, 0.7% to 10% for penicillin, 0.22% to 1% for radiocontrast media, and 0.5% to 5% after insect stings. There were 220 cases of anaphylaxis reported after exposure to latex [19]. As with other forms of anaphylaxis, the true incidence of idiopathic anaphylaxis is unknown, but some studies suggest that increasing numbers of cases are being seen in the United States with 6% to 31% of reported anaphylaxis cases classified as idiopathic [16, 20]. Patterson's study reasoned that they could therefore, by extrapolation of the cases of idiopathic anaphylaxis reported by the allergists surveyed (approximately 4000 allergists in the United States) estimate the number of cases of idiopathic anaphylaxis in the United States population as between 20,592 and 47,024 [20].

Rising Incidence of Anaphylaxis

The increasing incidence of atopy and allergic disease globally are possibly based on two paradigms; a) that there is the same amount of people with atopic disease but an increased presentation of episodes of allergic disease; or b) the underlying prevalence of predisposing allergic disease is increasing e.g. food allergy.

Incidence of anaphylaxis is rising in Australia [9] (Figure 1), the UK [10], and the US [21]. The youngest age group appears to have the most pronounced rise in the incidence of anaphylaxis with the most common trigger being food [9]. Recent reports suggest that this increase in food-induced anaphylaxis is consistent with the increased prevalence of food allergy in the general population [4]. Food as the primary trigger for anaphylaxis in Australia are reported to account for between 33.2-56% of all anaphylaxis cases [22]. The literature seems to support that some of the important drivers in the trend towards a relatively high and increasing incidence of food-induced anaphylaxis in young children may be early life factors [24]. Liew et al. [9], confirm that there has been an overall rise, in Australia, of 350% for anaphylaxis that is food-induced over the previous 11 years. In the UK, hospital admissions for anaphylaxis rose seven-fold from 50 to 360 per 100,000 population in a period of 13 years from 1990/1 to 2003/4. [10]

The highest rate of hospital admissions for food-induced anaphylaxis (9.4 per 100,000 population) occurred in children who were under five years old, and interestingly this age group also had the greatest increase in the rate of hospital admissions over time [9].

In the developed westernized countries the most common anaphylaxis presentation amongst the adult population was due to drug-induced anaphylaxis. Most deaths due to drug-induced anaphylaxis occur between the ages of 60-85 years [9], and it is estimated that in 2004/2005 there has been an increase of 150% in drug-induced anaphylaxis over an 8-year period to 2.6 per 100 000 population [9].

Time trends of fatal anaphylaxis were examined by Liew et al., (Figure 1) [9] and these suggested that despite the anaphylaxis rates increasing overall, fatal outcomes from food-induced anaphylaxis remain stable. Liew et al. also showed that in the past decade there has been a decrease in insect sting anaphylaxis fatalities of 88% (data on insect sting anaphylaxis admissions were not available) [9].

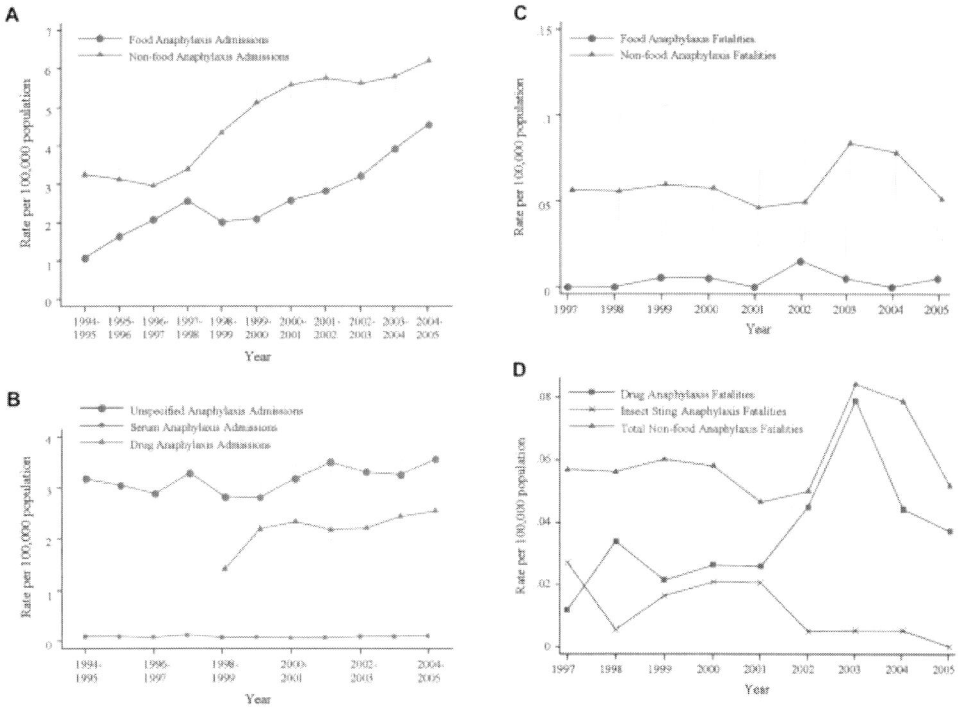

Figure 1. Time trends for food-induced and non–food–induced anaphylaxis admissions and fatalities in Australia. A, Time trends for food-induced and non–food-induced anaphylaxis admissions show increasing admission rates. B, Time trends for non–food-induced anaphylaxis admissions categorized by cause. C, Time trends for food-induced and non–food-induced anaphylaxis fatalities have remained stable despite increasing admissions. D, Time trends for non–food induced anaphylaxis fatalities, with drug-induced and insect sting–induced anaphylaxis deaths shown separately. Data show increasing drug-induced anaphylaxis deaths but decreasing insect sting–induced anaphylaxis deaths [9].

The juxtaposition between this and the fatality rates from drug induced anaphylaxis is of significant concern, with Liew et al. [9] noting that there had been more than a 300% increase in the death rates from drug-induced anaphylaxis in the last 10 years. This is greater than the rise in admissions for drug-induced anaphylaxis. The need for further research to improve on the diagnosis and management of drug allergy is highlighted by these figures [9].

In addition to Liew et al., others have also made the observation that whilst the 0-4 year old age group has the most admissions for food-induced anaphylaxis, teenagers and young adults have the highest mortality rate [9]. During Liew's study there were seven deaths in Australia, due to food-induced anaphylaxis [9]. All these deaths occurred in individuals who were aged between 5-34 years of age.

There is a marked disparity between this and hospital admissions for drug-induced anaphylaxis and deaths, which occur most commonly in adults, particularly in those over 55 years of age. Similarly all insect sting-induced anaphylaxis fatalities were aged 15 years or over [9]. Liew et al. also observed that most admissions were in males under 15 years, and after this age there was a distinct sex switch with women more commonly admitted among adults [9]. This gender switch has also been observed to occur in the underlying prevalence of both food allergies and other allergic conditions such as asthma [23].

Studies conducted in the US have found that, whilst food remains the primary culprit for anaphylaxis, insect stings are the second most common cause, accounting for 18.5% of anaphylactic reactions, followed by medications which account for 13.7% of anaphylactic cases [21].

Factors Associated with Increased Incidence of Anaphylaxis

Allergic disease, and thus by default anaphylaxis, appears to be more prevalent in 'Westernised countries'. There is one hypothesis which suggests that factors which are responsible for the changes in prevalence are those associated with progressive lifestyle changes [24]. The support for this hypothesis arises from the studies which show that allergic disease is occurring more rapidly in these Westernized countries than any possible changes to the genome could occur [24]. According to Prescott and Allen [24] there are a number of factors that are associated with this hypothesis, particularly in regards to the increase in food allergy, and these include: 'declining microbial exposure [25], an increased pro-inflammatory modern diet [26] and inhaled pollutants associated with motor vehicles and the rise in traffic.' An increase in asthma and inhalant sensitization has been associated with these factors yet there has been no definitive evidence to show these factors as contributory and this may be due to multifactorial lifestyle factors. The sequential differences in susceptibility to inhaled vs food related allergic diseases, or the rationale behind changing relationships between allergic disease persistence and severity are also not explained by these hypothesized factors [24]. Prescott and Allen suggest that whilst food allergy specifically continues to rise, there has been a plateauing and subsequent decline in asthma in highly Westernized areas, which may indicate that there are additional risk factors at play [24]

Because food allergy is more common in developed than developing countries and migrants seem to acquire the incident risk of allergy of their adopted country, it seems likely that the cause of the rise is linked to the "modern lifestyle." Although environmental factors including those associated with the hygiene hypothesis and dietary factors have been found to be associated with the development of eczema and atopy, there has been little investigation into whether they may also impact food allergy development [24].

In addition to factors previously linked to allergic disease in general there may well be some factors that are specific to food allergy. These might include changing methods of food manufacturing and preparation, the advent of widespread use of antacids and proton pump inhibitors, use of medicinal creams containing food allergens, or the introduction of allergenic foods at a later stage into the diet of infants [24].

The literature suggests that vitamin D insufficiency could be a lifestyle factor that may lead to an increased risk of food allergy and thus by default food-induced anaphylaxis. A number of studies have explored the relationship between anaphylaxis and latitude and their findings support this rationale [23]. In Australia Mullins et al. [27] explored the regional variation in the prescription of adrenaline auto injectors by studying emergency department visits in Australia. It became apparent that once demographic factors, such as socioeconomic status and access to medical care, including specialist allergy care were controlled, the Southern regions of Australia which have less sunlight year around, had a higher prescription rate of EpiPens when compared to the Northern regions [23, 27]. The regional differences were greater in children whose ages were less than 5 years, with the differences between far northern Queensland and far Southern Australia being six-fold (383 vs. 2318 per 100,000 population per year) [27]. Mullins et al. [27] further discussed how admissions for anaphylaxis in the southern regions had a higher incidence, with food induced anaphylaxis accounting for 42% of cases, but found that there was no statistical significance in the association between anaphylaxis admission rates and latitude [27]. The highest admission rates for anaphylaxis occurred in children who were less than 5 years of age. Children under the age of 5 years had the highest incidence of anaphylaxis admissions (22.3 per 100,000 population per year) [27], with 81% of admissions in this age group attributed to food [27]. Mullins' findings are consistent with a study by Carmargo et al. in 2007 [28], which explored the differences in EpiPen prescriptions by latitude in the United States. A recent study by Rudders et al. [29] described similar findings to those of Mullins and Carmargo [27, 28]. Rudders et al. [29], investigated acute allergic reactions (including anaphylaxis) emergency department visits and found that the North-Eastern regions (which have less sunlight) had a higher incidence of visits to the emergency department because of acute allergic reactions than the Southern regions, particularly among visits due to food-induced allergic reactions. This is an inverse association to the Southern hemisphere [27].

Factors Determining the Risk and Severity of Anaphylaxis

One of the most pronounced risk factors is age, with the incidence of anaphylaxis occurring most commonly in children less than 5 years of age. Hospitalization (suggesting more severe disease expression) due to food-induced anaphylaxis also occurs most frequently in this age group [6]. An important research priority should be working towards the recognition of risk factors for severe adverse reactions, including anaphylaxis [30]. Recently, using data from electronic medical records two large cohort studies confirmed that a significant risk factor for anaphylaxis was concominant asthma with those individuals with severe asthma demonstrating the highest risk of all [31].

Patients with other concomitant chronic respiratory disease also have increased risk [31]. Reported risk factors for either an increased risk or increase in the severity of anaphylaxis include, 'cardiovascular disease [7], mastocytosis or clonal mast cell disorders [7], [32], and severe atopic disease such as allergic rhinitis' [33]. Medications such as beta-adrenergic blockers and angiotensin-converting enzyme (ACE) inhibitors when taken concurrently might also increase the risk of anaphylaxis [34-38]. Additionally, defects in mediator degradation pathways leading to elevated bradykinin (because of low serum ACE activity) and a low serum platelet activation factor acetylhydrolase activity may be connected with episodes of severe, or fatal, anaphylaxis [33, 39, 40]. There are a number of co-factors which are reported to increase the risk of an anaphylaxis episode and these can include premenstrual status in females, emotional stress, upper respiratory tract infections and other acute intercurrent infections, fever, and disruptions in routine or travel [7].

Exercise is the most common and well known of the co-factors that may increase the risk of anaphylaxis [7]. As Simmons et al. [7] discuss, this often involves the ingestion of a specific food in conjunction with exercise, most commonly wheat/omega-5 gliadin, celery or shellfish. However diverse ranges of foods have been implicated in this syndrome. The concomitant ingestion of a non-steroidal anti-inflammatory drugs or ethanol may increase the risk of this syndrome as they can enhance intestinal permeability and allergen absorption thus increasing risk of anaphylaxis [11, 33].

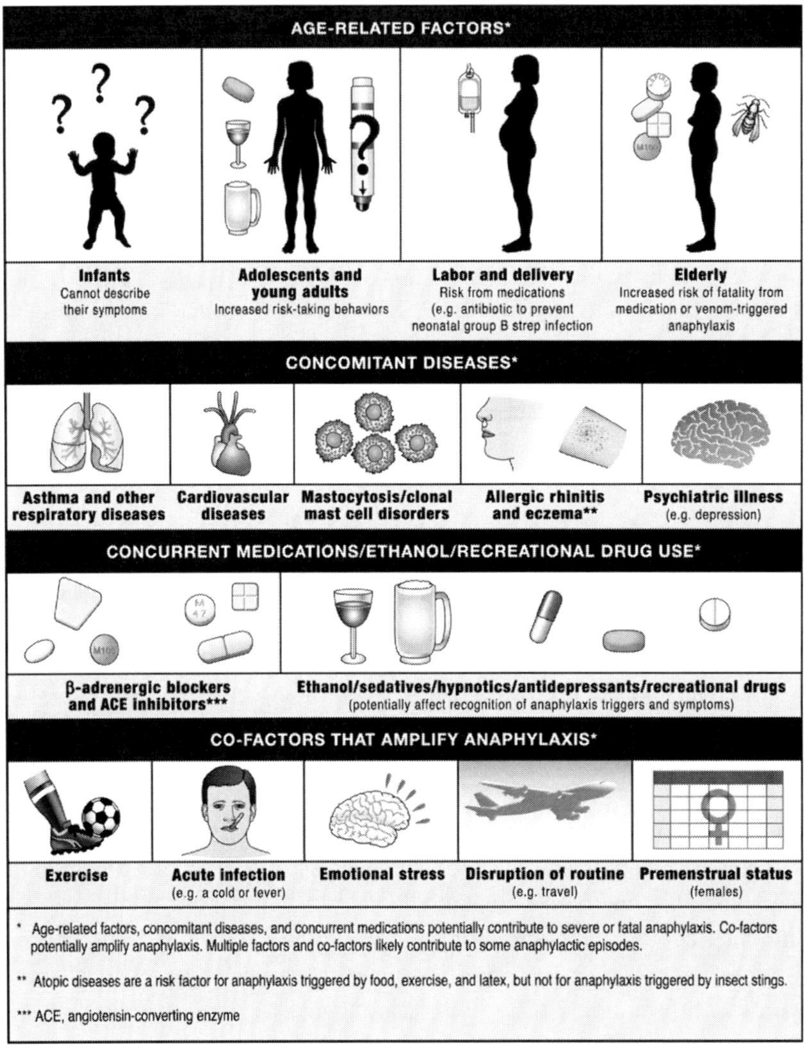

Figure 2. Patient factors that contribute to anaphylaxis. Age-related factors, concomitant diseases, and concurrent medications potentially contribute to severe or fatal anaphylaxis. Cofactors potentially amplify anaphylaxis. Multiple factors and cofactors likely contribute to some anaphylactic episodes. For relevant references, please see the Fig 1 legend published online at www.jacionline.org. Beta blockers, b-adrenergic blockers; ACE inhibitors, angiotensin-converting enzyme inhibitors [41].

One of the most challenging aspects of caring for patients who are at risk of anaphylaxis is our inability to predict who will or will not develop anaphylaxis. In the absence of either predictive factors or biomarkers the only historical factor at hand is that those with a history of a previous anaphylactic reaction are at higher risk of a further episode than those who have never had an episode. However one report describes a patient series in which 80% of those presenting with anaphylaxis had only ever had a mild reaction previously [17]. It would be unethical to prospectively challenge all patients to the point of anaphylaxis and events within the community are low enough that large population cohorts would need to be mounted in order to confidently characterize better predictors of anaphylaxis. As a result most clinicians continue to rely on a risk-management algorithm that errs on the side of caution. Additionally assessing the level of risk is further complicated because in a given individual this is not static but may change over time thus warranting ongoing assessment and review by the health care provider is needed for the individual with anaphylaxis.

A positive allergy test (whether serum specific IgE antibody or skin prick test) will not accurately indicate how severe the allergic reaction will be, simply how likely.

From a study undertaken in 2008 in Manchester, UK [33], collated data suggests that the severity of coexisting atopic disease could predict the likelihood of a patient having anaphylaxis to peanuts and tree nuts. A previous history of rhinitis was linked to increased risk of upper airway oedema during anaphylaxis; and patients with pre existing asthma were more likely to present with predominantly an asthmatic mode of anaphylaxis [3, 33]. A recent large population-based study by Gonzalez-Perez et al. [42] supported these findings that a person with asthma has an increased risk of anaphylaxis, and those with severe and/or poorly controlled asthma may have an even higher risk.

Data was collected through the examination of a UK health database of 2.1 million people for individuals aged between 10-79 years, who had had at least one health contact with their registered general practitioner in the year before entering the study and who had been registered with that general practitioner for at least 12 months. The study group all had an asthma diagnosis and consisted of 177,000 individuals. Of these, 45,103 were identified as having severe asthma (defined as either hospitalization or any of the following medication use in a 1-year period: prescriptions for oral corticosteroids, prescriptions for inhaled *b*2 agonists, or classes of asthma medications). The anaphylaxis incident rate was estimated at 34.4 per 100 000 person years with incidence higher in women than in men, double that in the group with-severe asthma and three-times greater in the group with severe asthma. The most common cause of anaphylaxis in this study was: drug allergies (27%), followed by food (24%), and insect stings (12%) [42].

Similar findings were reported in a study conducted by Iribarren et al. [43] in northern California. The data found that patients with asthma had a 5.2-fold higher incidence of anaphylaxis than those patients without asthma. This study also found a clear and significant relationship between groups with food-induced anaphylaxis and food-related anaphylaxis, with the non severe asthma group having a hazard ratio of 5.05 (95% confidence interval [CI] 4.39–5.80), and the severe asthma group having a hazard ratio of 8.23 (95% CI 6.59–10) [43] [23].

Finally Summers et al., in Manchester identified an additional and novel risk factor for predicting the severity of an anaphylactic reaction. They found that if a patient had a low serum concentration of angiotensin converting enzyme (ACE), life threatening pharyngeal oedema was more likely to develop during anaphylaxis [33].

The Role of Race and Gender in Anaphylaxis

Whilst gender disparities in the prevalence of some allergic disorders including allergic asthma have been well delineated [24], the relationship between food allergy and gender is less clear [44]. While asthma is more common in young boys, many studies have reported that a gender switch occurs around the time of puberty with asthma being more common and severe in women [45-46], perhaps due to hormonal changes occurring during puberty [45]. This gender switch is also evident in clinical presentations with food allergy, however this has not yet been formally explored at the population level [24].

Similarly, racial and ethnic differences in asthma prevalence have also been well described, whereas there have been fewer studies which have explored the impact that ethnicity has on the likelihood of developing allergy or anaphylaxis [24]. Even though there are lower rates of allergic disease in populous countries like Asia, it does not mean that these ethnic and racial groups are less susceptible to allergic disease. There is growing evidence that when living in a 'westernised environment' Asian populations may be more susceptible to allergic disease [47, 48, 24].

Lack et al. [47] in their 2003 article discussed how earlier studies of respiratory disease found that Asian Australians had a higher incidence of sensitisation and allergic symptoms than in non Asian Australians. An Australian study recently found a higher rate of food-sensitized eczema among children of Asian descent. On examination of risk factors for eczema development (a closely associated infantile allergic disease) the study found that Asian children were not only more likely to have eczema than their non-Asian counterparts but that their parents were less likely to have allergic disease than non-Asian parents [24].

Asian populations in particular appear to be highly susceptible to food allergy [48], suggesting that a Western environment can amplify an existing strong genetic propensity. This is consistent with earlier work indicating evolutionary differences in genetic polymorphisms affecting candidate genes [49]. Prescott and Allen state that this has major global implications as areas in Asia become more industrialized, urbanized and Westernized this may have a significant impact on the prevalence and incidence of allergic disease [24].

Causes and Triggers of Anaphylaxis

This section of the chapter will discuss the most common causes or triggers for anaphylaxis from an epidemiological viewpoint; these are discussed in further detail later in the book.

Triggers of anaphylaxis in specific age groups tend to be universal. In terms of immunological triggers of anaphylaxis there are three principal triggers (Figure 3) of anaphylaxis, these are foods, insect stings and drugs. The incidence rate of these triggers each contributes to the anaphylaxis figures in different regions will vary according to study population, design or geographical area [50]. In children, adolescents and young people the most common trigger of anaphylaxis is food; whilst in middle-aged and elderly adults, the commonest triggers are insect stings, medications and idiopathic anaphylaxis [7]. Whilst many of the specific triggers are universal, it is important to note that there are a number of specific geographical variations that have been reported (see Figure 3).

Food-Induced Anaphylaxis

The prevalence of food-induced anaphylaxis is increasing and at a global level food is one of the most common triggers for an allergic reaction. Anaphylactic cases that are food-induced vary by age, gender and region. The leading cause of anaphylaxis in most studies is food allergy [51], also comprising 30% of fatal cases [5]. Food allergic reactions also account for 33-50% of anaphylaxis presentation in North American, European, Asian and Australian emergency departments [52]. In Australia, the UK and US hospitalization due to food-induced anaphylaxis is most commonly due to peanuts, tree nuts, and seafood [53]. There have been increasing reports from many countries around the world, of episodes of anaphylaxis occurring to a more diverse range of foods which traditionally have not been commonly linked to anaphylaxis [23].

Asero et al. [54] investigated into incidence of anaphylaxis in an Italian population (age 12-79 years, mean = 31 years [n=1100]). Allergic reactions were diagnosed by clinical history and positive skin prick test (SPT) or serum specific IgE. The authors [54] reported that 5% of food allergic individuals experienced at least one episode of anaphylaxis with lipid transfer protein (LTP) being the commonest cause (n=19), closely followed by 10 and 9 cases of anaphylaxis due to shrimp and tree nuts respectively. It was interesting to note that there was only one case of peanut-induced anaphylaxis in this group [54].

Asero et al. [54] study also supports the paradigm that the scope of foods as triggers for allergic reactions, including anaphylaxis, can vary significantly from region to region and country to country. They found that LTP was an important allergen causing food- induced anaphylaxis in Italy, and the most common food causing food-induced anaphylaxis being peach [54]. There are a number of reports that suggests that lupin, which belongs to the legume family, is a newly emerging food allergen in Europe [54]. Producers are increasingly using lupin flour in the production of bakery products in France and Mediterranean countries. Whilst a number of cases of anaphylaxis due to the ingestion of lupin flour have been reported in these countries [55], the true prevalence in the general population is not known.

A recent Finish study [56] using SPT reported a sensitization rate of 1.6% (25 out of 1522) to lupin in patients presenting between 2005-2007 with a suspected food allergy. Eighteen of these patients were sensitized to other legumes such as pea, soy or peanut. A previous study carried out in Portugal reported a higher sensitization rate of 4.1% [57]. Other studies have shown that sesame seed in the Middle East [58-60], celeriac in Switzerland [61], and foods such as rice, buckwheat, birds nest soup and chickpea, in Asian countries have been linked to food induced allergic reactions [7]. The triggers of food related anaphylaxis can differ according to specific food exposures, local dietary habits and food preparation techniques, methods [7]. There is potential for future researchers using a sizeable unselected community population to systematically test for food allergy by employing the 'gold standard' of oral food challenges, to definitively and accurately assess prevalence of clinical IgE-mediated food allergy in this age group [62]. The main limitation of most studies thus far is that the data on prevalence is based on utilization of questionnaires using 'parental' or 'self reporting' which can potentially lead to overestimation. Some population studies have also used a SPT as a means of confirmation of food allergy, but there are very few large scale studies which have confirmed the prevalence of food allergy, objectively through the use of of oral food challenge/s [24].

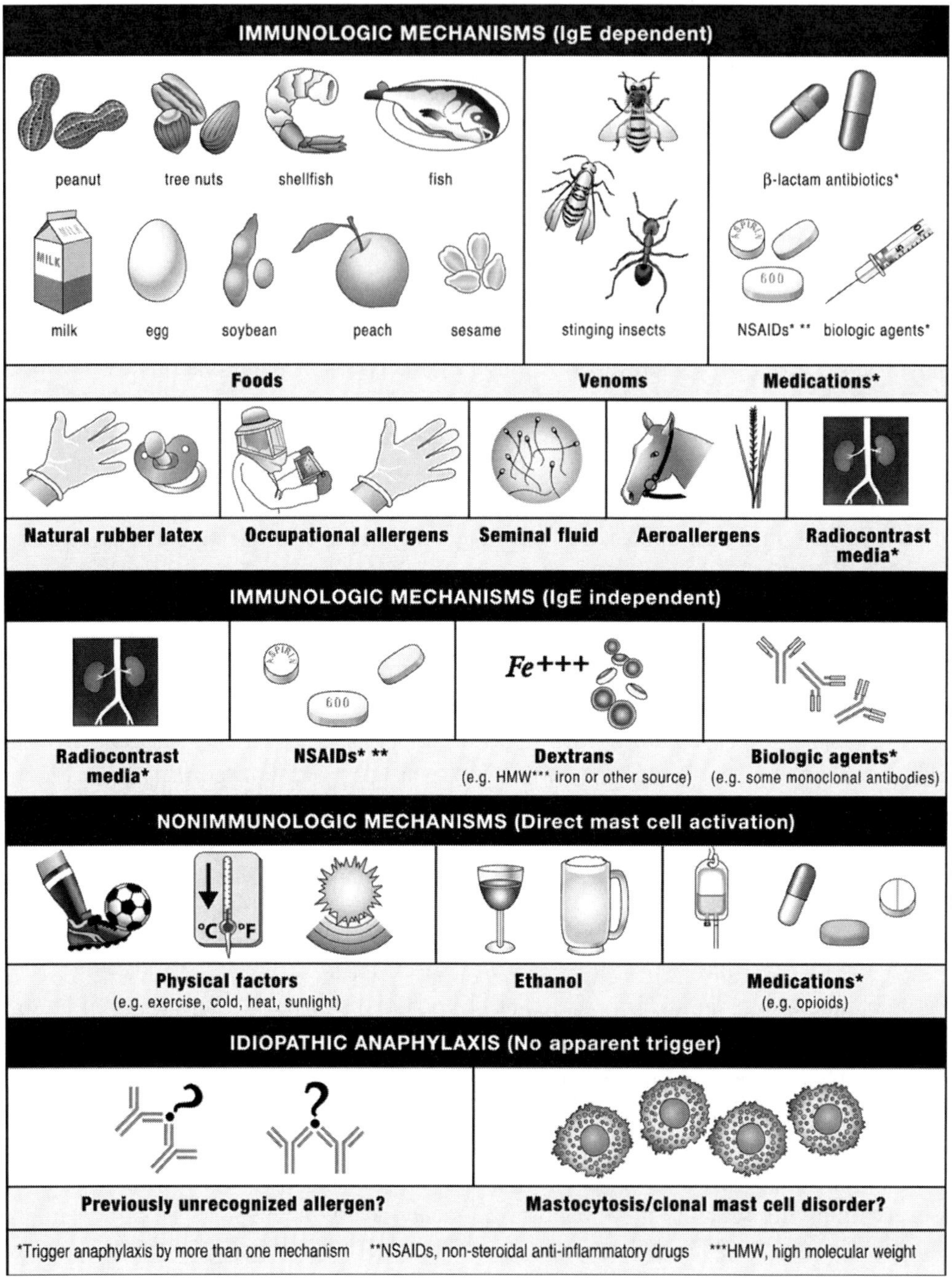

Figure 3. Anaphylaxis mechanisms and triggers. Anaphylaxis typically occurs through an IgE-dependent immunologic mechanism, most commonly triggered by foods, stinging insect venoms, or medications. Medications can also trigger anaphylaxis through an IgE-independent immunologic mechanism and through direct mast cell stimulation. Radiocontrast media can trigger anaphylaxis through both IgE dependent and IgE-independent mechanisms. In patients with idiopathic anaphylaxis, the possibility of a novel allergen trigger or of underlying mastocytosis or a clonal mast cell disorder should be considered. For relevant references, please see the Figure 2 legend published online at www.jaionline.org. HMW, High molecular weight; NSAID, nonsteroidal anti-inflammatory drug [41].

To date the Australian HealthNuts study is the only 'large-scale single-centre, population-based cross-sectional study of food allergy in 12-month-old' that has been conducted [24].

Current or accurate prevalence data is not available in most regions and there is a paucity of data in the age group most commonly impacted – infants and children under 3 years of age.

This study could be considered internationally unique, as the results were precise and unbiased due to the fact that it utilized a large population based sample (n=5300) and had a high community participation rate of 73% [24]. High rates of atopy were identified in the preliminary analysis of the first infants (n=2828), with 18% showing sensitization to food. Additionally up to 10% of the 12 month-old infants were found to have an IgE mediated food allergy that was proven by oral food challenge. Common allergens identified through the oral food challenges were egg and peanut occurring in 8.9% and 3.0% of the population respectively. This report confirmed that, even after adjusting for participation bias, Australia currently has a food allergy rate that is higher than has ever been reported previously [24].

Exercise-Induced Anaphylaxis

Exercise Induced Anaphylaxis (EIA) is rare. The prevalence of EIA, triggered purely by exercise, in comparison to food dependent EIA (FDEIA) that requires food and exercise is not known, although the latterhas been reported more frequently [63]. EIA is characterized by symptoms due to mast cell mediator release, which occurs within the setting of physical exertion. Most people with EIA still exercise regularly, however attacks of EIA are unpredicible and can occur irregularly [5]. Exercise, which is vigorous, such as jogging, dancing, and racquet sports, is most commonly associated with EIA, although even lower levels of exertion in an exercise regime, such as walking briskly may be a trigger in some people [64]. Once exercise ceases, or treatment is received there is usually an immediate improvement or symptoms will resolve over a number of hours. The incidence of fatal anaphylaxis in EIA is not known, although there has been a report of at least on death [65].

Important factors for FDEIA include ingestion of specific food followed by exercise within 4-6 hours of consumption [66]. Typically the person individually tolerates food and exercise independently [64]. Seafood, nuts, wheat and other grain types are the foods most commonly implicated [66], although over the past decade there has been an increase in the reporting of a diverse spectrum of foods associated with EIA, including, soy [in tofu] and peach [23].

Important co-factors include non-steroidal anti-inflammatory drugs (NSAIDS) [64, 67]; alcoholic beverages; menstruation [68]; or seasonal pollen exposure in pollen sensitized persons. According to Lieberman et al. [5] these events, and co-factors, when causing fatal anaphylaxis, are often under and misdiagnosed, resulting in a dearth of accurate statistics around EIA.

The majority of reports which have investigated the epidemiology of EIA on a population scale, have been conducted in Korea [69] and Japan [70, 71] as there is a high incidence of hospital admissions for anaphylaxis which have been accredited to EIA (up to 14%) [72]. It is indeterminate whether these reports reflect a higher prevalence of EIA in these countries when compared with other countries, or the increase in reporting is due to better awareness, and thus associated reporting, in Asian countries [23]. Females are more commonly affected by EIA than males, and the majority of cases of EIA occur in individuals <30 years of age [72,73].

Insect Stings

Similar to food there are differences in the native insect populations between continents and even between regions. As a result of these differences iand in types of exposure to different stinging or biting insects, the risk of anaphylaxis will also differ. The exposure to stinging insects, and thus the number of stings, is also seasonal and will differ between Northern and Southern hemispheres, for example in the UK fatal sting reactions occurs predominately May-November, peaking in August when the wasp population is at its highest [3]. Extensive studies of the relationship between stinging insects [order Hymenopetera] and anaphylaxis have only been conducted in Australia, Europe and North America. In Australia venom from the stings of bee's, ants and wasps are accountable for up to 18% of fatal anaphylactic reactions in the population [9]. There have been no studies that optimally investigate anaphylaxis triggered by biting insects such as mosquitoes (order Diptera) and ticks (order Acarnia) [30].

There are clinical differences in insect-induced anaphylaxis, which exist between children and adults [5]. In children, 60% will have cutaneous signs and symptoms as the sole manifestation whilst in adults it occurs in only 15% [74]. Individuals who are stung and experience a large localised reaction, or who are children with mild cutaneous reactions, will have a low [5-10%] chance of a systemic reaction to the sting. This will vary in adults to between 25% and 70% depending on the severity of previous sting reactions [75, 76]. Anaphylaxis to insect stings occurs in approximately 3% of adults and 1% of children within the population [77]. Respiratory signs and symptoms occur in 50% of both adults and children. Hypotension is uncommon in children but occurs in over 60% of adults, with over 50% of these experiencing a loss of consciousness [74].

Risk factors for anaphylaxis to honeybee or vespid stings were published by Rueff et al. [37] in 2009 from a multicenter study. The study found that within the study group there was a strong association with severe anaphylaxis for those people who had a higher baseline serum tryptase level. eg., Angiotensin converting enzyme inhibitors regardless of the individual's age, can increase the risk for insect-induced anaphylaxis occurring to honeybee or vespid stings [37]. Other factors includevespid venom allergy, male gender, older age, and a previous history of mild-moderate systemic reaction to a sting [37]

Between 2001-2006 a study was conducted by Rudders et al. [29] in Boston which investigated the characteristics and treatment requirements of patients [n=153] who had a hypersensitivity to stinging insects and who presented to one or more of 3 emergency departments. Both Rudders [29] and Liew et al. [9] in their respective studies found that fatal anaphylaxis from insect stings tends to occur in adults 35-84 years with more males than females affected. The median age in the study conducted by Rudders et al. was 33 years and they reported that males constituted 54% of the 153 cases [29], whilst Liew et al. stated that 19/20 [95%] of cases were male [9]

Medications

In 2011 Thong and Tan published a review of the epidemiology of drug allergy and found that the true incidence of drug allergy is unknown [78]. The majority of epidemiological studies, which are currently available, have not focused on drug allergy specifically but rather have been focused on adverse drug reactions (ADRs) [79]. Studies from Australia [9], the United Kingdom [80, 81] and New Zealand [82] have identified that the most common cause of fatal anaphylaxis in adults are drug induced.

The most common drug related anaphylactic triggers universally are: Antimicrobial, antiviral and antifungal agents, with variation among countries; for example, in countries where intramuscular penicillin is used for rheumatic fever it is a common trigger as are anti-tuberculosis medications relatively more common in some countries [30]. Non Steroidal Anti Inflammatory drugs (NSAID) can commonly trigger anaphylaxis that is medication specific within this pharmacological class, and is not related to other NSAID associated diseases such as asthma, rhinitis, and nasal polyps [30]. In their review Thong and Tan also identified that one of the most common causes of IgE-mediated anaphylaxis are drugs, in particular penicillin and general anaesthetic agents administered during peri-operative period [78]. The review also identified that common triggers for non allergic anaphylaxis are radio contrast media and NSAIDs [78].

In the review there were several limitations identified for obtaining an accurate picture on the epidemiology of medication-induced anaphylaxis. These included: differences in study populations (i.e., children, adults, ethnic differences) resulting in a limited comparability between studies. Many of the studies did not differentiate between the types of drug sensitivity (i.e., immunological vs non immunological) and there were a variety of methodologies reported (i.e., spontaneous vs. nonspontaneous reporting), and the diagnosis of drug allergy varied greatly from study to study with many studies not including validated *in-vivo* or *in-vitro* tests [23, 78].

Anaesthetic-Induced Anaphylaxis

Anaphylaxis to anaesthesia is a rare and serious adverse reaction [6]. In the summary article on the definition and management of anaphylaxis Sampson et al. [6] stated that the incidence of anaesthetic-induced anaphylaxis varies between 1:3500 and 1:20,000, the reported mortality rate is approximately 4% with an additional 2% surviving, but with severe brain damage [83].

Natural Rubber Latex [NRL]

In the last decade there has been a dramatic fall in incidence of new reported cases of NRL allergy and anaphylaxis. Current studies which have found low prevalence rates suggest that the peak of the latex allergy epidemic has already passed in health care workers (HCWs) [84]. Hospital-wide interventions which have impacted on prevalence rates have included strategies which require the use of low-allergen gloves to reduce sensitization and changing available gloves to nonlatex ones, or even using low-allergen latex gloves, appears to confer adequate secondary prevention [85].

The literature shows that spina bifida patients are at a high risk of becoming sensitised, and in turn allergic, to latex allergens [86]. Studies in the 1990's showed variations in prevalence of sensitization to NRL with reports that about half the children who had spina bifida had become sensitised to latex [87-89]. One study had a reported prevalence rate of latex sensitisation in children at 64.5% [90].

As a result of studies conducted in the 1990's the majority of hospitals and centres who treat children with spina bifida have implemented primary prevention programs, with a focus on latex-free surgical procedures as well as avoidance of latex in the general environment [85]. In recent years the few studies on latex sensitisation that have been published, report that sensitisation rates can be reduced if prevention strategies such as the use of powder-free latex gloves for health care workers are implemented [86, 91-93].

Vaccines and Anaphylaxis

Mild local reactions and fever after vaccinations are common and do not contraindicate future doses [94]. Although there are some adverse reactions to vaccines that constitute absolute contraindications to administration of future doses, most such reactions do not preclude subsequent immunization [95]. Anaphylactic reactions after vaccination are rare [94].

After reviewing the diagnostic codes from the medical encounters, in the United States, following the administration of more than 7.5 million doses of vaccines, the Vaccine Safety Data link estimated the risk of anaphylaxis post vaccination to be 0.65 to 1.53 per million doses [96].

Children with egg allergy can safely receive measles, mumps and rubella immunisation following changes to manufacturing of this vaccine although care is still needed for children with a history of egg anaphylaxis who wish to receive the influenza vaccine [95, 97].

Idiopathic Anaphylaxis

Idiopathic anaphylaxis is a diagnosis of exclusion. It is diagnosed when 'no trigger can be identified despite a detailed history of the episode, allergen skin tests, measurement of serum IgE levels to obvious and potentially hidden allergen triggers' [6, 41]. Idiopathic anaphylaxis exists in all age groups [98] but has some variation according to gender. Ditto et al. [99] in their literature review of over 335 cases of idiopathic anaphylaxis reported that that 65% of their cohort were women. Similar results were reported in a smaller study conducted by Tejedor et al. [100] with 68% of the 81 cases identified as women.

Mortality and Anaphylaxis

Data from national mortality reporting systems in the United Kingdom and Australia estimate the prevalence of anaphylaxis fatalities from all causes (including food, medication, insect sting, and idiopathic) to be 0.33 deaths per year per million population in the United Kingdom [101], with Australia reporting the highest rate of 0.64 deaths per year per million population [9] (Figure 4).

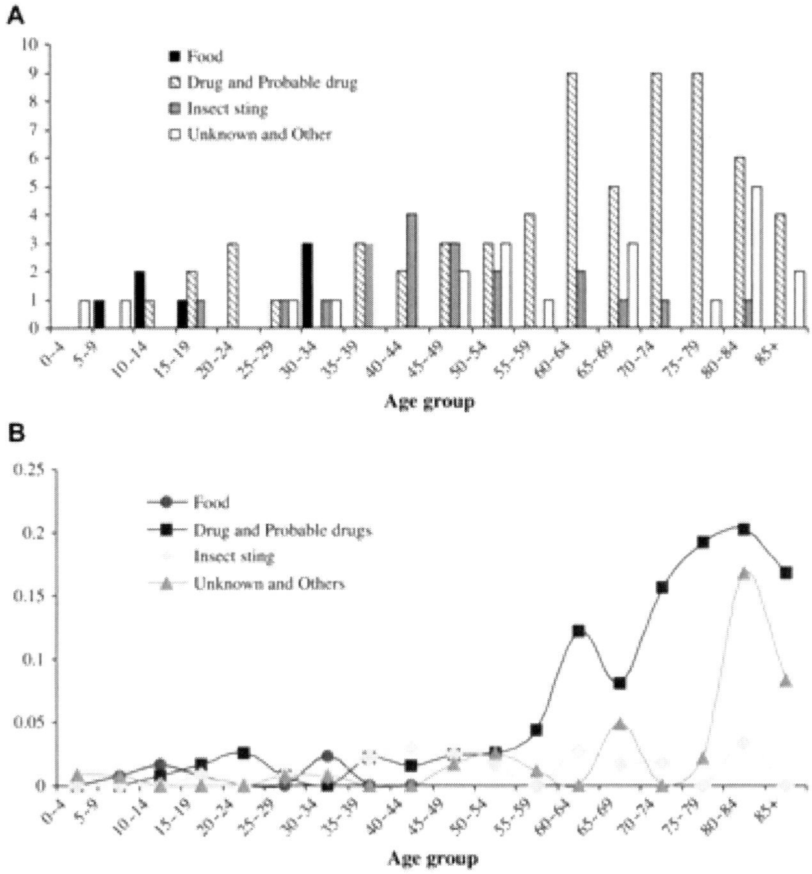

Figure 4. Anaphylaxis fatalities. A, Absolute number of anaphylaxis deaths by cause and age group. B, Anaphylaxis death rates by cause and age group [9].

For as yet undetermined reasons in Australia only 6% of anaphylaxis deaths are ascribed to food-induced anaphylaxis compared with 31% in the United Kingdom [2].

Risk factors for a poor outcome from an episode of anaphylaxis vary from trigger to trigger, but all includes age, gender and region/country. For example, with food-induced anaphylaxis, risk is highest in adolescence and young adults, and for anaphylaxis from honey bees, males with a median age of 33 are more at risk [29].

The common themes that have emerged specifically to fatal anaphylactic reactions to foods are:

- Anaphylactic reactions to food can occur after the first known exposure [72].
- Most victims are adolescents or young adults who typically have a known food allergy [5].
- Reactions commonly involve peanuts and tree nuts [52].
- Asthma is a risk factor for mortality, with severity of other atopic diseases also being a contributing factor [2, 9, 33]. In a study of fatal food allergic reactions the majority of patients had underlying asthma [102].
- Presentation of life threatening food-induced anaphylaxis may be characterized by only respiratory and cardiovascular symptoms, without any cutaneous manifestations showing [103].
- Bi-phasic reactions have been reported in 25% of fatal or near-fatal food-induced anaphylactic reactions, making this phenomenon more common in food-induced anaphylaxis than related to other causes [103].
- In most cases of food-induced anaphylaxis the serum tryptase has not been elevated [72].

Conclusion

In conclusion our understanding of anaphylaxis is constantly changing and evolving as ongoing studies elicit new data as to causes and triggers of this condition. The diversity between the statistical findings, in population studies of the epidemiology of anaphylaxis, will hopefully diminish as inclusion criteria and terminology becomes consistent at a global level. The last few years has seen an increased focus on better defining the prevalence of allergy and anaphylaxis and studies are now emerging that attempt to understand the drivers of the rise in prevalence. As for other allergic diseases, the cause of the rise in anaphylaxis is likely to be multifactorial. Improved precision about measurement of allergy outcomes and epidemiologic exposures and the advent of improved inclusion criteria and terminology is likely to accelerate the uncovering of alleged causative factors.

Clinical Pearls

- Clear figures on the incidence and prevalence of anaphylaxis are difficult to ascertain due to only recent consensus on a case definition
- The overall incidence of anaphylaxis has been estimated to be between 1-36 per 100,000 hospital admissions in Australia, the United Kingdom and the United States
- The prevalent cause of anaphylaxis is different in children and adults.
    - Children are more likely to have anaphylaxis due to food-related triggers
    - Adults more likely to have anaphylaxis triggered by drugs or idiopathic reasons
- There are regional variations of food triggers for anaphylaxis, depending on dietary and environmental factors

- Food-induced anaphylaxis appears to be increasing with the underlying increase of food allergy in general
- Asthma and adolescence are risk factors for mortality from anaphylaxis

Acknowledgment

Figures 1-4 reproduced with permission.

References

[1] Lieberman P, Camargo CA, Jr., Bohlke K, Jick H, Miller RL, Sheikh A, et al. Epidemiology of anaphylaxis: findings of the American College of Allergy, Asthma and Immunology Epidemiology of Anaphylaxis Working Group. *Ann. Allergy Asthma Immunol.* 2006 Nov; 97 (5):596-602.

[2] Allen KJ KJ. The Epidemiology of IgE-Mediated Food Allergy and Anaphylaxis. *Immunol. Allergy Clin. North Am.* 2012; 32:35-50.

[3] Pumphrey RS. An Epidemiological Approach to Reducing the Risk of Fatal Anaphylaxis. In: M C, editor. *Anaphylaxis and Hypersensitivity Reactions.* Ist edition ed. New York: Humana Press; 2011. p. 376 pages.

[4] Johansson SG, Bieber T, Dahl R, Friedmann PS, Lanier BQ, Lockey RF, et al. Revised nomenclature for allergy for global use: Report of the Nomenclature Review Committee of the World Allergy Organization, October 2003. *J. Allergy Clin. Immunol.* 2004 May; 113 (5): 832-6.

[5] Lieberman P, Nicklas RA, Oppenheimer J, Kemp SF, Lang DM, Bernstein DI, et al. The diagnosis and management of anaphylaxis practice parameter: 2010 update. *J. Allergy Clin. Immunol.* 2010 Sep; 126 (3):477-80 e1-42.

[6] Sampson HA, Munoz-Furlong A, Bock SA, Schmitt C, Bass R, Chowdhury BA, et al. Symposium on the definition and management of anaphylaxis: summary report. *J. Allergy Clin. Immunol.* 2005 Mar; 115 (3):584-91.

[7] Simons FER, Ardusso LRF, Bilò MB, El-Gamal YM, Ledford DK, Ring J, et al. World Allergy Organization anaphylaxis guidelines: summary. *The Journal of Allergy and Clinical Immunology.* 2011; 127 (3): 587-93.e1-22.

[8] Atkins D, Bock SA. Fatal anaphylaxis to foods: epidemiology, recognition, and prevention. *Curr. Allergy Asthma Rep.* 2009 May; 9 (3): 179-85.

[9] Liew WK, Williamson E, Tang ML. Anaphylaxis fatalities and admissions in Australia. *J. Allergy Clin. Immunol.* 2009 Feb; 123 (2): 434-42.

[10] Gupta R, Sheikh A, Strachan DP, Anderson HR. Time trends in allergic disorders in the UK. *Thorax.* 2007;62 (1): 91-6.

[11] Sampson HA, Munoz-Furlong A, Campbell RL, Adkinson JNF, Bock SA, Branum A, et al. Second symposium on the definition and management of anaphylaxis: Summary report--Second National Institute of Allergy and Infectious Disease/Food Allergy and Anaphylaxis Network symposium. *Journal of Allergy and Clinical Immunology.* 2006; 117 (2):391-7.

[12] Soar J, Pumphrey R, Cant A, Clarke S, Corbett A, Dawson P, et al. Emergency treatment of anaphylactic reactions--guidelines for healthcare providers. *Resuscitation.* 2008 May; 77 (2):157-69.
[13] Pumphrey RS, Stanworth SJ. The clinical spectrum of anaphylaxis in north-west England. *Clin. Exp. Allergy.* 1996 Dec; 26 (12):1364-70.
[14] Moneret-Vautrin DA, Kanny G. [Food-induced anaphylaxis. A new French multicenter survey]. *Annales de gastroenterologie et d'hepatologie.* 1995 Sep; 31 (4):256-63.
[15] Novembre E, Cianferoni A, Bernardini R, Mugnaini L, Caffarelli C, Cavagni G, et al. Anaphylaxis in children: clinical and allergologic features. *Pediatrics.* 1998 Apr; 101 (4):E8.
[16] Braganza SC, Acworth JP, McKinnon DR, Peake JE, Brown AF. Paediatric emergency department anaphylaxis: different patterns from adults. *Archives of disease in childhood.* 2006 Feb; 91 (2):159-63.
[17] Poulos LM, Waters AM, Correll PK, Loblay RH, Marks GB. Trends in hospitalizations for anaphylaxis, angioedema, and urticaria in Australia, 1993-1994 to 2004-2005. *J. Allergy Clin. Immunol.* 2007 Oct; 120 (4):878-84.
[18] Gaeta TJ, Clark S, Pelletier AJ, Camargo CA. National study of US emergency department visits for acute allergic reactions, 1993 to 2004. *Ann. Allergy Asthma Immunol.* 2007 Apr; 98 (4):360-5.
[19] Neugut AI, Ghatak AT, Miller RL. Anaphylaxis in the United States: an investigation into its epidemiology. *Arch. Intern. Med.* 2001 Jan 8; 161 (1):15-21.
[20] Patterson R, Hogan MB, Yarnold PR, Harris KE. Idiopathic anaphylaxis. An attempt to estimate the incidence in the United States. *Arch. Intern. Med.* 1995 Apr 24; 155 (8):869-71.
[21] Decker WW, Campbell RL, Manivannan V, Luke A, St Sauver JL, Weaver A, et al. The etiology and incidence of anaphylaxis in Rochester, Minnesota: a report from the Rochester Epidemiology Project. *J. Allergy Clin. Immunol.* 2008 Dec; 122 (6):1161-5.
[22] Gold MS. EpiPen epidemic or good clinical practice? *J. Paediatr. Child Health.* 2003 Jul; 39 (5):376-7.
[23] Koplin JJ, Martin PE, Allen KJ. An update on epidemiology of anaphylaxis in children and adults. *Current Opinion In Allergy And Clinical Immunology.* 2011; 11 (5):492-6.
[24] Prescott S, Allen KJ. Food allergy: riding the second wave of the allergy epidemic. *Pediatr. Allergy Immunol.* 2011 Mar; 22 (2):155-60.
[25] Strachan DP. Family size, infection and atopy: the first decade of the "hygiene hypothesis". *Thorax.* 2000 Aug;55 Suppl 1:S2-10.
[26] Black PN, Sharpe S. Dietary fat and asthma: is there a connection? *Eur. Respir. J.* 1997 Jan;10 (1):6-12.
[27] Mullins RJ, Clark S, Camargo CA, Jr. Regional variation in epinephrine autoinjector prescriptions in Australia: more evidence for the vitamin D-anaphylaxis hypothesis. *Ann. Allergy Asthma Immunol.* 2009 Dec; 103 (6):488-95.
[28] Camargo CA, Jr., Clark S, Kaplan MS, Lieberman P, Wood RA. Regional differences in EpiPen prescriptions in the United States: the potential role of vitamin D. *J. Allergy Clin. Immunol.* 2007 Jul; 120 (1): 131-6.
[29] Rudders SA, Espinola JA, Camargo CA, Jr. North-south differences in US emergency department visits for acute allergic reactions. *Ann. Allergy Asthma Immunol.* 2010 May;104 (5):413-6.

[30] Simons FE, Ardusso LR, Bilo MB, Dimov V, Ebisawa M, El-Gamal YM, et al. 2012 Update: World Allergy Organization Guidelines for the assessment and management of anaphylaxis. *Curr. Opin. Allergy Clin. Immunol.* 2012 Aug; 12 (4):389-99.

[31] Greenberger PA, Rotskoff BD, Lifschultz B. Fatal anaphylaxis: postmortem findings and associated comorbid diseases. *Ann. Allergy Asthma Immunol.* 2007 Mar; 98 (3):252-7.

[32] Brockow K, Jofer C, Behrendt H, Ring J. Anaphylaxis in patients with mastocytosis: a study on history, clinical features and risk factors in 120 patients. *Allergy.* 2008 Feb; 63 (2):226-32.

[33] Summers CW, Pumphrey RS, Woods CN, McDowell G, Pemberton PW, Arkwright PD. Factors predicting anaphylaxis to peanuts and tree nuts in patients referred to a specialist center. *Journal of Allergy and Clinical Immunology.* 2008; 121 (3): 632-8.e2.

[34] Lieberman P. Use of epinephrine in the treatment of anaphylaxis. Curr Opin Allergy Clin Immunol. 2003 Aug;3[4]:313-8.

[35] Müller U, Haeberli G. The problem of anaphylaxis and mastocytosis. *Current Allergy and Asthma Reports.* 2009; 9 (1):64-70.

[36] TenBrook J, John A., Wolf MP, Hoffman SN, Rosenwasser LJ, Konstam MA, Salem DN, et al. Should [beta]-blockers be given to patients with heart disease and peanut-induced anaphylaxis? A decision analysis. *Journal of Allergy and Clinical Immunology.* 2004 2004/5;113 (5): 977-82.

[37] Rueff F, Przybilla B, Bilo MB, Muller U, Scheipl F, Aberer W, et al. Predictors of side effects during the buildup phase of venom immunotherapy for Hymenoptera venom allergy: the importance of baseline serum tryptase. *J. Allergy Clin. Immunol.* 2010 Jul; 126 (1): 105-11 e5.

[38] Caviglia AG, Passalacqua G, Senna G. Risk of severe anaphylaxis for patients with Hymenoptera venom allergy: Are angiotensin-receptor blockers comparable to angiotensin-converting enzyme inhibitors? *J. Allergy Clin. Immunol.* 2010 May; 125 (5):1171; author reply -2.

[39] Schwartz LB. Diagnostic value of tryptase in anaphylaxis and mastocytosis. *Immunol. Allergy Clin. North Am.* 2006 Aug; 26 (3): 451-63.

[40] Komarow HD, Hu Z, Brittain E, Uzzaman A, Gaskins D, Metcalfe DD. Serum tryptase levels in atopic and nonatopic children. *J. Allergy Clin. Immunol.* 2009 Oct; 124 (4):845-8.

[41] Simons FE, Ardusso LR, Bilo MB, El-Gamal YM, Ledford DK, Ring J, et al. World Allergy Organization anaphylaxis guidelines: summary. *J. Allergy Clin. Immunol.* 2011 Mar; 127 (3):587-93 e1-22.

[42] Gonzalez-Perez A, Aponte Z, Vidaurre CF, Rodriguez LA. Anaphylaxis epidemiology in patients with and patients without asthma: a United Kingdom database review. *J. Allergy Clin. Immunol.* 2010 May; 125 (5):1098-104 e1.

[43] Iribarren C, Tolstykh IV, Miller MK, Eisner MD. Asthma and the prospective risk of anaphylactic shock and other allergy diagnoses in a large integrated health care delivery system. *Ann. Allergy Asthma Immunol.* 2010 May; 104 (5):371-7.

[44] Chen W, Mempel M, Schober W, Behrendt H, Ring J. Gender difference, sex hormones, and immediate type hypersensitivity reactions. *Allergy.* 2008 Nov; 63 (11):1418-27.

[45] Carey MA, Card JW, Voltz JW, Arbes SJ, Jr., Germolec DR, Korach KS, et al. It's all about sex: gender, lung development and lung disease. *Trends Endocrinol. Metab.* 2007 Oct; 18 (8):308-13.

[46] Almqvist C, Worm M, Leynaert B. Impact of gender on asthma in childhood and adolescence: a GA2LEN review. *Allergy.* 2008 Jan; 63 (1):47-57.

[47] Lack G, Fox D, Northstone K, Golding J. Factors associated with the development of peanut allergy in childhood. *N. Engl. J. Med.* 2003 Mar 13; 348 (11):977-85.

[48] Fox AT, Sasieni P, du Toit G, Syed H, Lack G. Household peanut consumption as a risk factor for the development of peanut allergy. *J. Allergy Clin. Immunol.* 2009 Feb; 123 (2):417-23.

[49] Strid J, Hourihane J, Kimber I, Callard R, Strobel S. Epicutaneous exposure to peanut protein prevents oral tolerance and enhances allergic sensitization. *Clin. Exp. Allergy.* 2005 Jun; 35 (6):757-66.

[50] Ben-Shoshan M, Clarke AE. Anaphylaxis: past, present and future. *Allergy.* 2011 Jan; 66 (1):1-14.

[51] Yocum MW, Butterfield JH, Klein JS, Volcheck GW, Schroeder DR, Silverstein MD. Epidemiology of anaphylaxis in Olmsted County: A population-based study. *The Journal of Allergy and Clinical Immunology.* 1999; 104 (2):452-6.

[52] Sampson HA. Anaphylaxis and emergency treatment. *Pediatrics.* 2003 Jun; 111 (6 Pt 3):1601-8.

[53] Pumphrey RS, Gowland MH. Further fatal allergic reactions to food in the United Kingdom, 1999-2006. *J. Allergy Clin. Immunol.* 2007 Apr; 119 (4):1018-9.

[54] Asero R, Antonicelli L, Arena A, Bommarito L, Caruso B, Colombo G, et al. Causes of food-induced anaphylaxis in Italian adults: a multi-centre study. *Int. Arch. Allergy Immunol.* 2009; 150 (3):271-7.

[55] Prieto A, Razzak E, Lindo DP, Alvarez-Perea A, Rueda M, Baeza ML. Recurrent anaphylaxis due to lupin flour: primary sensitization through inhalation. *J. Investig. Allergol. Clin. Immunol.* 2010; 20 (1):76-9.

[56] Hieta N, Hasan T, Makinen-Kiljunen S, Lammintausta K. Lupin allergy and lupin sensitization among patients with suspected food allergy. *Ann. Allergy Asthma Immunol.* 2009 Sep;103 (3):233-7.

[57] Reis AM, Fernandes NP, Marques SL, Paes MJ, Sousa S, Carvalho F, et al. Lupine sensitisation in a population of 1,160 subjects. *Allergol. Immunopathol.* (Madr). 2007 Jul-Aug; 35 (4):162-3.

[58] Dalal I, Binson I, Reifen R, Amitai Z, Shohat T, Rahmani S, et al. Food allergy is a matter of geography after all: sesame as a major cause of severe IgE-mediated food allergic reactions among infants and young children in Israel. *Allergy.* 2002; 57 (4): 362-5.

[59] Ben-Shoshan M, Harrington DW, Soller L, Fragapane J, Joseph L, St Pierre Y, et al. A population-based study on peanut, tree nut, fish, shellfish, and sesame allergy prevalence in Canada. *J. Allergy Clin. Immunol.* 2010 Jun; 125 (6):1327-35.

[60] Gangur V, Kelly C, Navuluri L. Sesame allergy: a growing food allergy of global proportions? *Ann. Allergy Asthma Immunol.* 2005 Jul; 95 (1):4-11; quiz -3, 44.

[61] Helbling A, Hurni T, Mueller UR, Pichler WJ. Incidence of anaphylaxis with circulatory symptoms: a study over a 3-year period comprising 940,000 inhabitants of the Swiss Canton Bern. *Clin. Exp. Allergy.* 2004 Feb; 34 (2):285-90.

[62] Allen KJ. Food allergy: is there a rising prevalence and if so why? *Med. J. Aust.* Jul 4; 195 (1):5-7.

[63] Sheffer AL, Soter NA, McFadden ER, Jr., Austen KF. Exercise-induced anaphylaxis: a distinct form of physical allergy. *J. Allergy Clin. Immunol.* 1983 Mar; 71 (3):311-6.

[64] Shadick NA, Liang MH, Partridge AJ, Bingham C, Wright E, Fossel AH, et al. The natural history of exercise-induced anaphylaxis: survey results from a 10-year follow-up study. *J. Allergy Clin. Immunol.* 1999 Jul; 104 (1):123-7.

[65] Ausdenmoore. RW. *Fatality in a Teenager Secondary to Exercise-Induced Anaphylaxis Pediatric Asthma, Allergy and Immunology.* 1991; 5 (1):21-4.

[66] Dohi M, Suko M, Sugiyama H, Yamashita N, Tadokoro K, Juji F, et al. Food-dependent, exercise-induced anaphylaxis: a study on 11 Japanese cases. *J. Allergy Clin. Immunol.* 1991 Jan;87 (1 Pt 1):34-40.

[67] Harada S, Horikawa T, Ashida M, Kamo T, Nishioka E, Ichihashi M. Aspirin enhances the induction of type I allergic symptoms when combined with food and exercise in patients with food-dependent exercise-induced anaphylaxis. *Br. J. Dermatol.* 2001 Aug; 145 (2): 336-9.

[68] Wade JP, Liang MH, Sheffer AL. Exercise-induced anaphylaxis: epidemiologic observations. *Prog. Clin. Biol. Res.* 1989; 297:175-82.

[69] Yang MS, Lee SH, Kim TW, Kwon JW, Lee SM, Kim SH, et al. Epidemiologic and clinical features of anaphylaxis in Korea. *Ann. Allergy Asthma Immunol.* 2008 Jan; 100 (1):31-6.

[70] Aihara Y, Takahashi Y, Kotoyori T, Mitsuda T, Ito R, Aihara M, et al. Frequency of food-dependent, exercise-induced anaphylaxis in Japanese junior-high-school students. *J. Allergy Clin Immunol.* 2001 Dec; 108 (6): 1035-9.

[71] Tanaka S. An epidemiological survey on food-dependent exercise-induced anaphylaxis in kindergartners, schoolchildren and junior high school students. *Asia Pac. J. Public Health.* 1994; 7 (1):26-30.

[72] Wang J, Sampson HA. Food anaphylaxis. *Clinical and Experimental Allergy.* 2007; 37 (5):651-60.

[73] Teo SL, Gerez IF, Ang EY, Shek LP. Food-dependent exercise-induced anaphylaxis - a review of 5 cases. *Ann. Acad. Med Singapore.* 2009 Oct; 38 (10): 905-9.

[74] Schuberth KC, Lichtenstein LM, Kagey-Sobotka A, Szklo M, Kwiterovich KA, Valentine MD. An epidemiologic study of insect allergy in children. I. Characteristics of the disease. *J. Pediatr.* 1982 Apr; 100 (4): 546-51.

[75] Graft DF, Schuberth KC, Kagey-Sobotka A, Kwiterovich KA, Niv Y, Lichtenstein LM, et al. A prospective study of the natural history of large local reactions after Hymenoptera stings in children. *J. Pediatr.* 1984 May;104 (5):664-8.

[76] Green AW, Reisman RE, Arbesman CE. Clinical and immunologic studies of patients with large local reactions following insect stings. *J. Allergy Clin. Immunol.* 1980 Sep; 66 (3):186-9.

[77] Golden DB, Moffitt J, Nicklas RA, Freeman T, Graft DF, Reisman RE, et al. Stinging insect hypersensitivity: a practice parameter update 2011. *J. Allergy Clin. Immunol.* 2011 Apr; 127 (4):852-4 e1-23.

[78] Thong BY, Tan TC. Epidemiology and risk factors for drug allergy. *Br. J. Clin. Pharmacol.* 2011 May;71 (5):684-700.

[79] Gomes ER, Demoly P. Epidemiology of hypersensitivity drug reactions. *Current Opinion In Allergy And Clinical Immunology*. 2005; 5 (4): 309-16.

[80] Pumphrey RS, Roberts IS. Postmortem findings after fatal anaphylactic reactions. *J. Clin. Pathol.* 2000 Apr; 53 (4):273-6.

[81] Pumphrey RS. Fatal anaphylaxis in the UK, 1992-2001. *Novartis Found Symp.* 2004; 257:116-28; discussion 28-32, 57-60, 276-85.

[82] Low I, Stables S. Anaphylactic deaths in Auckland, New Zealand: a review of coronial autopsies from 1985 to 2005. *Pathology.* 2006 Aug; 38 (4):328-32.

[83] Mertes PM, Laxenaire MC, Alla F. Anaphylactic and anaphylactoid reactions occurring during anesthesia in France in 1999-2000. *Anesthesiology.* 2003 Sep; 99 (3): 536-45.

[84] Gawchik SM. Latex allergy. *Mt. Sinai J. Med.* 2011 Sep-Oct; 78 (5): 759-72.

[85] Turjanmaa K, Alenius H, Reunala T, Palosuo T. Recent developments in latex allergy. *Curr. Opin. Allergy Clin. Immunol.* 2002 Oct; 2 (5): 407-12.

[86] Blumchen K, Bayer P, Buck D, Michael T, Cremer R, Fricke C, et al. Effects of latex avoidance on latex sensitization, atopy and allergic diseases in patients with spina bifida. *Allergy.* 2010; 65 (12):1585-93.

[87] Beaudouin E, Prestat F, Schmitt M, Kanny G, Laxenaire MC, Moneret-Vautrin DA. High risk of sensitization to latex in children with spina bifida. *Eur. J. Pediatr. Surg.* 1994 Apr; 4 (2):90-3.

[88] Niggemann B, Buck D, Michael T, Wahn U. Latex provocation tests in patients with spina bifida: who is at risk of becoming symptomatic? *J. Allergy Clin. Immunol.* 1998 Oct; 102 (4 Pt 1):665-70.

[89] Nieto A, Estornell F, Mazon A, Reig C, Garcia-Ibarra F. Allergy to latex in spina bifida: a multivariate study of associated factors in 100 consecutive patients. *J. Allergy Clin. Immunol.* 1996 Sep; 98 (3):501-7.

[90] Yassin MS, Sanyurah S, Lierl MB, Fischer TJ, Oppenheimer S, Cross J, et al. Evaluation of latex allergy in patients with meningomyelocele. *Ann. Allergy.* 1992 Sep;69[3]:207-11.

[91] Cremer R, Kleine-Diepenbruck U, Hering F, Holschneider AM. Reduction of latex sensitisation in spina bifida patients by a primary prophylaxis programme [five years experience]. *Eur. J. Pediatr. Surg.* 2002 Dec; 12 Suppl 1:S19-21.

[92] Nieto A, Mazon A, Pamies R, Lanuza A, Munoz A, Estornell F, et al. Efficacy of latex avoidance for primary prevention of latex sensitization in children with spina bifida. *J. Pediatr.* 2002 Mar; 140 (3): 370-2.

[93] Niggemann B, Buck D, Michael T, Haberl H, Wahn U. Latex allergy in spina bifida: at the turning point? *J. Allergy Clin. Immunol.* 2000 Dec; 106 (6):1201.

[94] Kelso JM, Greenhawt MJ, Li JT, Nicklas RA, Bernstein DI, Blessing-Moore J, et al. Adverse reactions to vaccines practice parameter 2012 update. *J. Allergy Clin. Immunol.* 2012 Jul; 130 (1):25-43.

[95] General recommendations on immunization --- recommendations of the Advisory Committee on Immunization Practices [ACIP]. *MMWR Recomm. Rep.* 2011 Jan 28; 60 (2):1-64.

[96] Bohlke K, Davis RL, Marcy SM, Braun MM, DeStefano F, Black SB, et al. Risk of anaphylaxis after vaccination of children and adolescents. *Pediatrics.* 2003 Oct; 112 (4):815-20.

[97] Mullins R, Kemp A, Gold M. Influenza vaccination of the egg-allergic individual. Medical Journal Australia. 2010 Sep;193(5):254-55.

[98] Krasnick J, Patterson R, Harris KE. Idiopathic anaphylaxis: long-term follow-up, cost, and outlook. *Allergy.* 1996 Oct; 51 (10):724-31.

[99] Ditto AM, Harris KE, Krasnick J, Miller MA, Patterson R. Idiopathic anaphylaxis: a series of 335 cases. *Ann. Allergy Asthma Immunol.* 1996 Oct; 77 (4):285-91.

[100] Tejedor Alonso MA, Sastre DJ, Sanchez-Hernandez JJ, Perez FC, de la Hoz Caballer B. Idiopathic anaphylaxis: a descriptive study of 81 patients in Spain. *Ann. Allergy Asthma Immunol.* 2002 Mar; 88 (3): 313-8.

[101] Pumphrey R. Anaphylaxis: can we tell who is at risk of a fatal reaction? *Curr. Opin. Allergy Clin. Immunol.* 2004 Aug; 4 (4):285-90.

[102] Bock SA, Munoz-Furlong A, Sampson HA. Further fatalities caused by anaphylactic reactions to food, 2001-2006. *J. Allergy Clin. Immunol.* 2007 Apr; 119 (4):1016-8.

[103] Lieberman P. Biphasic anaphylactic reactions. *Ann. Allergy Asthma Immunol.* 2005 Sep; 95 (3):217-26; quiz 26, 58.

In: Anaphylaxis: Principles and Practice
Editor: M. Thirumala Krishna

ISBN: 978-1-62618-688-0

Chapter II

Anaphylaxis: Clinical Approach and Differential Diagnosis

***Lavanya Diwakar*[1] *and S. Hasan Arshad*[2,*]**
[1]Department of Allergy and Clinical Immunology, Heartlands Hospital, Birmingham, UK
[2]Clinical and Experimental Sciences, University of Southampton,
The David Hide Asthma and Allergy Research Centre, Isle of Wight, UK

Abstract

The clinical presentation of anaphylaxis may be extremely diverse depending upon the nature and route of allergen exposure, age of the affected individual, and other physiological factors including co-morbidities and concomitant drug intake. A carefully elicited, detailed history is necessary for the diagnosis of anaphylaxis and to differentiate between many conditions that may present similarly. This is necessary in order to optimally manage this potentially fatal but often preventable condition.

In this chapter, we will discuss the clinical presentation and various conditions that can masquerade as anaphylaxis. The clinical and pathognomonic features and diagnostic investigations for these conditions will be presented. Clinical vignettes have been incorporated to illustrate the varied conditions and presentations outlined in the chapter.

Background

Charles Richet obtained the Nobel prize for medicine in 1913 for coining the term 'anaphylaxis' to describe the violent reactions observed following injection of a second dose of sea-anemone venom into dogs [1]. Anaphylaxis was considered the opposite of immunity (ana- anti; phylaxis- protection against infection) and while it was recognised quite early on

* Corresponding author: Prof. S.H. Arshad, MP: 810, Level F, South Block, Southampton General Hospital, Tremona Road, Southampton, SO16 7JB. +44 (0)23 8079 6148. +44 (0)23 8070 1771 (Fax). E-mail: S.H.Arshad@soton.ac.uk.

that histamine release may be responsible [2], it was many more years before IgE antibodies [3] and mast cells were implicated in the pathophysiology of this condition.

Given that its presentation can be very diverse and symptoms overlap with those of many other conditions, the diagnosis of anaphylaxis may sometimes be difficult. Detailed history with regards to symptoms, possible trigger factors, co-morbid conditions and a thorough clinical examination are important to establish the diagnosis. An accurate diagnosis is important not only to ensure timely and appropriate management, but also to enable better estimation of the incidence of this very serious condition [4].

Diagnosis of Anaphylaxis

Until recently, the lack of specific diagnostic criteria meant that thc condition was perhaps under-reported, incorrectly managed and there was heterogeneity in research conducted in this area [5, 6]. In the last few years, significant efforts have been made to consolidate expertise in this disease area and to define anaphylaxis in a simple, unambiguous manner. Currently accepted definitions include "A serious, life-threatening, generalised or systemic hypersensitivity reaction" [7] and "A serious allergic reaction that is rapid in onset and may cause death" [4]. The word 'anaphylaxis' is now used to describe both IgE and non-IgE mediated reactions and the use of the term 'anaphylactoid' is no longer recommended [8].

Clinical Manifestations

The diagnosis of anaphylaxis is based almost entirely on the clinical presentation of the patient. Whilst the clinical manifestations of anaphylaxis can be confused with other conditions (e.g. acute asthma, panic attack, myocardial infarction), early diagnosis is important since delay in instituting treatment with adrenaline can be fatal [9].

Typically, anaphylaxis can affect the cutaneous, gastrointestinal, respiratory and cardiovascular systems. The diagnostic criteria for anaphylaxis as stipulated by the World Allergy Organisation (WAO) are shown in table 1. It is recognised that about 80 percent of all individuals with anaphylaxis will manifest cutaneous and mucosal symptoms [4] while in the remaining, a combination of other systemic features such as respiratory distress, persistent gastrointestinal symptoms or hypotension predominate. Very rarely, single organ system involvement (e.g. hypotension) has been reported in isolation following known allergen exposure [10]. The degree and severity of systemic allergic symptoms can be graded using the Mueller classification (table 2).

Presentation of Anaphylaxis

Presentation can vary depending upon the age of the patient(11), route of allergen exposure [9], and also upon co-morbid factors (Table 3).

Age: Children generally present with respiratory compromise whilst cardiovascular symptoms appear to predominate in adults [12]. This may be a reflection of the higher incidence of asthma in the paediatric age group. In an Australian study, it was observed that while infants developed hives and vomiting, respiratory symptoms were more common in pre-school children. Compared with adults, cardiovascular symptoms are rarely reported in young children [11]. Adolescents and young adults have been found to be at a high risk for fatality with food related anaphylaxis [13], while the elderly have a higher fatality rate with insect venom anaphylaxis [14].

Table 1. WAO Guidelines for the diagnosis of Anaphylaxis [8]

Anaphylaxis is highly likely when any *one* of the following three criteria is fulfilled:
1. Acute onset of an illness (minutes to several hours) with involvement of the skin, mucosal tissue, or both (e.g. generalised hives, pruritis or flushing, swollen lips-tongue-uvula) And *at least one* of the following: • Respiratory compromise (dyspnoea, wheeze-bronchospasm, stridor, reduced PEF, hypoxemia) • Reduced BP or associated symptoms of end-organ dysfunction (eg, hypotonia [collapse], syncope, incontinence)
2. *Two or more* of the following that occur rapidly after exposure to a likely allergen for that patient (minutes to several hours): • Involvement of the skin-mucosal tissue (eg, generalized hives, itch-flush, swollen lips-tongue-uvula) • Respiratory compromise (eg, dyspnoea, wheeze-bronchospasm, stridor, reduced PEF, hypoxemia) • Reduced BP or associated symptoms (eg, hypotonia [collapse], syncope, incontinence) • Persistent gastrointestinal symptoms (eg, crampy abdominal pain, vomiting)
3. Reduced BP after exposure to known allergen for that patient (minutes to several hours): • Infants and children: low systolic BP (age specific) or greater than 30% decrease in systolic BP * • Adults: systolic BP of less than 90 mm Hg or greater than 30% decrease from that person's baseline

PEF: Peak expiratory flow; *BP*: blood pressure.

Adapted from Simons, E et al. 2011.

* Low systolic blood pressure for children is defined as less than 70 mm Hg from 1 month to 1 year, less than (70 mm Hg + [2 x age]) from 1 to 10 years, and less than 90 mm Hg from 11 to 17 years.

Table 2. Mueller classification of systemic allergic reactions

Grade	Symptoms
I	Generalized urticaria, itching, malaise and anxiety
II	Any of the above plus two or more of: angioedema, chest constriction, nausea, vomiting, diarrhea, abdominal pain, dizziness
III	Any of the above plus two or more of: dyspnoea, wheezing, stridor, dysarthria, hoarseness, weakness, confusion, feeling of impending disaster
IV	Any of the above plus two or more of: fall in blood pressure, collapse, loss of consciousness, incontinence, cyanosis

Table 3. Anaphylaxis presentation following exposure to common allergens [&&1]

Organ system	Symptoms	Usual allergens
Skin and mucous membranes	• Flushing, itching, urticaria (hives), angioedema, morbilliform rash, piloerection • Periorbital itching, erythema and edema; conjunctival erythema, tearing • Itching of lips, tongue, palate, and external auditory canals; and swelling of lips, tongue, and uvula • Itching of genitalia, palms, and soles	• All *
Respiratory	• Nasal itching, congestion, rhinorrhoea, sneezing • Throat itching and tightness, dysphonia, hoarseness, stridor, dry staccato cough • Lower airways: increased respiratory rate, shortness of breath, chest tightness, deep cough, wheezing/bronchospasm, decreased peak expiratory flow • Cyanosis • Respiratory arrest	• Food • Sublingual immunotherapy • Subcutaneous immunotherapy • Asthmatics [$]
Gastrointestinal	• Abdominal pain, nausea, vomiting (stringy mucus), diarrhoea, dysphagia	• Food • Oral drugs
Cardiovascular system	• Chest pain • Tachycardia, bradycardia (less common), other arrhythmias, palpitations • Hypotension, feeling faint, urinary or fecal incontinence, shock • Cardiac arrest	• Insect venom • Intravenous drugs • Subcutaneous immunotherapy • Mastocytosis ** • Food
Central nervous system	• Aura of impending doom, uneasiness (in infants and children, sudden behavioral change, eg. irritability, cessation of play, clinging to parent); throbbing • headache (pre-epinephrine), altered mental status, dizziness, confusion, tunnel vision	• Insect venom • Food • Drugs
Other	• Metallic taste in the mouth • Cramps and bleeding due to uterine contractions in females	• All [£]

[1] Adapted from the WAO guidelines for anaphylaxis [87].

[&&] There is a significant overlap between symptoms caused by various allergens. This table discusses the most common presentations due to specific allergens given a certain route of exposure (e.g. oral vs intravenous).

* > 80% of all anaphylactic reactions (irrespective of the offending allergen) present with cutaneous symptoms.

[$] Generally following food related anaphylaxis but can occur with any allergen.

** Mostly described with insect venom and radio contrast media but can occur with any allergen.

[£] These are rare but described.

Route of exposure: Route of allergen exposure is also known to affect the presentation in anaphylaxis. This may be illustrated by the finding that injection immunotherapy may occasionally cause severe systemic reactions, these are extremely rare with sublingual immunotherapy regimens [15].

In an Italian study, investigators found that children with food induced anaphylaxis presented more frequently with cutaneous, respiratory and gastrointestinal symptoms while cardiovascular involvement was rare; whereas in exercise induced anaphylaxis cutaneous and respiratory symptoms appeared to predominate [16]. Similarly, a study from the UK demonstrated that cardiovascular collapse was more frequent in patients who succumbed to drug or insect sting related systemic reactions as compared to those with fatal food induced anaphylaxis [9].

Co-morbid conditions: Atopic patients are recognised to have a higher risk of anaphylaxis [10]. Asthma is associated with an increased incidence of fatal allergic symptoms [17]. Asthmatics, especially those with poorly controlled disease, are at a higher risk of adverse reactions during immunotherapy [15].

Patients being treated with beta blockers are at a higher risk of developing severe and protracted anaphylactic reactions that do not respond to adrenaline therapy [18]. There have also been reports of protracted allergic reactions due to ACE (Angiotensin converting enzyme) inhibitor therapy [19] as well as alpha blockers [20]. Pre-existing cardiovascular disease is also considered an independent risk factor for developing severe anaphylaxis [21].

Some drugs which reduce the individual's (and physician's) ability to detect anaphylaxis (such as alcohol, recreational drugs, sedatives and hypnotics) can also increase the probability of fatal reactions [22].

Mastocytosis (discussed in detail later in this chapter) is also known to predispose to severe anaphylactic episodes following exposure to various allergens [23], particularly insect venom [24].

Other factors that play an important role in the severity of presentation include strenuous exercise, aspirin [25], severity of and time elapsed since recent allergic reaction [22].

Biphasic Reactions

Following the characteristic immediate hypersensitivity response to allergen, about 1-20% of patients can develop further symptoms related to anaphylaxis [26]. A biphasic reaction is characterized by symptoms similar to that of anaphylaxis which occur without any further exposure to the allergen, usually between 1-24 hours (but can occur up to 72 hours) after apparent resolution of the symptoms of the index episode [27].

Symptoms can range from being milder to more severe compared with the index reaction [26], with fatal reactions occasionally reported [28].

Biphasic reactions are often not considered by emergency room doctors [29] and consequently patients may be discharged early following their anaphylactic reaction, exposing them to a risk of death due to a delayed reaction.

It is recommended that patients should be admitted for observation for at least 24 hours following their index reaction [26], but this is often ignored. It is not currently possible to accurately estimate a given individual's risk of developing biphasic reactions. However, a few risk factors have been proposed in the literature. These include:

1. Severity of index reaction: Severe anaphylactic reactions resulting in hypotension or laryngeal oedema have been reported to increase the risk of developing biphasic reactions [30].
2. Adrenaline usage: Biphasic reactions are thought to be more likely in individuals who require greater amounts of adrenaline for resuscitation during the initial reaction, likely signifying severe reactions [27]. Some authors have reported increased frequency of delayed reactions following under treatment with adrenaline and steroids [31].
3. Age: Biphasic reactions occur more frequently in adults compared with children [32, 33]. The reason for this is unknown but it appears to hold true for reactions secondary to unplanned allergen exposure as well as those following allergen immunotherapy.
4. Corticosteroids: So far, data on the importance of corticosteroids in the prevention of biphasic reactions have been inconclusive. Some authors have reported a reduction in the frequency and severity of biphasic reactions following administration of steroids for the index reaction [34], while others reported no significant benefit [35].
5. Other: Few researchers have reported other features predisposing to biphasic reactions. These include female sex [32], administration of intravenous fluid bolus during initial resuscitation [27] and a history of previous biphasic reactions [30].

Differential Diagnosis

Many conditions are known to mimic anaphylaxis (table 4). A good history and documentation of clinical findings at presentation are important in differentiating between this and other conditions that show various degrees of overlap clinically. Photographic documentation of the rash can be very useful where direct observation is not possible. Scrutiny of previous medical and emergency room records may be necessary.

Conditions That Closely Mimic Anaphylaxis

Scombroid poisoning: Scombroid poisoning is the most common toxicity (icthyotoxicosis) associated with fish consumption worldwide [36]. Fish belonging to the family Scomberesocidae (which include mackerel, tuna, skipjack and bonito [37]) contain large quantities of histidine which is converted to histamine by the enteric bacteria in spoilt fish resulting in the characteristic features of this condition [38]. Non-scombroid fish such as blue fish, salmon, sardines, anchovies as well as some types of cheese have also been implicated in this condition [39].

Patients describe an oral burning or peppery sensation, hives, nausea, vomiting, diarrhoea, flushing, dizziness within a few minutes of ingesting the culprit food [40]. Occasionally, bronchospasm and respiratory distress may occur.

Table 4. Differential diagnosis of anaphylaxis

1. Flush syndromes
    - Carcinoid syndrome
    - Mastocytosis
    - Phaeochromocytoma
    - Medullary carcinoma of thyroid
    - Vasoactive intestinal peptide (VIP) related tumors
    - Other: Monosodium glutamate and sulfite induced flushing
2. Disorders affecting the upper/ lower respiratory tract
    - Acute severe asthma
    - Vocal cord dysfunction
    - Foreign body aspiration
    - Acute bronchiolitis (croup)
3. Disorders affecting the cardiovascular system
    - Cardiogenic shock
    - Vasovagal syndrome
    - Kounis syndrome
4. Conditions that present similarly to anaphylaxis
    - Scombroid toxins
    - Amniotic fluid embolism
    - Undifferentiated somatoform idiopathic anaphylaxis

Adapted from the WAO guidelines [87].

Symptoms generally subside after a few hours and respond very well to antihistamines [39], although adrenaline may be needed in the acute management of a few patients. The condition may be confused with acute allergy to fish but high urine methylhistamine content within the first four hours without raised tryptase [40] and negative allergy tests can help in the diagnosis.

Amniotic fluid embolism: Amniotic fluid embolism (AFE) is a very serious peripartum condition associated with high maternal and perinatal mortality rates [41]. It is often clinically indistinguishable from allergic anaphylaxis during anaesthesia [42]. Patients may present with cardiovascular collapse, hypotension, hypoxia and cyanosis, coagulopathy, dyspnoea, respiratory arrest, pulmonary oedema, generalised rash and sometimes angioedema [42-44].

Patients may report premonitory symptoms such as breathlessness, light headedness, panic, nausea, feeling cold, pins and needles sensation in extremities [43]. Definitive diagnosis is only possible in cases where foetal squames and lanugo are found in the mother post-mortem. Markers such as sialyl Tn antigen, zinc coproporphyrin which are normally found in foetal tissue may be detected in maternal circulation in AFE [43] although no definitive serological marker has been recognised. Complement C3, C4 may be reduced. Serum tryptase may be raised in some instances, prompting the hypothesis that AFE is an anaphylactic reaction to foetal proteins [45]. Acute management is supportive and can be similar to that of intra-operative anaphylaxis. Diagnosis is difficult but skin and serum tests to anaesthetic agents are likely to be negative in these patients [42].

Table 5. Diagnostic Criteria for an Undifferentiated Somatoform Disorder*

A. One or more physical complaints (e.g., fatigue, loss of appetite, gastrointestinal or urinary complaints).
B. Either (1) or (2):
   (1) after appropriate investigation, the symptoms cannot be fully explained by a known general medical condition or the direct effects of a substance (e.g., a drug of abuse, a medication)
   (2) when there is a related general medical condition, the physical complaints or resulting social or occupational impairment is in excess of what would be expected from the history, physical examination, or laboratory findings
C. The symptoms cause clinically significant distress or impairment in social, occupational, or other important areas of functioning.
D. The duration of the disturbance is at least 6 months.
E. The disturbance is not better accounted for by another mental disorder (e.g., another Somatoform Disorder, Sexual Dysfunction, Mood Disorder, Anxiety Disorder, Sleep Disorder, or Psychotic Disorder).
F. The symptom is not intentionally produced or feigned (as in Factitious Disorder or Malingering).

* From the Diagnostic and Statistical Manual of Mental Disorders, Fourth Edition, Text Revision, Washington DC, American Psychiatric Association, 2000.

Undifferentiated somatoform idiopathic anaphylaxis (US-IA): Of the individuals diagnosed with idiopathic angioedema, a few may be classified as having US-IA. These patients have history that is similar to that of idiopathic anaphylaxis. However, there is paucity of physical findings and the individuals do not respond well to conventional therapy for anaphylaxis. In addition, they satisfy the Diagnostic and Statistical Manual of Mental disorders (DSM-4) criteria for an undifferentiated somatoform disorder (table 5) [46]. Diagnosis generally involves extensive scrutiny of the patients' medical records to look for clinical signs of anaphylaxis (urticaria, angioedema, bronchospasm, hypotension). Patients should be encouraged to attend the hospital during an acute episode so that detailed, objective assessments can be made. It is important to consider the diagnosis early so that psychiatric support can be instituted. These patients are generally more difficult to evaluate and manage, present on many occasions to the outpatient and accident and emergency setting and result in high costs to the health care system [7]. Some authors have suggested algorithms for diagnosis and management of these patients [48].

Flushing Syndromes

Systemic Mastocytosis (SM): Mastocytosis is a condition characterised by clonal increase in mast cells and accumulation in one or more organs [49]. This condition is highly heterogenous and the clinical course may vary from asymptomatic to highly aggressive. Seven disease variants are described as per the WHO consensus document [50].

Patients may present with paroxysms of flushing, hypotension with or without syncope, diarrhoea, headaches and bone pain. In addition to mimicking anaphylaxis, mastocytosis is known to increase the predisposition to idiopathic anaphylaxis and also anaphylaxis due to other allergic triggers [23, 51, 52]. The criteria for diagnosis of SM are described in table 11, chapter-12. Elevated serum alpha tryptase is a useful marker, although pro-beta tryptase levels may be more sensitive in the diagnosis [53].

Carcinoid Syndrome: Carcinoid tumours are the most common neuroendocrine tumours of the gut and are often asymptomatic. In about 10% of patients vasoactive amines, principally serotonin, are secreted from the non-GI tumour sites causing the triad of symptoms considered typical of this condition i.e, flushing, gastrointestinal hypermotility and cardiac involvement [54]. Myopathy, bronchospasm and skin hyperpigmentation are less commonly seen [55]. Symptoms can follow exposure to triggers such as cheese, alcohol, coffee or exercise.

Carcinoid syndrome (CS) is an important diagnosis to consider in individuals with intermittent generalised flushing [56]. Hypotension, bronchoconstriction and GI disturbances (such as cramps, diarrhoea) are often associated making the distinction between CS and anaphylaxis difficult. Diagnosis will require careful elicitation of history and trigger factors. Laboratory findings that aid diagnosis include elevated 24 hour urinary levels of 5- hydroxy indole acetic acid (5-HIAA), which is a metabolite of serotonin. Serum chromogranin A is a useful test [57] and neuro-specific enolase, although useful, is not readily available.

Phaeochromocytoma: Phaeochromocytomas are "catecholamine-producing neuroendocrine tumours arising from chromaffin cells of the adrenal medulla or extra-adrenal paraganglia" [58]. Some genetic conditions (such as neurofibromatosis) can predispose to these tumors. In the general population, however, phaeochromocytomas are rare.

This condition has a very heterogenous presentation and the diagnosis is often delayed or missed [59]. Signs and symptoms may include paroxysms of hypertension, headache, palpitations, sweating, anxiety/ panic and pallor. Chest pain and GI symptoms such as nausea or vomiting may also be associated. Flushing may also occur [56]. Blood pressure may be normal between episodes. Episodes are often unpredictable but certain drugs, foods or tumour manipulation during surgery can precipitate a paroxysm [58].

24 hour urinary measurement of metanephrine and normetanephrine is a sensitive and reliable test for the diagnosis of this condition. 24 hour vanillyl mandelic acid is aspecific test for the condition while being less sensitive and is, therefore, not suitable for initial screening [60].

Other causes of flushing: These include common causes such as fever/ infection, anxiety and much rarer conditions such as Medullary Carcinoma of thyroid, Pancreatic cell tumour secreting vasoactive intestinal peptide, renal cell carcinoma, certain drugs (eg disulfiram, chlorpropamide) [56]. Good history and a high index of suspicion can usually help in the identification of these conditions and in differentiating them from anaphylaxis.

Cardiovascular Involvement

Kounis syndrome: Kounis syndrome or allergic angina refers to a condition where a patient develops clinical and laboratory features of classical angina pectoris secondary to inflammatory mediators released during an allergic reaction. This condition has been described after exposure to various allergens and in individuals of all age groups [61-63]. Typically, these patients present concurrently with chest pain and with symptoms characteristic of an allergic reaction, display elevated tryptase and troponin I levels which often reverse with timely management of the anaphylaxis. Prolonged, untreated episodes may result in myocardial infarction [64].

Two variants of this syndrome have been described:

a. Type 1 where the affected individual has normal coronary arteries [61, 65]
b. Type 2 resulting from plaque disruption in atheromatous coronary vasculature [66]

Treatment of this condition is often tricky given the adverse effects of adrenaline and H1 antagonists on the myocardium and therefore a high index of suspicion is necessary for optimal management [67].

Cardiogenic shock: In some instances, severe allergic reaction to a substance may manifest as transient cardiomyopathy and cardiogenic shock [68, 69]. On one occasion, the cardiac symptoms manifested a few hours after apparent cessation of the allergic reaction [69]. Although described separately in the literature, these vignettes are indistinguishable from Kounis syndrome.

Vasovagal reactions: Vasovagal reactions (VVR) presenting with hypotension and pallor can occasionally be confused with anaphylaxis [70]. This has been particularly reported in cases of suspected local anaesthetic allergy following dental procedures [71]. Bradycardia is one of the key presenting features in VVR (unlike tachycardia in anaphylaxis) and symptoms often recover quickly when patients are made to lie in a supine position. However, it is important to note that relative bradycardia during anaesthesia may reflect the Bezold-Jarisch reflex and does not rule out anaphylaxis [72].

Respiratory Involvement

Vocal cord dysfunction: Vocal cord dysfunction (VCD) is a condition characterised by "paroxysmal periods of true vocal cord adduction during inspiration, non-phonatory expiration, or both" [73]. It has been reported from age three years upwards although most patients first present between the second and fourth decades of life [74]. Patients generally present with sudden onset (and cessation) of flushing, inspiratory stridor, breathing difficulties, dysphonia. Symptoms are generally localised to the throat region. A variety of triggers may be identified by the affected individuals such as chemicals, dust, smoke, certain odours [74] as well as exercise, especially in adolescents [75]. Most individuals are diagnosed and managed as having asthma [76]. Early diagnosis is important to avoid unnecessary treatments (such as steroids, adrenaline) and tracheal intubation.

VCD patients have an increased incidence of psychiatric illness suggesting a functional component to this condition. Gastro-oesophageal reflux disease is also strongly associated with the condition [77] and the use of proton-pump inhibitors or, in extreme cases, surgical intervention may be indicated [78]. Gold standard for diagnosis is direct observation during an attack by laryngoscopy. Flattening of the inspiratory loop of the flow-volume loops during an attack (unlike that of the expiratory loop in asthma) is suggestive of this condition [74]. Management involves speech therapy and psychological therapy, where indicated.

Other: Two other conditions that present similarly to VCD are foreign body aspiration and acute bronchiolitis (or croup). Good history is important in distinguishing between these conditions and management is specific to the diagnosis.

Acute severe asthma: Distinguishing between asthma and an allergic reaction can occasionally be difficult. Anaphylaxis, unlike asthma, is generally accompanied by skin and/ or gastrointestinal, cardiovascular manifestations. However since most anaesthetic drugs can not only induce bronchospasm or anaphylaxis but also result in flushing due to non-specific histamine release, clear distinction between the two diagnoses may not be possible [79].

Rare Causes of Anaphylaxis

Anisakis: Anisakidae is a family of nematode parasites that primarily affect fish such as hake, anchovy and cod. Humans are aberrant hosts to these parasites and get infected when they eat raw or undercooked infected fish. Anisakis simplex, the most common parasite in this family is known to induce IgE mediated allergic reactions in humans. Patients generally present with urticaria and abdominal pain a few minutes to hours after ingestion of raw or undercooked fish; some may develop respiratory symptoms and few may present with anaphylaxis [80]. On many occasions, patients do not link the ingestion of fish to the onset of symptoms and indeed, they are able to eat the same kind of fish later without any allergic symptoms [81]. A detailed history followed by skin and serum specific IgE tests to A. simplex will help confirm the diagnosis. Allergy tests to fish are generally negative [82]. Eosinophilia and increased serum IgE may also be present. Typical findings on gastroscopy may also help with diagnosis [83]. Mebendazole is the treatment of choice.

Hydatid: Hydatid cysts are caused by larval forms of cestode parasites belonging to the genus Echinococcus. These cysts have a host derived fibrous ectocyst and an inner parasite derived endocyst.

The germinal layer of the endocyst gives rise to new daughter cysts and brood capsules that freely float within the clear cyst fluid [84]. Release of these parasitic proteins within the host either due to spontaneous or surgical cyst disruption is a well recognised cause of anaphylaxis [85]. There have been reports of anaphylaxis even in individuals with unruptured cysts [86]. Asymptomatic hydatid cysts should be considered as a differential diagnosis for intra-operative anaphylaxis, especially in endemic areas.

Clinical Cases

1. A Case of Salmon Allergy

A 65 years old man (AR) developed chest tightness, hypotension and collapsed within 15 minutes of a having a meal in a restaurant. He was taken to the emergency department where he was found to have ST depression in the lateral leads (Figure 1). Symptoms and ECG changes improved rapidly with aspirin, clopidogrel, morphine and oxygen therapy. Troponin I level was elevated at 450 ng/L. A diagnosis of non ST elevation myocardial infarction (NSTEMI) was made and he was discharged home after observation on the coronary care unit with a provisional diagnosis of coronary artery disease pending further investigations. However, subsequently cardiac investigations failed to confirm significant coronary artery obstruction.

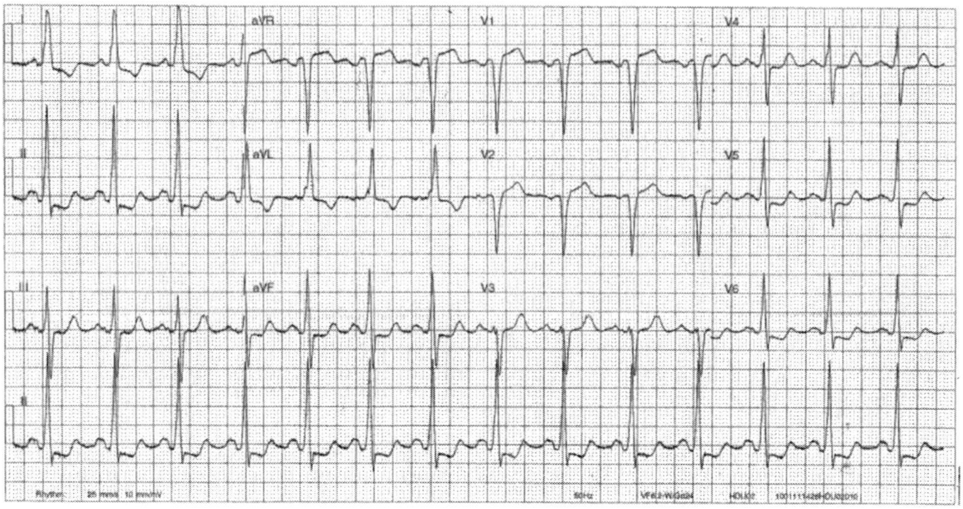

Figure 1. ECG showing ST depression in the lateral leads.

A few days later, he had a small amount of baked salmon at home and stopped eating as he developed swelling of the lips, mouth and urticaria. He managed this reaction with antihistamine that he had at home. Later, he consulted his GP who referred AR to the allergy clinic. A careful history revealed that the restaurant meal had salmon and AR did feel unwell with nausea, flushing and generalised itching immediately after the meal but ignored these symptoms as "he did not wish to make a fuss". Skin prick tests to salmon was positive with a large reaction of 10 x 12 mm. He had smaller reactions to tuna and prawn. Specific IgE was also positive to salmon at 18 KU/L. Oral challenge was not considered appropriate given his clear history and evidence of sensitisation.

The original diagnosis of myocardial infraction was revised in favour of anaphylaxis due to fish allergy. The presentation with myocardial infarction was likely to represent type 1 Kounis syndrome in this case (see text).

2. Allergy to Tuna or Was It?

A 24 year old university graduate (RH) presented to the allergy clinic complaining of an allergic reaction to tuna. She bought cous cous from supermarket and added tomato, pesto and tuna steak for her dinner. About 20 minutes after eating the meal, she developed headache, palpitations, angioedema and shortness of breath. The reaction settled in 3-4 hours without needing specific treatment. Skin prick test was negative to sea-food panel (tuna, cod, salmon, mackerel, shrimp, crab and mussels), nut panel and other foods such as tomato and lupin. She had a negative oral challenge to tuna. The final diagnosis was scombroid poisoning and this was explained to the patient.

3. An Unusual Presentation

A 62 year old lady was referred to the allergy unit for investigation following 1 year history of recurrent anaphylaxis. She gave history of sudden episodes of generalised rash, dizziness, breathing difficulty associated with cramping abdominal pain and profuse, watery diarrhoea. Frequency of episodes was steadily increasing and she experienced between 1-2 episodes every 2 weeks at the time of referral. Although most episodes occurred after meal times, no specific trigger factor could be identified and she was labelled as having idiopathic anaphylaxis and was prescribed an emergency management kit by her general practitioner, which included self injectable adrenaline device and H1 inhibitors. She also had a medic-alert bracelet. At the time of consultation in the allergy clinic, she appeared anxious and tired. She reported having lost about 7 kgs in the last year, which she attributed to the stress caused by her condition. Photographs which she had taken on her mobile phone showed flushing (rather than a rash). Further questioning revealed that alcohol and cheese often made her feel unwell and could sometimes precipitate her 'anaphylactic' symptoms. Clinical examination was normal apart from a vague mass in the umbilical region of the abdomen.

Ultrasound scan of the abdomen revealed a small bowel mass with hypoechoic lesions in the liver, which were confirmed on an MRI scan. Ultrasound guided liver biopsy was performed and histological examination established that this was a neuro-endocrine tumour. Plasma chromogranin A was elevated and 24 hour urine test revealed raised 5-hydroxy indole acetic acid, confirming a diagnosis of Carcinoid syndrome. The patient was referred to surgeons for resection of the tumor.

Conclusion

Anaphylaxis is a serious, life threatening condition which is rapid in onset. It may or may not be IgE mediated. Diagnosis of anaphylaxis is clinical and should be made based on the World Allergy Organisation (WAO) criteria. Presentation is varied, based upon a number of factors, and may overlap with various other conditions as discussed in this chapter. A few conditions can predispose to anaphylaxis. Biphasic reactions can sometimes occur and whilst these cannot be predicted with certainty, it is important to observe all patients with anaphylaxis for at least 24 hours before discharge.

Clinical Pearls

- Anaphylaxis is a serious condition that is very diverse in its presentation.
- Most patients with anaphylaxis present with cutaneous features but occasionally, only either respiratory or cardiovascular systems may be involved.
- There are established criteria for the diagnosis of anaphylaxis laid down by the World Allergy Organisation (WAO).
- Biphasic reactions may occur in a proportion of patients and these can range from being less severe to more severe compared to the index reaction

- Biphasic reactions are often unpredictable, but some risk factors have been identified; patients should be observed in hospital for at least 24 hours following presentation with anaphylaxis.
- Some conditions (such as asthma, mastocytosis) increase the risk of anaphylaxis, while others closely mimic anaphylaxis in their presentation.
- Diagnosis is mainly based on meticulous history taking, while skin and blood tests can assist in confirmation of the clinical suspicion.

Conflict of Interest

The authors declare that they have no conflicts of interest.

References

[1] Richet C. An Address on Ancient Humorism and Modern Humorism. *British Medical Journal* 1910; 2(2596):921-6.

[2] Farmer L. Histamine in anaphylaxis and allergy. *Bulletin of the New York Academy of Medicine* 1940; 16(10):618.

[3] Layton LL. Passive transfer of human atopic allergies into lemurs, lorises, pottos, and galagos: possible primate-ordinal specificity of acceptance of passive sensitization by human atopic reagin. *J. Allergy* 1965 Nov-Dec; 36(6):523-31.

[4] Sampson HA, Munoz-Furlong A, Campbell RL, Adkinson NF, Allan Bock S, Branum A, et al. Second Symposium on the Definition and Management of Anaphylaxis: Summary Report of Second National Institute of Allergy and Infectious Disease/Food Allergy and Anaphylaxis Network Symposium. *Annals of emergency medicine* 2006; 47(4):373.

[5] Bohlke K, Davis RL, DeStefano F, Marcy SM, Braun MM, Thompson RS. Epidemiology of anaphylaxis among children and adolescents enrolled in a health maintenance organization. *J. Allergy Clin. Immunol.* 2004 Mar; 113(3):536-42.

[6] Lieberman P, Camargo CA, Jr., Bohlke K, Jick H, Miller RL, Sheikh A, et al. Epidemiology of anaphylaxis: findings of the American College of Allergy, Asthma and Immunology Epidemiology of Anaphylaxis Working Group. *Ann. Allergy Asthma Immunol.*2006Nov;97(5):596-602.

[7] Johansson SG, Bieber T, Dahl R, Friedmann PS, Lanier BQ, Lockey RF, et al. Revised nomenclature for allergy for global use: Report of the Nomenclature Review Committee of the World Allergy Organization, October 2003. *J. Allergy Clin. Immunol.* 2004 May; 113(5): 832-6.

[8] Simons FE, Frew AJ, Ansotegui IJ, Bochner BS, Golden DB, Finkelman FD, et al. Risk assessment in anaphylaxis: current and future approaches. *Journal of Allergy and Clinical Immunology*2007Jul;120(1Suppl):S2-24.

[9] Pumphrey. Lessons for management of anaphylaxis from a study of fatal reactions. *Clinical and Experimental Allergy* 2000; 30(8):1144.

[10] Pumphrey RSH, Stanworth SJ. The clinical spectrum of anaphylaxis in north-west England. *Clinical and Experimental Allergy* 1996; 26(12): 1364.

[11] Rudders SA, Banerji A, Clark S, Camargo CA, Jr. Age-related differences in the clinical presentation of food-induced anaphylaxis. *Journal of Pediatrics* 2011 Feb; 158(2): 326-8.

[12] Braganza SC, Acworth JP, McKinnon DR, Peake JE, Brown AF. Paediatric emergency department anaphylaxis: different patterns from adults. Arch Dis Child2006 Feb;91(2):159-63.

[13] Bock SA, Munoz-Furlong A, Sampson HA. Fatalities due to anaphylactic reactions to foods. *J. Allergy Clin Immunol.* 2001 Jan; 107(1): 191-3.

[14] Guenova E, Volz T, Eichner M, Hoetzenecker W, Caroli U, Griesinger G, et al. Basal serum tryptase as risk assessment for severe Hymenoptera sting reactions in elderly. *Allergy* 2010; 65(7): 919-23.

[15] Calabria C, Chacko T, Finegold I, Nelson M, Weber R, Reviewers TF, et al. Allergen immunotherapy: a practice parameter third update. *J. Allergy Clin. Immunol.* 2011.

[16] Novembre E, Cianferoni A, Bernardini R, Mugnaini L, Caffarelli C, Cavagni G, et al. Anaphylaxis in children: clinical and allergologic features. *Pediatrics* 1998 Apr; 101(4):E8.

[17] Tse Y, Rylance G. Emergency management of anaphylaxis in children and young people: new guidance from the Resuscitation Council (UK). *Archives of disease in childhood* - Education and practice edition 2009 August 1, 2009; 94(4):97-101.

[18] Toogood JH. Beta-blocker therapy and the risk of anaphylaxis. *CMAJ: Canadian Medical Association Journal* 1987; 136(9):929.

[19] Stumpf JL, Shehab N, Patel AC. Safety of angiotensin-converting enzyme inhibitors in patients with insect venom allergies. *The Annals of pharmacotherapy* 2006; 40(4): 699-703.

[20] Yilmaz Ä, Dogan S, Tutar N, Kanbay A, Buyukoglan H, Demir R. Biphasic anaphylaxis to gemifloxacin. *Asia Pacific Allergy*; 2(4):280.

[21] Mueller UR. Cardiovascular disease and anaphylaxis. *Current opinion in allergy and clinical immunology* 2007; 7(4):337-41.

[22] Simons F, Frew AJ, Ansotegui IJ, Bochner BS, Golden DBK, Finkelman FD, et al. Risk assessment in anaphylaxis: current and future approaches. *Journal of allergy and clinical immunology* 2007; 120(1):S2-S24.

[23] Brockow K, Jofer C, Behrendt H, Ring J. Anaphylaxis in patients with mastocytosis: a study on history, clinical features and risk factors in 120 patients. *Allergy* 2008; 63(2):226-32.

[24] Rueff F, Placzek M, Przybilla B. Mastocytosis and Hymenoptera venom allergy. *Current opinion in allergy and clinical immunology* 2006; 6(4): 284-8.

[25] Harada S, Horikawa T, Ashida M, Kamo T, Nishioka E, Ichihashi M. Aspirin enhances the induction of type I allergic symptoms when combined with food and exercise in patients with food dependent exercise induced anaphylaxis. *British Journal of Dermatology* 2001; 145(2):336-9.

[26] Lieberman P. Biphasic anaphylactic reactions. *Annals of allergy, asthma and immunology: official publication of the American College of Allergy, Asthma, and Immunology* 2005; 95(3):217.

[27] Mehr S, Liew WK, Tey D, Tang MLK. Clinical predictors for biphasic reactions in children presenting with anaphylaxis. *Clinical and Experimental Allergy* 2009; 39(9):1390.

[28] Sampson HA, Mendelson L, Rosen JP. Fatal and Near-Fatal Anaphylactic Reactions to Food in Children and Adolescents. *New England Journal of Medicine* 1992; 327(6):380-4.

[29] Krugman SD, Chiaramonte DR, Matsui EC. Diagnosis and management of food-induced anaphylaxis: a national survey of pediatricians. *Pediatrics* 2006; 118(3):e554-e60.

[30] Choo KJL, Simons FE, Sheikh A. Glucocorticoids for the treatment of anaphylaxis. *Cochrane Database Syst. Rev.* 2012;4.

[31] Ellis AK, Day JH. Incidence and characteristics of biphasic anaphylaxis: a prospective evaluation of 103 patients. Annals of Allergy, Asthma andamp; *Immunology* 2007; 98(1):64.

[32] Scranton SE, Gonzalez EG, Waibel KH. Incidence and characteristics of biphasic reactions after allergen immunotherapy. *J. Allergy Clin. Immunol.* 2009 Feb; 123(2): 493-8.

[33] De Swert LFA, Bullens D, Raes M, Dermaux AM. Anaphylaxis in referred pediatric patients: demographic and clinical features, triggers, and therapeutic approach. *European Journal of pediatrics* 2008; 167(11): 1251-61.

[34] Stark BJ, Sullivan TJ. Biphasic and protracted anaphylaxis. *Journal of Allergy and Clinical Immunology* 1986; 78(1, Part 1):76.

[35] Popa VT, Lerner SA. Biphasic systemic anaphylactic reaction: three illustrative cases. *Ann. Allergy* 1984 Aug; 53(2):151-5.

[36] Bagnis R, Berglund F, Elias PS, van Esch GJ, Halstead BW, Kojima K. Problems of toxicants in marine food products. 1. Marine biotoxins. *Bull. World Health Organ* 1970; 42(1):69-88.

[37] Hughes JM, Merson MH. Current concepts fish and shellfish poisoning. *The New England Journal of medicine* 1976 Nov 11; 295(20):1117-20.

[38] Morrow JD, Margolies GR, Rowland J, Roberts LJ. Evidence That Histamine Is the Causative Toxin of Scombroid-Fish Poisoning. *New England Journal of Medicine* 1991; 324(11):716-20.

[39] Taylor SL, Stratton JE, Nordlee JA. Histamine Poisoning (Scombroid Fish Poisoning): An Allergy-Like Intoxication. *Clinical Toxicology* 1989; 27(4-5):225-40.

[40] Sanchez-Guerrero IM, Vidal JB, Escudero AI. Scombroid fish poisoning: A potentially life-threatening allergic-like reaction. *The Journal of allergy and clinical immunology* 1997; 100(3):433.

[41] Conde-Agudelo An, Romero R. Amniotic fluid embolism: an evidence-based review. *American Journal of Obstetrics and Gynecology* 2009; 201(5):445.e1.

[42] Harboe T, Benson MD, Oi H, Softeland E, Bjorge L, Guttormsen AB. Cardiopulmonary distress during obstetrical anaesthesia: attempts to diagnose amniotic fluid embolism in a case series of suspected allergic anaphylaxis. *Acta Anaesthesiologica Scandinavica* 2006; 50(3):324.

[43] Lewis Ge. Saving Mothers' Lives: reviewing maternal deaths to make motherhood safer - 2003-2005. *The Seventh Report on Confi dential Enquiries into Maternal Deaths in the United Kingdom*. London: CEMACH2007.

[44] Tuffnell DJ, Hamilton S. Amniotic fluid embolism. *Obstetrics, Gynaecology andamp; Reproductive Medicine* 2008; 18(8):213.

[45] Farrar SC, Gherman RB. Serum tryptase analysis in a woman with amniotic fluid embolism. *A case report. J. Reprod. Med.* 2001 Oct; 46(10): 926-8.

[46] Patterson R, Stoloff RS, Greenberger PA, Grammer LC, Harris KE. Algorithms for the diagnosis and management of idiopathic anaphylaxis. *Annals of allergy* 1993; 71(1):40.

[47] Patterson R, Tripathi A, Saltoun C, Harris KE. Idiopathic anaphylaxis: variants as diagnostic and therapeutic problems. *Allergy and Asthma Proceedings* 2000; 21: 141-4.

[48] Choy AC, Patterson R, Patterson DR, Grammer LC, Greenberger PA, McGrath KG, et al. Undifferentiated somatoform idiopathic anaphylaxis: nonorganic symptoms mimicking idiopathic anaphylaxis. *Journal of Allergy and Clinical Immunology* 1995 Dec; 96(6 Pt 1):893-900.

[49] Patnaik MM, Rindos M, Kouides PA, Tefferi A, Pardanani A. Systemic Mastocytosis: A Concise Clinical and Laboratory Review. *Archives of Pathology and Laboratory Medicine* 2007 2007/05/01; 131(5):784-91.

[50] Valent P, Akin C, Escribano L, Födinger M, Hartmann K, Brockow K, et al. Standards and standardization in mastocytosis: Consensus Statements on Diagnostics, Treatment Recommendations and Response Criteria. *European Journal of Clinical Investigation* 2007; 37(6):435-53.

[51] Oude Elberink JNG, de Monchy JGR, Kors JW, van Doormaal JJ, Dubois AEJ. Fatal anaphylaxis after a yellow jacket sting, despite venom immunotherapy, in two patients with mastocytosis. *Journal of Allergy and Clinical Immunology* 1997; 99(1):153-4.

[52] Greenhawt M, Akin C. Mastocytosis and allergy. *Curr. Opin. Allergy Clin. Immunol.* [Review]. 2007 Oct;7(5):387-92.

[53] Caughey GH. Tryptase genetics and anaphylaxis. *Journal of Allergy and Clinical Immunology* 2006; 117(6):1411-4.

[54] McCormick D. Carcinoid tumors and syndrome. *Gastroenterology nursing : the official journal of the Society of Gastroenterology Nurses and Associates.* [Case Reports Review]. 2002 May-Jun;25(3):105-11.

[55] Läuffer JM, Zhang T, Modlin IM. Review article: current status of gastrointestinal carcinoids. *Alimentary pharmacology and therapeutics* 1999; 13(3):271-87.

[56] Izikson L, English JC, 3rd, Zirwas MJ. The flushing patient: differential diagnosis, workup, and treatment. *Journal of the American Academy of Dermatology.* [Research Support, Non-U.S. Gov't Review]. 2006 Aug; 55(2):193-208.

[57] Ramage JK, Davies AHG, Ardill J, Bax N, Caplin M, Grossman A, et al. Guidelines for the management of gastroenteropancreatic neuroendocrine (including carcinoid) tumours. *Gut* 2005 June 1, 2005; 54(suppl 4):iv1-iv16.

[58] Lenders JWM, Eisenhofer G, Mannelli M, Pacak K. Phaeochromocytoma. *The Lancet* 2005; 366(9486):665-75.

[59] Lo CY, Lam KY, Wat MS, Lam KS. Adrenal pheochromocytoma remains a frequently overlooked diagnosis. *American Journal of surgery.* [Comparative Study]. 2000 Mar; 179(3):212-5.

[60] Lenders JW, Pacak K, Eisenhofer G. New advances in the biochemical diagnosis of pheochromocytoma: moving beyond catecholamines. *Annals of the New York Academy of Sciences.* [Review]. 2002 Sep; 970:29-40.

[61] Biteker M, Ekşi Duran N, Sungur Biteker F, Ayyıldız Civan H, Kaya H, Gökdeniz T, et al. Allergic myocardial infarction in childhood: Kounis syndrome. *European Journal of Pediatrics* 2010; 169(1):27.

[62] Kogias JS, Sideris SK, Anifadis SK. Kounis syndrome associated with hypersensitivity to hymenoptera stings. *Int. J. Cardiol.* 2007 Jan 8; 114(2): 252-5.

[63] Wada T, Abe M, Yagi N, Kokubu N, Kasahara Y, Kataoka Y, et al. Coronary vasospasm secondary to allergic reaction following food ingestion: a case of type I variant Kounis syndrome. *Heart and vessels* 2010; 25(3):263-6.

[64] Pfister CW, Plice SG. Acute myocardial infarction during a prolonged allergic reaction to penicillin. *Am. Heart J.* 1950 Dec; 40(6):945-7.

[65] Kounis NG, Zavras GM. Histamine-induced coronary artery spasm: the concept of allergic angina. *Br. J. Clin. Pract.* 1991 Summer;45(2):121-8.

[66] Kounis GN, Hahalis G, Soufras GD, Mazarakis A, Niarchos C, Kounis NG. Kounis syndrome and simultaneous multivessel acute coronary syndromes after successful drug-eluting stent implantation. International *Journal of Cardiology* 2008; 127(1):146.

[67] Cevik C, Nugent K, Shome GP, Kounis NG. Treatment of Kounis syndrome. *International Journal of Cardiology* 2010;143(3):223.

[68] Suk EH, Kim DH, Kweon TD, Na SW, Shin JA. Stress-induced cardiomyopathy following cephalosporin-induced anaphylactic shock during general anesthesia. *Can. J. Anaesth.* 2009 Jun; 56(6):432-6.

[69] Hartmann M, Bode C, Zirlik A. Anaphylactic shock-associated cardiomyopathy. *International Journal of Cardiology* 2008;127(3): e136.

[70] Garvey LH, Roed-Petersen J, Husum B. Anaphylactic reactions in anaesthetised patients – four cases of chlorhexidine allergy. *Acta Anaesthesiologica Scandinavica* 2001; 45(10):1290.

[71] Jacobsen RB, Borch JE, Bindslev-Jensen C. Hypersensitivity to local anaesthetics. *Allergy* 2005; 60(2):262.

[72] Simon MR. Anaphylaxis associated with relative bradycardia. *Annals of allergy* 1989; 62(6):495-7.

[73] Powell DM, Karanfilov BI, Beechler KB, Treole K, Trudeau MD, Forrest LA. Paradoxical vocal cord dysfunction in juveniles. *Arch. Otolaryngol. Head Neck Surg.* 2000 Jan; 126(1):29-34.

[74] Brugman SM, Newman K. Vocal cord dysfunction. *Med/Sci Update* 1993; 11:1-6.

[75] Kayani S, Shannon DC. Vocal cord dysfunction associated with exercise in adolescent girls. *CHEST Journal* 1998;113(2):540-2.

[76] Meltzer EO, Orgel HA, Kemp JP, Welch MJ, Ostrom NK, Park SM, et al. Clinical Acumen: Vocal Cord Dysfunction in a Child with Asthma. *Journal of Asthma* 1991; 28(2):141-5.

[77] Tilles SA. Vocal cord dysfunction in children and adolescents. *Current allergy and asthma reports* 2003; 3(6):467-72.

[78] Deveney CW, Benner K, Cohen J. Gastroesophageal reflux and laryngeal disease. *Archives of Surgery* 1993; 128(9):1021.

[79] Hepner DL. Propofol-Induced Bronchoconstriction: Asthma or Allergy? *Anesthesia and Analgesia* 2002 April 1, 2002; 94(4):1045.

[80] Choi S-J, Lee J-C, Kim M-J, Hur G-Y, Shin S-Y, Park H-S. The Clinical Characteristics of Anisakis Allergy in Korea. Korean *J. Intern. Med.* 2009; 24(2):160.

[81] Audicana M, García M, Del Pozo MD, Díez J, Muñoz D, Fernández E, et al. Clinical manifestations of allergy to Anisakis simplex. *Allergy* 2000; 55(Supp59):28.

[82] Kimura S, Takagi Y, Gomi K. IgE response to Anisakis compared to seafood. *Allergy* 1999; 54(11):1225.

[83] Repiso Ortega A, Alcantara Torres M, Gonzalez de Frutos C, de Artaza Varasa T, Rodriguez Merlo R, Valle Munoz J, et al. Gastrointestinal anisakiasis. Study of a series of 25 patients. *Gastroenterologia y hepatologia* 2003; 26(6):341-6.

[84] Langer JC, Rose DB, Keystone JS, Taylor BR, Langer B. Diagnosis and management of hydatid disease of the liver. A 15-year North American experience. *Annals of surgery* 1984; 199(4):412.

[85] Boyano T, Moldenhauer F, Mira J, Joral A, Saiz F. Systemic anaphylaxis due to hepatic hydatid disease. *Journal of investigational allergology and clinical immunology: official organ of the International Association of Asthmology (INTERASMA) and Sociedad Latinoamericana de Alergia e InmunologÃ-a* 1994; 4(3):158.

[86] Gelincik A, Ozseker F, Buyukozturk S, Colakoglu B, Dal M, Alper A. Recurrent anaphylaxis due to non-ruptured hepatic hydatid cysts. *International archives of allergy and immunology* 2007; 143(4):296-8.

[87] Simons FE, Ardusso LR, Bilo MB, El-Gamal YM, Ledford DK, Ring J, et al. World Allergy Organization anaphylaxis guidelines: summary. *J. Allergy Clin. Immunol.* 2011 Mar; 127(3):587-93 e1-22.

In: Anaphylaxis: Principles and Practice
Editor: M. Thirumala Krishna

ISBN: 978-1-62618-688-0

Chapter III

Biomarkers of Anaphylaxis

Gabriel K. Wong and Aarnoud P. Huissoon*
Department of Allergy and Clinical Immunology, Birmingham Heartlands Hospital, Bordesley Green East, Birmingham, UK

Abstract

The measurement of histamine and tryptase have become firmly established to aid the diagnosis of allergic reactions and anaphylaxis. However both have their limitations in the acute setting, being either impractical or insensitive in a number of important clinical scenarios including food allergy and post mortem diagnosis. Baseline or resting measurements are also of limited value in disease diagnosis and in predicting the likelihood and severity of anaphylaxis. For this reason novel markers have been sought for allergy diagnosis and prognostication. A number of candidate molecules and genetic polymorphisms have emerged which may find their way into the diagnostic armamentarium. Most of these are still in the early stages of development, and will require extensive testing to establish their sensitivity and specificity against the wide range of alternative presentations that may masquerade as allergy. While the clinical presentation remains paramount, the diagnosis and management of this devastating and unpredictable condition may soon be augmented by a new array of biomarkers. Alone or in combination, these should help to provide guidance and reassurance to patients and their physicians alike.

Introduction

Biomarkers are usually considered to be protein, molecular or other biological signatures of the presence, progress or severity of a disease. To this can be added their use in

* Corresponding author: Dr. Aarnoud Huissoon; Address: Department of Allergy and Clinical Immunology, Birmingham Heartlands Hospital, Bordesley Green East, Birmingham, B9 5SS, United Kingdom; Tel:0121 424 0185; Fax: 0121 424 3229; Email: aarnoud.huissoon@heartofengland.nhs.uk.

prognostication, which may include the likelihood of a condition occurring or of response to specific therapies.

Anaphylaxis describes a combination of extreme and potentially harmful multisystem physiological responses to mast cell degranulation into the systemic circulation. [1] It is becoming clear that several cell types are involved in mediating and modulating the features of anaphylaxis. Furthermore, anaphylactic pathways may be triggered through IgE (classical) or via non-IgE mediated (alternative) mechanisms. [2]

Knowledge of the signature mechanisms of the anaphylactic process has lead to the identification of biomarkers such as histamine and tryptase, which can be measured clinically as indices of mast cell burden or activation. These can be helpful when the distinction between anaphylaxis and other causes of collapse is not clear, for example during general anaesthetic allergy when cardiovascular collapse can occur in isolation prior to any detectable mucocutaneous signs of anaphylaxis [3].

Measurement of laboratory biomarkers are therefore now routinely recommended in conjunction with the clinical assessment of patients with suspected anaphylaxis, [4] and a wider range of markers may offer more sophisticated tools for the diagnosis of anaphylaxis.

Biomarkers associated with the effector mechanisms of anaphylaxis may also provide information that will help with assessing the risk of future reactions and their likely severity. This may in turn lead to better individualised management plans for patients who suffer from allergies, many of whom may be unnecessarily concerned about the risk of future severe reactions.

In this chapter we will discuss an array of molecules (Table 1) relating to anaphylaxis mostly in human studies, the historical and current clinical applications of some of these biomarkers and finally some of the potential future markers that are likely to help in the diagnosis and management of anaphylaxis.

Biomarkers in Humans and Animal Models of Anaphylaxis

Mast cell degranulation is considered to have a pivotal role in the pathogenesis of anaphylaxis and numerous intracellular and extracellular molecules were shown to be associated with this mechanism.

When mast cells are activated, usually via cross-linking of surface IgE (IgE mediated reaction), they release pre-formed cytoplasmic granules containing histamine, prostaglandins, leukotrienes, tryptase, chymase, cathepsin G, and carboxypepitdase A3 [5, 6] into the circulation and surrounding tissues within seconds to minutes. A late phase response may follow 8-72 hours after the primary reaction, when the synthesis of eicosanoids and other inflammatory mediators, platelet activation, recruitment of other effector cells, and activation of the renin-angiotensin-bradykinin system manifest as recurrence of angioedema, bronchospasm and hypotension [7, 8].

While IgE-mediated mast cell activation is the best understood mechanism of anaphylaxis, non IgE-mediated reactions can also occur and may be facilitated via neutrophils, eosinophils and the complement system.

Table 1. Biomarkers in anaphylaxis

	Diagnosis	Prognosis	Notes
Histamine	Y	N	Short half-life. Serum needs to be frozen promptly
Tryptase	Y	Y	Stable, clinically useful kinetics. May lack sensitivity in some situations.
N-methyl histamine	Y	N	Measured in urine. May be increased in a variety of non-allergic conditions, and with bacterial contamination of urine sample.
Prostaglandins	Y	N	Specificity for anaphylaxis uncertain
Leukotrienes	Y	N	Specificity for anaphylaxis uncertain
Cathepsin G	?	N	Only preliminary data published
Carboxypeptidase A3	Y	N	Only preliminary data published
Diamine oxidase activity	N	?	No relationship with anaphylaxis established to date
Platelet activating factor	Y	N	PAF raised in anaphylaxis. Sample collection difficult.
PAF acetyl hydrolase	N	Y	Activity inversely correlated with severity.
Dipeptidylpeptidase	Y	N	Non-specific – expressed in many other cells.
Bradykinin	?	N	Bradykinin measurement requires special sampling conditions. Byproducts of bradykinin pathway may be more clinically useful.
Angiotenson converting enzyme	N	Y	Reduced ACE activity associated with increased risk of angioedema.

Histamine

Histamine was first identified and synthesised over 100 years ago, and was immediately recognised as one of the key mediators of allergic symptoms and anaphylaxis. Histamine synthesis is regulated by histidine decarboxylase [9] and is degraded by N-methyl transferase and diamine oxidase. [10, 11] Evidence of histamine involvement in anaphylaxis was best demonstrated by the occurrence of anaphylaxis following the direct infusion of histamine in humans. [12] Moreover, the clear beneficial effects of H1 histamine antagonists in allergy and anaphylaxis, demonstrated in the 1920s, further consolidated histamine as an important mediator in these conditions. However it is only relatively recently with the development of the histidine decarboxylase knockout mouse, which lacks the capacity to synthesise histamine, that it has been possible to more clearly delineate which features of an experimental model of anaphylaxis were directly attributable to histamine. [13] This showed that reduction of body temperature and respiratory modulation were attributable to histamine, but that hypotension occurred independently of histamine. If this is also true in humans, then this might help to explain why anti-histamines fail to reduce the severity of anaphylaxis, for example in the context of venom immunotherapy, while effectively treating local reactions. [14] Impaired degradation of histamine by reduced diamine oxidase activity might enhance anaphylaxis.

In humans, diamine oxidase activity has been linked to atopic eczema and histamine intolerance, and gene polymorphisms have been associated with enzyme activity, but it's role in anaphylaxis, if any, is not clear [15, 16, 17].

Mast Cell Proteases

The proteases (mainly tryptase, chymase and carboxypeptidase A3 and dipeptidylpeptidase) make up a large proportion of total mast cell protein [18]. Tryptases (α and β) are serine-endopeptidases that have trypsin-like activities including inhibition of fibrinogen, activation of endothelial cells and chemokines, in particular IL-8 which promotes the migration of neutrophils and eosinophils towards the sites of inflammation. [19, 20] The relevance of this in human asthma was supported by the finding that a tryptase inhibitor was able to inhibit the late asthmatic response. [21] Like histamine, these proteases are found within the pre-formed granules of mast cells and basophils. When mast cells are activated, proteases are released and exert their effects mainly via activation of the complement, coagulation and kallikrein-kinin pathways [22].

Chymase is also located within the secretory granules of mast cells and can augment allergic inflammation. Similar to the action of angiotensin converting enzyme (ACE), it converts angiotensin I into angiotensin II. Furthermore, it augments the allergic inflammatory response by increasing the level of IL-1 beta, a potent inflammatory cytokine. However, the function of chymase may be more complex and it has been shown to have anti-inflammatory properties by inhibiting bradykinin, neuropeptide VIP and substance P [23-26].

Of all mast cell proteases, Carboxypeptidase A3 is probably the most specific for mast cells since it is not found in basophils. [27] It is predominantly found in mast cells that are located in the gastrointestinal tract and skin (MCTC). It converts angiotensin I into angiotensin II and degrades neuropeptidase. [27-29] Carboxypeptidase A3 is not elevated during exacerbations of asthma which may make it a suitable biomarker for anaphylaxis. [11, 30] It may also have a role in the laboratory diagnosis of drug allergy and post-mortem examination of anaphylaxis [31, 32].

Dipeptidylpeptidase I (Cathepsin C) is also abundant in mast cells, and elevated levels have been reported to correlate well with objective allergic reactions in food challenges [31]. However, both this enzyme and cathepsin G are present in many other cell types, and may therefore not be helpful as specific markers of mast cell degranulation [18].

Eicosanoids

Derivatives of arachidonic acids are key inflammatory mediators of allergic disorders. Lipooxygenase facilitates the breakdown of arachidonic acid into various forms of leukotrienes while cycloxygenase mediates the synthesis of prostaglandins [33].

Prostaglandin has a range of physiological effects - it regulates contraction and relaxation of smooth muscles, inhibits platelet aggregation and recruits neutrophils and eosinophils. [34-

36] Prostaglandin can be broadly divided into PGD2, PGE2 and PGF2 which can be detected both in urine as well as serum either in their naïve forms or as metabolites. The involvement of prostaglandins in the pathogenesis of anaphylaxis and other allergic disorders is undisputed.

Intradermal injection of PGD2 leads to vasodilatation and increased vascular permeability, [37] and elevated PGD2 has been detected in bronchial and nasal secretions of patients with asthma and rhinitis. [38, 39] More specifically, 9alpha, 11beta-PGF2 can be significantly elevated during anaphylaxis. [40] However, there are studies to suggest that the release of prostaglandins is not confined to anaphylaxis and elevated urinary PGD2 could also be found in aspirin-intolerant asthma and even with physical agitation of lung tissues. [41, 42] No effective anti-prostaglandin agent exists for human use.

Leukotrienes exert a chemotactic effect on migrating neutrophils and also regulate bronchoconstriction and vascular permeability. [43, 44] Cysteinyl leukotrienes such as LTC4, LTD4 and LTE4 exhibit their effects by binding to leukotriene receptors (CysLT1 and CysLT2). Leukotrienes have been extensively studied in the context of asthma and bronchial inflammation. Leukotriene receptor antagonists such as montelukast are now widely used for treatment of chronic asthma and rhinitis. In addition there is increasing evidence to support its role in eosinophillic inflammation by attracting and activating eosinophils at inflammatory sites. [45] In vitro release of sulfidoleukotrienes by cellular antigen stimulation test (CAST) has been shown in patients with a history of beta lactam allergy and anaphylaxis, [46] but direct measurements in vivo have not been performed. Administration of low concentration of histamine and cysteinyl leukotrienes can cause significant systemic and coronary haemodynamic effects [47].

The combined assessment of prostaglandins and leukotrienes may increase the diagnostic specificity as a recent study has shown that elevation in both urinary leukotriene E4 and prostaglandin D2 metabolites were specific for anaphylaxis and were not found in asthmatic patients and healthy controls [40].

Renin-Angiotensin System and the Kallikrein-Bradykinin Pathway

Bradykinin is the end product of the kallikrein-bradykinin pathway. It binds bradykinin beta2 receptors expressed on a range of tissues and exerts potent physiological effects such as vasodilatation and increased vascular permeability, [48] and is inactivated by angiotensin converting enzyme. [49] Bradykinin is an important mediator for angioedema and hypotension during anaphylaxis. Increased plasma bradykinin can be seen during IgE-mediated allergic reactions, in patients receiving angiotensin converting enzyme inhibitor (ACE-I) therapy, and during an acute attack of C1 esterase inhibitor deficiency. Angioedema as a result of excess bradykinin has the potential to lead to life-threatening laryngeal obstruction and is a medical emergency.

The conversion of angiotensinogen into its active form is an important result of mast cell activation and degranulation. Genetic polymorphisms of angiotensinogen have been found to influence the potency of the renin-angiotensin system. The polymorphism AGTp.M235T occurs more frequently in patients with insect venom anaphylaxis than in healthy individual and is associated with an increased risk of grade IV anaphylactic reactions. [50] Renin can also be released by mast cells, especially cardiac mast cells [51].

Bradykinin is broken down by angiotensin-converting enzyme (ACE), carboxypeptidase N and aminopeptidase P. [52] In a series of patients with severe nut allergy, low serum ACE levels were associated with an increased risk of severe pharyngeal oedema, whereas aminopeptidase P levels showed no association with any features of anaphylaxis [53]. The substantial overlap of ACE levels between the patient groups in this study means that the prospective determination of ACE levels is unlikely to be a useful predictor of reaction severity in individual patients. Nevertheless, the observed association does emphasise the role of bradykinin in the pathogenesis of angioedema in anaphylaxis due to food allergy. Despite much circumstantial evidence for its role in eliciting angioedema during allergic responses, more recent specific studies of the role of bradykinin in human anaphylaxis are lacking [54, 55].

This is mainly due to the difficulties in measuring this very labile component *ex vivo*. Samples need to be appropriately prepared within seconds of venepuncture, and stored routine serum or plasma samples are useless for bradykinin measurement. Products of the contact activation system can be measured, giving indirect evidence for bradykinin production [55].

Platelet Activation: PAF and Its Relationship with PAF Acetyl Hydrolase

Platelet activating factor (PAF) is a proinflammatory phospholipid synthesised by mast cells, basophils, macrophages and monocytes. [56, 57] The PAF-receptor is expressed on platelets, neutrophils, monocytes and macrophages. [58] PAF has multiple actions and the ligation of PAF onto its receptor triggers platelet aggregation, inflammation, oxidative burst, chemotaxis as well as mast cell degranulation. [58-60] Mast cell degranulation occurs within seconds following PAF:PAF-receptor binding and this process is dependent on extracellular Ca2+. [61] In addition, PAF can induce bronchoconstriction, increase vascular permeability leading to shock, and promote neutrophil transmigration. [62-64].

In view of its potent activities in anaphylaxis, PAF and its regulatory enzyme PAF-acetyl hydrolase have recently been the focus of research interest. A number of studies have now showed that plasma PAF levels are elevated during human anaphylaxis. [57, 58] Vadas and colleagues first showed that serum PAF is correlated with the severity of anaphylaxis and high levels may be found in almost all patients with severe anaphylaxis, even in the absence of an elevated tryptase. [65] This ability to reflect severity of anaphylaxis provides an additional dimension to the current standard investigation of anaphylaxis.

PAF is degraded by PAF acetylhydrolase in the circulation and PAF acetylhydrolase activity is inversely correlated with severity of anaphylaxis in peanut allergic patients. [57] These observations suggest that PAF is more than simply a passive marker of mast cell degranulation and support its role as an important mediator in human anaphylaxis.

This is further supported in animal models. A PAF receptor knockout mouse was found to be generally healthy but resistant to anaphylaxis. [66] In a murine nut allergy model fatal anaphylaxis was prevented by blocking PAF and histamine. [67] However a range of PAF antagonists have had disappointing clinical effects in asthma.

The administration of PAF acetyl hydrolase also markedly reduced anaphylaxis mortality in a dose dependent manner in a mouse model. [59] This last observation could even have therapeutic implications for management of anaphylaxis in humans.

Complement C3a, C5a and sC5-9

Activation of the complement system releases anaphylotoxins such as C3a, C4a and C5a which can have a direct amplification effect on mast cell activity. [68] C5a causes rapid release of histamine and tryptase from human mast cells. [47] In addition, soluble C5-9 complex can augment the process of anaphylaxis by inducing platelet activation. [69] In both murine and human allergic model, peanut extracts can activate mast cells and basophils via C3a. [62] However, attempts to identify polymorphisms in the complement control system associated with severity of peanut anaphylaxis failed to find any link [70]. Although the activation of the complement system and the release of anaphylotoxins are closely associated with anaphylaxis they are by no means confined to this scenario and their role as biomarkers is likely to be limited.

IgG / FCγRIII - Mediated Anaphylaxis

In addition to IgE, anaphylaxis may be mediated via IgG / immune complexes and FCγRIII and the majority of the evidence is derived from murine studies. [71] This mechanism may be facilitated via activation of neutrophils and basophils instead of mast cells. [56, 72] Immune complexes may actually block the classical (IgE mediated) pathway of anaphylaxis but promote this alternative pathway. [73] Upon IgG activation basophils can release platelet activating factor (PAF) resulting in anaphylaxis. [56] The classical pathway of anaphylaxis may increase plasma IL-4, soluble IL-4Ra and IL-4Ra expression on T cells but this is not seen in alternative pathway activation. [71] There is currently no direct evidence of involvement of this alternative pathway of anaphylaxis in humans.

Cytokines

Given the wide range of cellular activation that occurs during anaphylaxis, it is not surprising that increases in systemic levels of a number of cytokines are detectable. A recent study by Stone et al. showed that IL-2, IL-6, IL-10 and TNF receptor I all increased significantly during anaphylaxis, and correlated with the severity of the reaction. [74] A range of plasma kinetics was observed for these cytokines, but most peaked within the first 10 hours after the reaction. These cytokines are known to be increased in other inflammatory reactions and infections, so may lack specificity for anaphylaxis in complex presentations. Interestingly, IL-4, IL-5 and IL-13, cytokines generally associated with T helper 2 responses and allergic phenomena, were only slightly raised, with no correlation with the severity of the reaction. In common with many biomarkers, such studies are limited by the fact that cytokine changes detected in peripheral blood may not accurately reflect the cytokine environment in the local milieu of the tissues involved in the reaction.

IL-33 is a relatively recently discovered IL-1 related cytokine released following cell lysis. Receptors of IL-33, orphan receptor ST2, are expressed on mast cells and Th2 T cells and IL-33 has been linked to the pathophysiology of asthma, atopic eczema and anaphylaxis.

[75, 76] Reports of IL-33's role as a significant mediator of anaphylaxis require independent confirmation.

Clinical Application of Biomarkers

We have discussed a number of mediators that trigger or are released during anaphylaxis as well as markers associating with an increased risk of anaphylaxis. Detection of these markers could support a clinical diagnosis of anaphylaxis. For an analyte to be suitable for routine clinical measurement, it needs to be stable in vitro, easy to collect and have a relatively long plasma half-life to allow clinicians a flexible window period for sample acquisition, having first stabilised the patient. Also the assay should be accurate and reproducible, and be subject to adequate internal and external quality measures. Unfortunately very few of the biomarkers discussed above would fulfil these criteria. Many are labile or cumbersome to use clinically and are currently only measured in the research setting. Tryptase, and to a lesser degree histamine, are exceptions.

Histamine and N-Methyl Histamine

The measurement of plasma histamine levels is an obvious candidate for the diagnosis of allergic reactions or anaphylaxis. It correlates well with urticaria and wheeze. [77] Unfortunately it is difficult to employ in routine clinical practise, since histamine levels peak within 5-10 minutes of anaphylaxis, and levels return to baseline within an hour (Figure 1). This largely limits its utility to experimental or induced situations such as insect venom sting challenge procedures, where blood can reliably be taken within a short interval of the onset of symptoms. This is not feasible for the majority of clinical anaphylaxis scenarios where primary treatment and investigation usually take place in the community or a busy emergency department. Furthermore, histamine is rapidly degraded *ex vivo*, and samples must be placed on ice as soon as possible after sampling to obtain a reliable result.

Because of timing and special sample requirements, blood-based histamine measurements are of little practical use as markers of anaphylaxis. In the few situations where histamine measurement is possible, it may be more sensitive than tryptase. [77, 78] The combined measurement of histamine and tryptase seems to offer superior sensitivity [79].

Systemic histamine is metabolised by the enzyme histamine N-methyltransferase to produce N-methyl histamine, which is excreted in the urine. This product is relatively stable, and urine samples taken soon after an allergic episode, and compared with a baseline sample taken more than 24 hours afterwards, can give indirect evidence of systemic histamine release. Urinary methyl histamine is also raised in mastocytosis, and has been used to monitor this disease. [80] It is also the only test which may give positive diagnostic information in scombroid fish poisoning, where histamine absorbed from spoiled fish such as tuna and mackerel causes allergic symptoms without mast cell or basophil activation. [81] Allergy testing or measurement of other mast cell mediators such as tryptase are of no help, but the finding of a transiently raised urine methyl histamine supports the diagnosis.

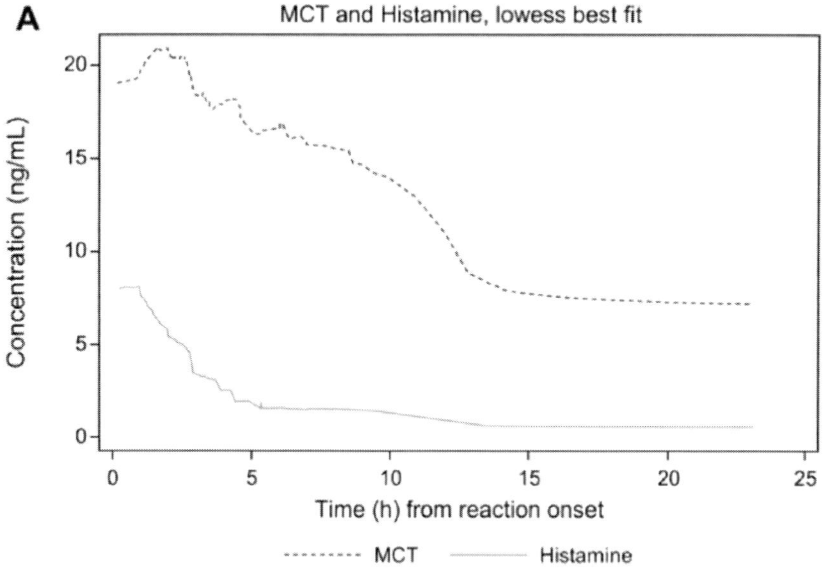

Figure 1. Serum levels of mast cell tryptase (MCT) and histamine from time of onset of anaphylaxis (reproduced with permission from Stone et al 2009 [74]).

Urinary methyl histamine is also elevated in a few other situations, including interstitial cystitis, some myeloproliferative disorders, carcinoid syndrome, phaeochromocytoma, ingestion of monoamine oxidase inhibitors and with bacterial contamination of the urine sample. The levels of N-methyl histamine in these cases are often modest compared with those seen in severe anaphylaxis, and comparison with a baseline sample can also be informative. However, since some of these conditions may mimic allergy and anaphylaxis, care must be taken in the interpretation of this test. Where the test is used for monitoring mastocytosis, patients should avoid histamine-rich foods for 24 hours prior to collection.

Mast Cell Tryptase

Mast cell tryptase has become the most widely used laboratory marker for anaphylaxis in the clinical setting and can be measured in either serum or plasma. It has a relatively long plasma half-life (approximately 2 hours) making it a more suitable analyte than histamine. [82] Frozen samples are stable for up to a year although it may start to degrade if left at room temperature for 2 days. It exists in α and β isoforms; α-tryptase is constitutively expressed and correlates with the total body mast cell load of an individual. Elevated α-tryptase may be found in all forms of systemic mastocytosis ranging from indolent systemic mastocytosis to mast cell leukaemia. [83] In contrast, β-tryptase is released into the circulation during acute mast cell degranulation, and is therefore suitable as a marker of anaphylaxis. Commercial assays do not differentiate between α and β tryptases and therefore measurement of both baseline and acute tryptase levels is necessary for the correct interpretation of the results. Serial samples should be taken in order to capture the rise and fall of serum tryptase level, and a recent review and guideline has analysed the evidence for this practice [4]. The first sample is ideally taken as soon as possible after the onset of the anaphylactic episode (but after treatment has started), and a further sample should be taken within 1-2 hours but no later than 4 hours. The baseline tryptase level should be measured ≥24 hours after the episode (in practice this is often in the allergy clinic after referral for assessment). A persistently elevated tryptase level, usually above 11.4 ng/ml, suggests an underlying mast cell disorder which needs to be investigated appropriately [84]. Mast cell disorders, indicated by an elevated resting tryptase, may contribute to the patient's susceptibility to anaphylaxis and therefore this forms part of the risk assessment in determining the patient's further management.

The "normal range" cut-off for tryptase is controversial, and different authors have suggested ways of assessing a significant rise in tryptase levels during the acute episode, even when this is below the commonly-quoted upper 95th centile for normal volunteers. In a recent review, the minimal elevation of the acute total tryptase level that is considered to be clinically significant was suggested to be 2 + 1.2 x baseline tryptase levels. [85] The specificity of tryptase has been established in many potentially confounding clinical scenarios: vasovagal reactions, septic shock, seizures, myocardial shock, benign flushing, or carcinoid syndrome are not associated with elevation of blood tryptase.

Serum tryptase is usually measured by Enzyme Immuno Assay (EIA). It is reliable, automated and quality control is robust. However, in common with all EIAs, inaccurate results may be obtained due to antigen excess and interference from other plasma proteins. False positive results may be seen in the presence of rheumatoid factor, cryoglobulinaemia, infliximab treatment, HIV (due to non-specific binding) as well as heterophile antibodies. [86] Tryptase may also be elevated in end-stage renal failure or with the use of vancomycin [83, 87].

Not all anaphylactic events will be accompanied by raised tryptase [88, 89] and its sensitivity has been reported to vary from 35% to 93%. [4] A normal result therefore does not exclude anaphylaxis. This is especially important in anaphylaxis due to food allergy, where serum tryptase levels may not be increased [88, 90]. The sensitivity of the test may be improved by assessing acute rises in serum total tryptase levels within the normal diagnostic range. [91] Measurement of mature (β) tryptase may also offer superior sensitivity and diagnostic performance but is only available as a research tool [92].

Tryptase may be helpful in the post-mortem diagnosis of anaphylaxis. However samples need to taken from the femoral vein, since cardiac samples show elevated tryptase levels in death from a wide range of causes. The result should be interpreted with caution, and a higher 'cut-off' value is likely to be required than for samples taken in life. [93] Raised tryptase has been found in patients dying from asphyxia, aspirin overdose, coronary heart disease and after abdominal surgery [94].

Mastocytosis Risk Assessment

Mastocytosis describes a heterogeneous group of disorders defined by abnormal growth and accumulation of clonal mast cells. The clinical spectrum varies from simple urticaria pigmentosa in children to aggressive mast cell leukaemia. [95] Patients with mastocytosis are intrinsically at greater risk of both IgE and non-IgE mediated anaphylaxis. Moreover, patients may develop anaphylaxis to insect venom on their first exposure in the absence of IgE sensitisation. [95] cKit (CD117) is the receptor for stem cell factor (SCF), which regulates mast cell differentiation, survival, priming, and activation. [96] The D816V mutation of cKit, which leads to a gain of function, can be detected in up to 80% of patients with systemic mastocytosis and can lead to dysregulated mast cell clonal expansion. [97] Increase in total body mast cell load is reflected in serum α-tryptase which is constitutively secreted by mast cells. Therefore an elevated baseline tryptase level can be used as a screening tool for systemic mastocytosis. Occasionally mastocytosis can concur with eosinophilia with FIP1L1-PDGFRA fusion gene. [98] Other peptidases have not been evaluated for their utility in this condition.

Potential Future Biomarkers

Tryptase and histamine, the two widely-available biomarkers of anaphylaxis, suffer from limited sensitivity in many scenarios, and other markers are sought to increase the reliable identification of anaphylaxis.

Promising research data relating to PAF and PAF acetyl-hydrolase activity make this an exciting area for future clinical development. These are currently the only biomarkers that may provide prognostic information on disease severity. However in the acute diagnostic setting PAF and PAF acetyl-hydrolase are unstable and the sample needs to be frozen immediately after venesection for accurate results. This makes it impractical for the clinician to collect the sample correctly as very little time can be devoted to collecting a blood sample when managing a patient with acute anaphylaxis. Also it is currently only measured in a few laboratories and transporting frozen samples will increase the cost of the assay. When these obstacles are overcome PAF and PAF acetyl-hydrolase activity do have promise in anaphylaxis diagnosis and management in the future.

LTE4 and PGD2 have received attention as possible biomarkers, but have several limitations. Clearance of prostaglandin from the systemic circulation is rapid, and elevated serum levels of PGD2 are generally difficult to detect [78]. Its metabolite, 11β-PGF2α, may however be measured in the urine with reasonable ease and accuracy. The concomitant use of non-steroidal anti-inflammatory drugs (NSAIDs) interferes with prostaglandin assays. It may offer superior diagnostic performance, particularly in its sensitivity, when compared to urinary histamine [99, 100]. Its exact sensitivity, specificity, and predictive values will also need to be determined in larger cohorts prior to its application. The power of urinary Leukotriene E4 to distinguish between anaphylaxis and other parallel allergic disorders makes it another potential clinical marker for anaphylaxis. [40] However there is conflicting evidence regarding this finding. The combined use of Leukotriene E4 and Prostaglandin D2/F2 might be more specific. With the possible exception of their use in aspirin sensitivity, the measurement of eicosanoids in isolation seems unlikely to be useful in routine clinical practice.

The ability of carboxypeptidase A3 to differentiate between asthma and anaphylaxis as well as its extended plasma half-life post-anaphylaxis make it an attractive candidate as an anaphylaxis biomarker in situations where plasma tryptase is not elevated. [29, 97] Preliminary data, published only in abstract form, in 181 patients with suspected anaphylaxis showed that their carboxypeptidase A3 levels were significantly higher than the control group. Moreover raised carboxypepitase A3 levels were detectable in 70% of patients with a negative tryptase [30] which suggests that the combined use of tryptase and carboxypeptidase may improve the sensitivity of laboratory detection of anaphyaxis. It may also have a role in the laboratory diagnosis of drug allergy and post-mortem diagnosis of anaphylaxis. [31, 32] Further studies will be required to clarify the clinical ultility of carboxypeptidase A3 in anaphylaxis of various causes, and to confirm its ability to discriminate anaphylaxis from common confounding conditions. While measurement of one or more biomarkers has shown promise in experimental situations, ultimately the simultaneous assessment of a larger panel of biomarkers may offer the best approach in the diagnosis and prognostication of anaphylaxis. For instance, a combination of markers may be used to estimate the relative contributions of histamine, PAF and kinin-related features, or even to assess whether IgG or IgE-mediated effector mechanisms predominate. This might enable a more tailored approach to the prevention and management of future reactions. Such multi-parameter diagnostic approach will require careful studies of these markers in a wide range of well-characterised patients with anaphylaxis and similar conditions.

Clinical Cases

Case 1

A 26-year-old woman suffered a reaction 10 minutes after induction of anaesthesia for surgery for open elbow fracture. The anaesthetic notes recorded that she had a '...generalised red rash' and that her systolic blood pressure fell to 60mm Hg. She was rescuscitated with fluids and adrenaline (epinephrine), and the surgery was later completed under regional anaesthesia. Tryptase levels 1 hour after the onset of the reaction were modestly elevated at 35 mcg/L (normal range 2-14). A baseline tryptase checked the following day was 8 mcg/L. A diagnosis of anaphylaxis was made and she was referred for allergy testing.

Skin tests and specific IgE (sIgE) tests to neuromuscular blocking agents, latex and chlorhexidine were negative. She had been given amoxicillin intravenously during the surgery, preceding the anaphylactic reaction. Skin tests to penicillin major and minor determinant, benzylpenicillin and amoxicillin were negative as were serum specific IgE for penicillin V/G and amoxicillin. An oral challenge test to amoxicillin was carried out, and at a dose of 50 mg she developed a generalised itchy skin rash and her systolic blood pressure dropped to 74mm Hg from a baseline of 110mm Hg. However, her serum tryptase 1 hour after the amoxicillin challenge reaction was not elevated, at 9 mcg/L. Penicillin allergy was diagnosed as the likely cause of the peri-operative reaction.

This case illustrates that an increase in tryptase does not always follow an anaphylactic reaction. Some authors have observed that anaphylaxis following oral exposure to an allergen is less likely to result in raised tryptase as was illustrated in this patient.

Case 2

A 28-year-old man was investigated after he had suffered 3 episodes of urticarial rash with symptoms of hypotension. On each occasion he had developed sudden-onset urticaria and dizziness and on one occasion he had collapsed, requiring resuscitation by paramedics. One episode occurred while he was cycling, one while driving his car, and the third and most severe episode 15 minutes after taking 400mg of ibuprofen and 2 co-codamol tablets for back pain. Serum tryptase measured 5 hours after this episode was 54 mcg/L.

No likely allergic triggers were identified, and a provisional diagnosis of spontaneous urticaria and anaphylaxis with possible opiate or NSAID sensitivity was made. Daily prophylactic cetirizine was commenced, he was instructed in the management of anaphylaxis and provided with chlorphenamine and adrenaline (epinephrine) for emergency use.

Investigations showed a raised baseline serum tryptase of 19-27 mcg/L on repeated measurements. Bone marrow biopsy showed no evidence of abnormal mast cell proliferation or CD25 expression, and testing for D816V mutation of the c-kit gene was negative.

A diagnosis of mast cell activation syndrome was made. Ketotifen successfully prevented further attacks and serum tryptase monitoring over a 2 year period remained stable. He was advised of the increased risk of reactions to opioids, contrast media, anaesthetic agents, hymenoptera stings and other physical and emotional stimuli.

This case illustrates the use of tryptase both to aid diagnosis and to inform management of disease. Even in the absence of a diagnosis of systemic mastocytosis, the presence of a raised tryptase is associated with an increased risk of severe reactions to a number of triggers, and appropriate advice can be given about behaviours and avoidances.

Conclusion

While tryptase and histamine measurement will retain an important place, a selection of new biomarkers is emerging that may improve the diagnosis and stratification of patients with allergies and anaphylaxis. PAF is probably the most advanced in its development. It shares some of the limitations that make routine use of histamine measurements difficult in practice, but it does offer improved sensitivity. Leukotrienes and prostaglandins may find a role in assessment of aspirin sensitivity, and perhaps beyond. Other biomarkers such as carboxypeptidase A3 and dipeptidylpeptidase I are early in their development as clinical tools, but show promise.

The prospect of better prediction of anaphylaxis risk is also exciting. PAF-AH and, to a lesser degree, ACE levels, may be able to offer some quantification of the likely severity of a reaction.

Ultimately it is unlikely that any one or few factors will be sufficient to make clinically robust decisions about the patient's risk. A large number of variables, including allergy history, comorbidities, specific IgE levels (including component-resolved diagnostics) may be added to molecular and genetic biomarkers to assess the overall risk that might inform the treatment strategy. The unpredictability of anaphylaxis represents one of the most challenging aspects of allergy management. These uncertainties may lead physicians to err on the side of caution, leading to over-emphasis of the risk of recurrence, unnecessary prescription of emergency management tools and unnecessary anxiety for a proportion of these patients. While reliable prognostic markers are still some distance from the clinic, progress in this area holds out hope of more rational management plans for these vulnerable patients. In the end, however, the details of the clinical presentation are key in the diagnosis of anaphylaxis, and biomarkers currently only provide support to this diagnosis and may in time inform its management.

Clinical Pearls

1. Blood tryptase and, to a lesser degree, histamine measurement are readily available and recommended in the evaluation of all cases of possible anaphylaxis.
2. An elevated baseline tryptase level is a marker of mast cell burden, including mastocytosis, and constitutes a risk factor for anaphylaxis in insect venom allergy.
3. Investigation of platelet activating factor (PAF) and its degradation by PAF-acetyl hydrolase may in future help in the diagnosis, treatment and prognostication of anaphylaxis
4. Further clinical studies are needed to establish the usefulness of other mast cell products such as proteases and eicosanoids in the diagnosis and management of anaphylaxis.

The authors have declared no conflicts of interest.

References

[1] Sampson HA, Munoz-Furlong A, Campbell R, et al. Second symposium on the definition and management of anaphylaxis: summary report. *J. Allergy Clin. Immunol.* 2006; 117:391-7.

[2] Simons FE. Anaphylaxis. *J. Allergy Clin. Immunol.* 2008;121 (2 Suppl): S402-7.

[3] Clark AT and Ewan PW. The prevention and management of anaphylaxis in children. *Curr. Paediatr.* 2002; 12:370–5.

[4] Dzingina M, Stegenga H, Heath M, et al. Assessment and referral after emergency treatment of a suspected anaphylactic episode: summary of NICE guidance. *BMJ.* 2011; 343:d7595.

[5] Levy,JH. Biomarkers in the diagnosis of anaphylaxis: making nature disclose her mysteries. *Clinical and Experimental Allergy*. 2009; 39 (1):5-7.

[6] Simons FE. Anaphylaxis pathogenesis and treatment. *Allergy.* 2011; 66(Suppl 95):31-4.

[7] Yang PC, Berin MC, Yu L, et al. Mucosal pathophysiology and inflammatory changes in the late phase of the intestinal allergic reaction in the rat. *Am. J. Pathol.* 2001; 158:681.

[8] Choi IW, Kim YS, Kim DK, et al. Platelet activating factor-mediated NF-kappaB dependency of a late anaphylactic reaction. *J. Exp. Med.* 2003; 198:145.

[9] Ichikawa A, Sugimoto Y, Tanaka S. Molecular biology of histidine decarboxylase and prostaglandin receptors. *Proc. Jpn. Acad. Ser. B Phys. Biol. Sci.* 2010; 86(8): 848-66.

[10] Maintz L, Schwarzer V, Bieber T, et al. Effects of histamine and diamine oxidase activities on pregnancy: a critical review. *Hum. Reprod. Update.* 2008; 14(5):485-95.

[11] Simons FE, Frew AJ, Ansotegui IJ, et al. Risk assessment in anaphylaxis: current and future approaches. *J. Allergy Clin. Immunol.* 2007; 120(1 Suppl):S2-24.

[12] Kaliner M, Sigler R, Summers R, et al. Effect of infused histamine: anaylsis of the effects of H1 and H2 histamine receptor antagonists on cardiovascular and pulmonary responses. *J. Allery Clin. Immunol.* 1981; 68:365-71.

[13] Yoko Makabe-Kobayashi, Yoshio Hori, Tetsuya Adachi, et al. The control effect of histamine on body temperature and respiratory function in IgE-dependent systemic anaphylaxis. *J. Allergy Clin. Immunol.* 2002; 110(2):298-303.

[14] Reimers A, Hari Y, Muller U. Reduction of side-effects from ultrarush immunotherapy with honeybee venom by pretreatment with fexofenadine: a double-blind, placebo-controlled trial. *Allergy.* 2000; 55:484–8.

[15] Maintz L, Benfadal S, Allam JP, et al. Evidence for a reduced histamine degradation capacity in a subgroup of patients with atopic eczema. *J. Allergy Clin. Immunol.* 2006; 117(5):1106-12.

[16] Jarisch R andWantke F. Wine and headache. *Int. Arch. Allergy Immunol.* 1996; 110(1):7-12.

[17] Maintz L. Yu CF. Rodriguez E. Baurecht H. Bieber T. Illig T. Weidinger S. Novak N. Association of single nucleotide polymorphisms in the diamine oxidase gene with diamine oxidase serum activities. *Allergy* 2011. 66(7):893-902.

[18] Trivedi NN. Caughey GH. Mast cell peptidases: chameleons of innate immunity and host defense. *American Journal of Respiratory Cell and Molecular Biology* 2010. 42(3):257-67.

[19] Hopsu VK and Glenner GG. A histochemical enzyme kinetic system applied to the trypsin-like amidase and esterase activity in human mast cells. *J. Cell Biol.* 1963; 17:503.

[20] Mullan CS, Riley M, Clarke D, et al. b-Tryptase Regulates IL-8 Expression in Airway Smooth Muscle Cells by a PAR-2–Independent Mechanism. *Am. J. Respir. Cell Mol. Biol.* 2008; 38(5):600-608.

[21] Krishna MT, Chauhan A, Little L, Sampson K, Hawksworth R, Mant T, Djukanovic R, Lee T, HolgateS. Inhibition of mast cell tryptase by inhaled APC 366 attenuates allergen-induced late-phase airway obstruction in asthma. *J. Allergy Clin. Immunol.* 2001; 107(6):1039-1045.

[22] Lieberman PL. Anaphylaxis. In: *Middleton's allergy: Principles and practice,* 7th ed, Adkinson NF, Bochner BS, Busse WW, et AL (Eds), Mosby, St. Louis 2009. p.1027.

[23] Wintroub BU, Schechter NB, Lazarus GS, et al. Angiotensin I conversion by human and rat chymotryptic proteinases. *J. Invest. Dermatol.* 1984; 83:336.

[24] Reilly CF, Schechter NB, Travis J. Inactivation of bradykinin and kallidin by cathepsin G and mast cell chymase. *Biochem. Biophys. Res. Commun.* 1985; 127:443.

[25] Caughey GH, Leidig F, Viro NF, et al. Substance P and vasoactive intestinal peptide degradation by mast cell tryptase and chymase. *J. Pharmacol. Exp. Ther.* 1988; 244:133.

[26] Mizutani H, Schechter N, Lazarus G, et al. Rapid and specific conversion of precursor interleukin 1 beta (IL-1 beta) to an active IL-1 species by human mast cell chymase. *J. Exp. Med.* 1991; 174:821.

[27] Irani AM, Goldstein SM, Wintroub BU, et al. Human mast cell carboxypeptidase. Selective localization to MCTC cells. *J. Immunol.* 1991; 147:247.

[28] Weidner N and Austen KF. Heterogeneity of mast cells at multiple body sites. Fluorescent determination of avidin binding and immunofluorescent determination of chymase, tryptase, and carboxypeptidase content. *Pathol. Res. Pract.* 1993; 189:156.

[29] Reynolds DS, Gurley DS, Austen KF. Cloning and characterization of the novel gene for mast cell carboxypeptidase A. *J. Clin. Invest.* 1992; 89:273.

[30] Zhou XY, Buckley MG, Lau LC, et al. Mast Cell Carboxypeptidase as a New Clinical Marker for Anaphylaxis. *J. Allergy Clin. Immunol.* 2006; 117(2) Supplement: pS85.

[31] Brown TA, Whitworth HS, Zhou XY, et al. Mast Cell Carboxypeptidase as a Confirmatory and Predictive Marker in Allergic Reactions to Drugs. *J. Allergy Clin. Immunol.* 2011; 127(2) Supplement: pAB143.

[32] Zhou X, Buckley MG, Lucas J, et al. Anaphylactic Mechanisms in Sudden Unexpected Infant Death: Elevated Concentrations of Mast Cell Carboxypeptidase in the Serum. *J. Allergy Clin. Immunol.* 2007; 119(1) Supplement:pS148.

[33] Huang MK and M Peters-Golden. Eicosanoid Lipid Mediators in Fibrotic Lung Diseases: Ready for Prime Time? *Chest.* 2008; 133(6): 1442–1450.

[34] Hardy CC, Robinson C, Tattersfield AE, et al. The bronchoconstrictor effect of inhaled Prostaglandin D2 in normal and asthmatic men. *N. Engl. J. Med.* 1984; 311:209.

[35] Goetzl EJ. Oxygenation products of arachidonic acid as mediators of hypersensitivity and inflammation. *Med. Clin. North Am.* 1981; 65:809.

[36] Raible DG, Schulman ES, DiMuzio J, et al. Mast cell Mediators Prostaglandin-D2 and histamine activate human eosinophils. *J. Immunol.* 1992; 148:3536.

[37] Flower RJ, Harvey EA and Kingtons WP. Inflammatory effects in prostaglandin D2 in rat and human skin. *Br. J. Pharmocol.* 1976; 56:229.

[38] Murray JJ, Tonnel AB, Brush AR, et al. Release of prostaglandin D2 into human airways during acute antigen challenge. *N. Engl. J. Med.* 1986; 315:800.

[39] Knani J, Campbell A, Enander L, et al. Indirect evidence of nasal inflammation assessed by titration of inflammatory mediators and enumeration of cells in nasal secretions of patients with chronic rhinitis. *J. Allergy Clin. Immunol.* 1992; 90:880.

[40] Ono E, Taniguchi M, Mita H, et al. Increased production of cysteinyl leukotrienes and prostaglandin D2 during human anaphylaxis. *Clin. Exp. Allergy.* 2009; 39:72-80.

[41] Higashi N, Mita H, Ono E, et al. Profile of eicosanoid generation in aspirin-intolerant asthma and anaphylaxis assessed by new biomarkers. *J. Allergy Clin. Immunol.* 2010; 125(5):1084-91.

[42] Piper PJ and Walker JL. The release of spasmogenic substances from human chopped lung tissue and its inhibition. *Br. J. Pharmacol.* 1973; 47(2):291-304.

[43] Austen, KF. The cysteinyl leukotrienes: where do they come from? What are they? Where are they going? *Nat. Immunol.* 2008; 9(2):113-115.

[44] Juhlin L and Hammarstrom S. Effects of intradermally injected leukotriene C4 and histamine in patients with urticaria and psoriasis and atopic dermatitis. *Br. J. Dermatol.* 1982;107 Suppl23;106.

[45] Nagata M and Saito K. The role of cysteinyl leukotrienes in eosinophilic inflammation of asthmatic airways. *Int. Arch. Allergy Immunol.* 2003; 131 Suppl 1:7-10.

[46] Garcia-Aviles C, Sanz ML, Gamboa P, et al. Antigen specific quantification of sulfidoleukotrienes in patients allergic to Betalactam antibiotics. *J. Investig Allergol. Clin. Immunol.* 2005; 15(1):37-45.

[47] Marone G, Bova M, Detoraki A, et al. The human heart as a shock organ in anaphylaxis. *Novartis Found Symp*. 2004 discussion 149-60, 276-85 257 133-149.
[48] Campbell DJ. The kallikrein-kinin system in humans. *Clin. Exp. Pharmacol. Physiol.* 2001; 28(12):1060-5.
[49] Kuoppala A, Lindstedt KA, Saarinen J, et al. Inactivation of bradykinin by angiotensin-converting enzyme and by carboxypeptidase N in human plasma. *Am. J. Physiol. Heart Circ. Physiol.* 2000; 278(4):H1069-74.
[50] Niedoszytko M, Ratajska M, Chelminska M, et al. The angiotensinogen AGT p.M235T gene polymorphism may be responsible for the development of severe anaphylactic reactions to insect venom allergens. *Int. Arch. Allergy Immunol.* 2010; 153(2): 166-72.
[51] Mackins CJ, Kano S, Seyedi N, et al. Cardiac mast cell-derived renin promotes local angiotensin formation, norepinephrine release and arrhythmias in ischaemia/ reperfusion. *J. Clin. Invest.* 2006; 116:1063.
[52] Kaplan AP. Kinins, airway obstruction, and anaphylaxis. *Chem. Immunol. Allergy.* 2010; 95:67-84.
[53] Summers CW, Pumphrey RS, Woods CN, et al. Factors predicting anaphylaxis to peanuts and tree nuts in patients referred to a specialist center. *J. Allergy Clin. Immunol.* 2008; 121(3):632-638.
[54] Dawson W, West GB. The importance of bradykinin in anaphylactic shock. *Journal of Pharmacy and Pharmacology* 1965. 17(4); 246–247s.
[55] van der Linden PW, Hack CE, Eerenberg AJ, Struyvenberg A, van der Zwan JK. Activation of the contact system in insect-sting anaphylaxis: association with the development of angioedema and shock. *Blood* 1993;82:1732-9.
[56] Karasuyama H, Tsujimura Y, Obata K, et al. Role for basophils in systemic anaphylaxis. *Chem. Immunol. Allergy*. 2010; 95:85-97.
[57] Vadas P. Gold M, Perelman B, et al. Platelet-activating factor, PAF acetylhydrolase, and severe anaphylaxis. *N. Engl. J. Med.* 2008; 358(1): 28-35.
[58] Vadas P, Gold M, Liss GM, et al. PAF acetylhydrolase deficiency predisposes to fatal anaphylaxis. *J. Allergy Clin. Immunol.* 2003; 111: S206.
[59] Fukuda Y, Kawashima H, Saito K. et al. Effect of human plasma-type platelet-activating factor acetylhydrolase in two anaphylactic shock models. *Eur. J. Pharmacol.* 2000; 390:203-207.
[60] Montrucchio G, Alloatti G and Camussi,G. Role of platelet-activating factor in cardiovascular pathophysiology. *Physiol Rev.* 2000; 80(4): 1669-1699.
[61] Kajiwara N, Sasaki T, Bradding P, et al. Activation of human mast cells through the platelet-activating factor receptor. *J. Allergy Clin. Immunol.* 2010; 125(5):1137-1145.
[62] Khodoun M, Strait R, Orekov T, et al. Peanuts can contribute to anaphylactic shock by activating complement. *J. Allergy Clin. Immunol.* 2009; 123(2)342-351.
[63] Smith LJ. The role of platelet activating factor in asthma. A*m. Rev. Respir. Dis.* 1991; 143:S100.
[64] Zimmerman GA, McIntyre TM and Prescott SM. Adhesion and signaling in vascular cell—cell. *J. Clin. Invest.* 1996; 98:1699.

[65] Vadas P, Perelman B, Liss G, et al. Platelet-activating factor, histamine, and tryptase levels in human anaphylaxis. *J. Allergy Clin. Immunol.* 2012 Oct 2. pii: S0091-6749(12)01377-2.

[66] Ishii S, Kuwaki T, Nagase T, et al. Impaired Anaphylactic Responses with Intact Sensitivity to Endotoxin in Mice Lacking a Platelet-activating Factor Receptor. *J. Exp. Med.* 1998; 187:1779-1788.

[67] Arias K, Baig M, Colangelo M, et al. Concurrent blockade of platelet-activating factor and histamine prevents life-threatening peanut-induced anaphylactic reactions. *J. Allergy Clin. Immunol.* 2009; 124:307-14.

[68] Metcalfe DD, Peavy RD and Gilfillan AM. Mechanisms of mast cell signaling in anaphylaxis. *J. Allergy Clin. Immunol.*2009;124(4):639-646.

[69] Andersen AJ, Hashemi SH, Andresen TL, et al. Complement: alive and kicking nanomedicines. *J. Biomed. Nanotechnol.* 2009; 5(4):364-372.

[70] Menikou S, Patel MP, Rose KL, Botto M, Warner JO, Pickering MC, Boyle RJ. Relationship between complotype and reported severity of systemic allergic reactions to peanut. *J. Allergy Clin. Immunol.* 2012; 129(5): 1398-1400.

[71] Khodoun MV, Strait R, Armstrong L, et al. Identification of markers that distinguish IgE- from IgG-mediated anaphylaxis. *Proc. Nat. Acad. Sci. USA.* 2011 108(30):12413-12418.

[72] Jonsson F, Mancardi,DA, Kita Y, et al. Mouse and human neutrophils induce anaphylaxis. *J. Clin. Invest.* 2011; 121(4):1484-1496.

[73] Strait R, Morrist SC and Finkelman FD. Cytokine enhancement of anaphylaxis. *Novartis Found Symp.* 2004discussion 91-100, 276-85 257 80-91.

[74] Stone SF, Cotterell C, Isbister GK, et al. Elevated serum cytokines during human anaphylaxis: Identification of potential mediators of acute allergic reactions. *Allergy Clin. Immunol.* 2009; 124(4):786-92.

[75] Liew FY, Pitman NI and McInnes IB. Disease-associated functions of IL-33: the new kid in the IL-1 family. *Nat. Rev. Immunol.* 2010; 10(2): 103-110.

[76] T. Ohno, H. Morita, K. Arae, K. Matsumoto, S. Nakae. Interleukin-33 in allergy. *Allergy* 2012; 67: 1203–1214.

[77] Lin RY, Schwartz LB, Curry A, et al. Histamine and tryptase levels in patients with acute allergic reactions: An emergency department-based study. *J. Allergy Clin. Immunol.* 2000; 106:65-71.

[78] van der Linden PW, Hack CE, Poortman J, et al. Insect-sting challenge in 138 patients: relation between clinical severity of anaphylaxis and mast cell activation. *J. Allergy Clin. Immunol.* 1992; 90:110.

[79] Brown SG, Blackman KE, Heddle RJ. et al. Can serum mast cell tryptase help diagnose anaphylaxis? *Emerg. Med. Australas.* 2004; 16(2): 120-4.

[80] van Doormaal JJ, van der Veer E, van Voorst Vader PC, et al. Tryptase and histamine metabolites as diagnostic indicators of indolent systemic mastocytosis without skin lesions. *Allergy.* 2012; 67(5):683-90.

[81] Morrow JD, Margolies GR, Rowland J, et al. Evidence that histamine is the causative toxin of scombroid-fish poisoning. *N. Engl. J. Med.* 1991; 324(11):716-20.

[82] Laroche D, Vergnaud MC, Sillard B, et al. Biochemical markers of anaphylactoid reactions to drugs. Comparison of plasma histamine and tryptase. *Anesthesiology.* 1991; 75(6):945-9.

[83] JournSchwartz, LB. Diagnostic value of tryptase in anaphylaxis and mastocytosis. *Immunol. Allergy Clin. North Am.* 2006; 26(3):451-463.

[84] Valent P, Horny HP, Triggiani M, et al. Clinical and laboratory parameters of mast cell activation as basis for the formulation of diagnostic criteria. *Int. Arch. Allergy Immunol.* 2011; 156(2):119-27.

[85] Valent P, Akin C, Arock M, et al. Definitions, criteria and global classification of mast cell disorders with special reference to mast cell activation syndromes: A consensus proposal. *Int. Arch. Allergy Immunol.* 2012; 157(3):215-25.

[86] van Toorenenbergen AW, Hooijkaas H, Heerenbrink GK, et al. Heterophilic antibody interference in a tryptase immunoassay. *Clin. Biochem.* 2008; 41:331.

[87] Veien M, Szlam F, Holden JT, et al. Mechanism of nonimmunological histamine and tryptase release from human cutaneous mast cells. *Anaesthesiology.* 2000; 92: 1074-81.

[88] Sampson HA, Mendelson L and Rosen JP. Fatal and near-fatal anaphylactic reactions to food in children and adolescents. *N. Engl. J. Med.* 1992; 327:380-4.

[89] Sampson HA and Jolie PL. Increased plasma histamine concentrations after food challenges in children with atopic dermatitis. *J. Allergy Clin. Immunol.* 1984;311:372-6.

[90] Ohtsuka T, Matsumaru S, Uchida K, et al. Time course of plasma histamine and tryptase following food challenges in children with suspected food allergy. *Ann. Allergy* 1993;71:139-46.

[91] Borer-Reinhold M, Haeberli G, Bitzenhofer M, et al. An increase in serum tryptase even below 11.4 ng/mL may indicate a mast cell-mediated hypersensitivity reaction: a prospective study in Hymenoptera venom allergic patients. *Clin. Exp. Allergy.* 2011; 41(12):1777-83.

[92] Caughey GH. Tryptase genetics and anaphylaxis. *J. Allergy Clin. Immunol.* 2006; 117:1411-4.

[93] Pumphrey RS and Roberts IS. Postmortem findings after fatal anaphylactic reactions. *J. Clin. Pathol.* 2000; 53(4):273-6.

[94] Edson E, Eriksson O and van Hage M. Mast cell tryptase in postmortem serum-reference values and confounders. *Int. J. Legal Med.* 2007; 121: 275-80.

[95] Akin,C. Anaphylaxis and mast cell disease: what is the risk? *Curr. Allergy and Asthma Rep.* 2010; 10(1):34-38.

[96] Bachelet I, Munitz A, Berent-Maoz B, et al. Suppression of normal and malignant kit signaling by a bispecific antibody linking kit with CD300a. *J. Immunol.* 2008; 180(9):6064-6069.

[97] Jensen BM, Akin C and Gilfillan AM. Pharmacological targeting of the KIT growth factor receptor: a therapeutic consideration for mast cell disorders. *Br. J. Pharmacol.* 2008; 154(8):1572-1582.

[98] Valent P, Sperr WR, Schwartz LB, et al. Diagnosis and classification of mast cell proliferative disorders: delineation from immunologic diseases and non-mast cell hematopoietic neoplasms. *J. Allergy Clin. Immunol.* 2004; 114:3.

[99] Dombrowicz D, Brini AT, Flamand V, et al. Anaphylaxis mediated through a humanized high affinity IgE receptor. *J. Immunol.* 1996; 157(4):1645-1651.

[100] Butterfield JH and Weiler CR. Prevention of mast cell activation disorder-associated clinical sequelae of excessive prostaglandin D(2) production. *Int. Arch. Allergy Immunol.* 2008; 147:338.

In: Anaphylaxis: Principles and Practice
Editor: M. Thirumala Krishna

ISBN: 978-1-62618-688-0

Chapter IV

Management of Anaphylaxis

Priyanka Saxena Lall and Karen Demuth*
Emory University School of Medicine,
Atlanta, GA, US

Abstract

Anaphylaxis requires immediate medical treatment. At the present time, the mainstays of therapy include educating patients and their caregivers to strictly avoid allergens, recognize early symptoms, and to self-administer injectable epinephrine. In a hospital setting the initial management of anaphylaxis includes a focused examination, procurement of a stable airway and intravenous access, and administration of epinephrine with antihistamines and steroids often used as adjuncts. Interventions include high-flow oxygen, cardiac monitoring, and intravenous access. Certain drugs, such as beta-blockers and angiotensin-converting enzyme (ACE) inhibitors, may hinder the successful treatment of an anaphylactic reaction and glucagon infusion can be considered inpatients on the former. A period of in hospital observation between 2 and 24 hours is recommended following stabilization due to concerns of biphasic anaphylaxis.

Anaphylaxis is a clinical diagnosis but measurement of serial plasma tryptase in the acute phase is an useful adjunct. In patients with anaphylaxis attributed to an IgE-mediated allergy, sensitization can be confirmed by allergy skin testing and/or measurement of allergen specific IgE levels in serum. People prone to anaphylaxis are advised to have an "allergy action plan", and parents are advised to inform schools of their children's allergies and what to do in case of an anaphylactic emergency. The action plan usually includes use of epinephrine auto-injector, recommendation to wear a medical alert bracelet, and counseling on avoidance of triggers.

---

* Correspondance: Karen A. DeMuth, MD, MPH; Emory University School of Medicine, 2015 Uppergate Drive, Atlanta, GA, 30322, US; Tel: 585-309-6907; Email: kdemuth@emory.edu.

Acute Management of Anaphylaxis

Immediate evaluation and management are critical in anaphylaxis, as respiratory or cardiac arrest, and death can occur within minutes if immediate action is not taken [1-3]. Initial assessment should be rapid and include determining whether history and physical findings are compatible with anaphylaxis. Evaluation should include level of consciousness, upper and lower airways, cardiovascular system, skin and gastrointestinal system. The cornerstones of the initial management of anaphylaxis are the following, and they should be instituted concurrently [4]:

- Removal of the inciting antigen, if possible.
- Call for help (summon a resuscitation team in the hospital setting, call 911 or an equivalent service in the community setting).
- Advanced Cardiac life support and basic life support concentrating on airway, breathing and circulation as well as adequacy of mentation is paramount.
- All patients who have had an anaphylactic reaction should be monitored as soon as possible with pulse oximetry, non-invasive blood pressure and 3-lead ECG.

Table 1. Pharmacologic considerations of epinephrine

Pharmacological particulars	• Sterile aqueous medication used to treat severe life-threatening allergic reactions, or cardiac arrest. • Store at < 77° Fahrenheit • Comes in 1:10,000 (intravenous use) and 1:1,000 (intramuscular) vials. Autoinjectors (1:1,000, 0.30 mg and 1:2,000, 0.15 mg) for use in emergencies. Administer intramuscularly. • Also available as a racemic version for inhalation.
Mechanisms of action:	• Acts on nearly all body tissues • Nonselective agonist of all adrenergic receptors, including the major subtypes ($\alpha1$, $\alpha2$, $\beta1$, $\beta2$, and $\beta3$).
Precautions for use	• Epinephrine is intended for use in the event of life-threatening situations so the following warnings and precautions are only relative. • Consider cautious administration to those at risk for cardiac complications (elderly, those with ischaemic heart disease, hypertension) as they may develop angina when coronary insufficiency is present. Also use caution in administration in patients with diabetes mellitus, hyperthyroidism, closed angle glaucoma, or psychoneurosis. • Use with extreme caution in patients with long-standing bronchial asthma and emphysema who have developed degenerative heart disease.
Medication Interactions	• Effects can be potentiated by tricyclic antidepressants, volatile liquid anaesthetics, digoxin, quinidine, fluorohydrocarbons or cocaine, ergot alkaloids or oxytocin • May cause hyperglycaemia in diabetic patients treated with hypoglycemic agents. • Reverses the antihypertensive effects of adrenergic neuron blockers such as guanethidine, which may result in severe hypertension.
Adverse Reactions	• Palpitations, tachycardia, arrhythmia, anxiety, jitteriness, headache, tremor, hypertension, and acute pulmonary edema.

Clear	• Food Allergy (IgE Mediated) • Exercise Induced Anaphylaxis • Food Dependent Exercise Induced Anaphylaxis • Venom Allergy • Systemic Mastocytosis • Idiopathic Anaphylaxis
Less Clear	• Oral Allergy Syndrome • Large Local Reactions to Vespids
No indication	• Drug Allergy • Others

Table 1 is from the 'Guidelines for the Management of Anaphylaxis', and outlines the acute management. Although treatment recommendations are always subject to physician discretion with physician judgment based on variations in sequence and performance, the cornerstone of treatment for anaphylaxis is rapid administration of the correct route and dose of epinephrine.

Epinephrine

Prompt administration of epinephrine is 'key' to favorable outcome and failure or delay has been associated with fatal anaphylaxis [1, 2].

Method of Action

Epinephrine has several pharmacological properties (Table 2) and its actions vary by tissue type and expression of adrenergic receptors. For example, binding to alpha adrenergic receptors causes increased vasoconstriction, peripheral resistance and decreased vascular permeability. Whilst binding through beta-1 adrenergic leads to increased ionotropy and, chronotropy, beta-2 receptors mediate increased bronchodilation and decreased release of mediators of inflammation from mast cells and basophils. Adverse reactions to adrenaline include anxiety, restlessness, headache, dizziness, palpitations, pallor, hypertension and tremor and may occur in patients of all ages.

Table 2. Notable effects of Epinephrine by system

Heart	• Increased heart rate (tachycardia), and vasoconstriction.
Blood Pressure	• Increased systolic BP/decreased diastolic BP.
Lungs	• Increased respiratory rate (tachypnea), and bronchodilation.
Liver	• Gluconeogenesis
Other	• Hypokalemia

Table 3. Available epinephrine autoinjectors and directions for administration

Appearance	Name	Administration
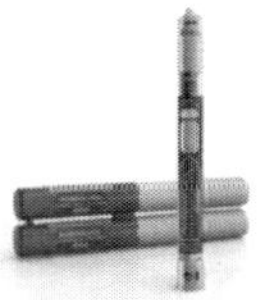	Adrenaclick 0.15 and 0.3	• Pull apart cylindrical carrying case • Slide out the pen • Pull off GRAY end cap with the [1]; you will now see a RED tip. Never put thumb, finger, or hand over the RED tip. • Pull off GRAY end cap with [2]. • Put the *RED* tip against the middle of the outer side of your thigh (upper leg). It can go through clothes. • Press down hard until the needle enters your thigh (upper leg) through your skin. Hold it in place while slowly counting to 10. • Remove the Adrenaclick from your thigh. • Check the RED tip. If the needle is exposed you received the dose. If needle is not visible, repeat Step B.
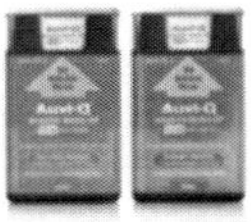	Auvi-Q 0.15 and 0.3	• Pull off red safety guard • Place black end against outer thigh, then press firmly and hold for 5 seconds
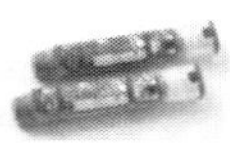	EpiPen (0.3) EpiPen Jr (0.15)	• Flip open yellow or green cap of the device's carrier tube • Remove the device by tipping and sliding it out of the carrier tube • Grasp the unit with the orange tip pointing downward • Form fist around the unit (orange tip down). • With your other hand, pull off the blue safety release. • Hold orange tip near outer thigh • Swing and firmly push against outer thigh until it clicks so that unit is perpendicular (at 90° angle) to the thigh • Hold firmly against thigh for approximately 10 seconds to deliver drug. (The injection is now complete. The window on the auto-injector will be obscured). • Remove unit from the thigh (the orange needle cover will extend to cover needle) and massage injection area for 10 seconds.
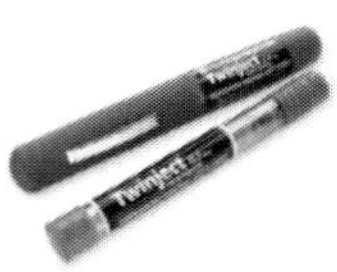	Twinject	• Pull apart cylindrical carrying case • Slide out the pen *First Dose* • Pull to remove GREEN caps labeled "1" and "2." • Place rounded tip against the middle of the outer thigh. • The needle may be injected through clothing. • Press down hard until auto-injector fires. • Hold in place while slowly counting to 10. *Second Dose* • If symptoms have not improved within about 10 minutes after the first injection, a second dose is needed. • Unscrew RED rounded tip. • Pull syringe from barrel, and slide YELLOW collar off plunger. • Put needle into thigh. • Push plunger down all the way.

Considerations for Dosing/Administering Epinephrine

Community Setting

The most common way to administer epinephrine in the community setting is by auto-injector intramuscularly into the mid-anterolateral thigh. These are available only in 0.15 mg and 0.3mg doses (Table 3).

Children weighing less than 25 Kg should receive the 0.15 mg dose [5, 6]. These devices simplify dosing and administration of epinephrine. Every person at risk of developing anaphylaxis should always have immediate access to an epinephrine auto-injector. However, many do not carry their epinephrine auto-injectors with them. In an evaluation of food allergic children being seen at an allergy-immunology clinic only 59% had an epinephrine auto-injector available [7]. Training in use of epinephrine auto-injector was significantly associated with increased odds of having an epinephrine auto-injector immediately available [7].

Epinephrine autoinjectors are widely available, but this has not solved all the problems confronting those at risk of a life-threatening reaction including patients not having access to their epinephrine. Some studies have shown that the physicians prescribing the device lacked knowledge of its use [8] and others noted that patients did not receive formal training [9].

Needle length may be a consideration in administration of epinephrine. Those with significantly elevated Body Mass Index (BMI) may require longer needle lengths to ensure intramuscular administration of the medication.

Clinic/in-Patient Setting (Table 4)

There are different forms and methods for administration including multidose vials, intramuscular, intravenous, inhaled/nebulised and intratracheal. The typical dosing is aqueous Epinephrine 1:1000 dilution (1mg/mL), 0.2-0.5 ml in adults or 0.01 mg per kilogram in children and is usually injected subcutaneously or intramuscularly into the mid-anterolateral thigh or less frequently the arms [10, 11]. Several studies have demonstrated that that intramuscular (IM) route is recommended over subcutaneous since the former consistently provides a more rapid increase in the plasma and tissue concentrations of epinephrine [11, 12].

Epinephrine for parenteral administration is available in two dilutions. For intramuscular injection 1 in 1,000 dilution containing 1 mg/ml is employed. The dose may be repeated at 5 min intervals as per clinical indication [11, 12]. Intramuscular epinephrine injections into the thigh is the preferred method of administration since this has been reported to provide more rapid absorption and higher plasma levels in both children and adults than subcutaneous injections administered in the arm [7], [13]. However, similar studies comparing intramuscular with subcutaneous injections in the thigh have not yet been done.

Patients who do not respond to intramuscular injection of epinephrine and fluid resuscitation may not be adequately perfusing muscle tissues if severe hypotension is present. These patients may benefit from a slow IV infusion with 1:10,000 dilution [may also be labeled 100 mcg per mL]. For adults, the initial dose for IV epinephrine is 2 to 10 micrograms per minute and 0.1 to 1 mcg per kilogram per minute for infants and children titrated to effect on blood pressure. Patients requiring IV epinephrine require cardiac monitoring because of potential arrhythmias and ischaemia.

Alternative routes of administration have been anecdotally successful. These include, for example, inhaled or nebulised epinephrine in the presence of laryngeal edema or sublingual administration if an intravenous route cannot be obtained. Endotracheally administered dosages have also been proposed for use when intravenous access is not available in intubated patients experiencing cardiac arrest. There is no data to support the use of epinephrine in anaphylaxis through a nonparenteral route.

Adjunctive Therapies: The evidence base for use of these second line medications in the initial management of anaphylaxis, is extrapolated mainly from their use in treatment of other diseases such as urticaria (antihistamines) or acute asthma (beta-2 adrenergic agonists and glucocorticoids) [14-16].

Inhaled beta-2 agonists: Inhaled beta-2 agonists are known to relieve bronchoconstriction. This reduces ventilation-perfusion (VQ) mismatching, improves oxygenation and relieves dyspnoea. Asthma *per se* is an independent 'risk factor' for 'fatal anaphylaxis' in food allergy [17].

H1-antihistamines: In contrast to the consensus about epinephrine, there is no agreement among available anaphylaxis guidelines with regard to the use of H1-antihistamines or glucocorticoids in the treatment of anaphylaxis [18]. The evidence base for use of these second line medications in the initial management of anaphylaxis, is extrapolated from their use in treatment of other diseases such as urticaria (antihistamines) or acute asthma (beta-2 adrenergic agonists and glucocorticoids). H_2-antihistamines are not mentioned in most guidelines [19].

A systematic review of the literature was unable to show any randomized controlled trials that support the use of H1 antihistamines in anaphylaxis. H1 receptor antagonist serves to reduce or eliminate effects mediated by histamine. These agents are useful adjuncts and relieve pruritus and hives. For parenteral treatment, only first-generation agents are available: for adults, consider diphenhydramine 25 to 50 mg IV, may be repeated up to a maximum daily dose of 400mg per 24 hrs. For children weighing less than 40 kg, consider diphenhydramine 1mg per kg (maximum 40 mg) IV, which may be repeated up to a maximum daily dose of 5 mg per kg.

For oral treatment, second-generation H1 anti-histamines offer distinct advantages over first-generation agents. They are less likely to impair cognition or psychomotor performance or cause sedation. Second generation H1 antihistamines are not available in parenteral formulations. The onset of action of antihistamines, even diphenhydramine given by injection is slow to provide any immediate benefit. Orally administered cetirizine acts within one hour.

H2-antihistamines: There is minimal evidence to support the use of H2 antihistamines in conjunction with H1 antihistamines in the emergency treatment of anaphylaxis. Consider ranitidine, 50 mg in adults and 12.5 to 50 mg (1 mg/kg) in children, which may be diluted in 5% dextrose to a total volume of 20 mL and injected intravenously over 5 minutes. However, these agents have a much slower onset of action than epinephrine and should never be used alone in the treatment of anaphylaxis. Both singly and in combination, these agents are second-line therapy to epinephrine [19].

Beta-agonists: Persistent respiratory distress or wheezing requires additional measures. Nebulized beta-adrenergic agents such as albuterol (Proventil) or terbutaline may be administered. Endotracheal intubation may be needed to secure the airway.

Corticosteroids: Even though the exact benefit of corticosteroids has not been established, most experts support their administration. The onset of action of glucocorticoids takes several hours, therefore these medications do not reduce the primary symptoms and signs of anaphylaxis. Their benefit may not be apparent for 6-12 hours after administration, the rationale for giving them is to avoid biphasic reaction so their primary role may be in prevention of recurrent or protracted anaphylaxis.

Table 4. Treatment of acute anaphylaxis

Treatment of acute anaphylaxis	
First Line Treatment	• Epinephrine IM (antero-lateral thigh) (auto-injector or 1:1,000 solution - Weight 10-25 kg: 0.15 mg - Weight > 25 kg: 0.30 mg • Epinephrine (1:1,000) 0.01mg/kg/dose • Dose may be repeated every 5-15 min. as needed
Adjunctive Treatment	• Bronchodilator ($\beta 2$ agonist) MDI (child 4-8 puffs, adult 8 puffs) • Nebulized (child 1.5mL; adult 3mL) q 20 min or continuous if needed. • H1 blocker (Diphenhydramine)1-2 mg/kg/dose. Maximum dose 50mg IV/oral liquid • Supplemental O2 therapy • IV fluids in large volume if hypotensive/orthostatic • Recumbent positioning

Methylprednisolone at a dose of 1 to 2 mg per kilogram per day is sufficient. If glucocorticoid treatment is instituted, it can be stopped after three days without a taper, since all biphasic reactions reported to date have occurred within 72 hours. Oral administration of glucocorticosteroids (e.g., prednisone, 0.5 mg/kg) might be sufficient for less critical anaphylactic episodes [20-21].

Glucagon: Glucagon infusion can be considered in those receiving beta-blockers since these patients may be resistant to treatment with epinephrine and can develop refractory hypotension and bradycardia. In these situations, glucagon should be administered because it has inotropic and chronotropic effects that is not mediated through beta-receptors. Therefore, glucagon, 1 mg intravenous bolus, followed by an infusion of 1 to 5 mg per hour, may improve hypotension in one to five minutes, with a maximal benefit at five to fifteen minutes (The U.S. Food and Drug Administration has not approved glucagon for this use). Nausea and vomiting may limit therapy with glucagon [22].

Other Considerations

Treatment of Respiratory Symptoms

Individuals with anaphylaxis may develop dyspnoea, wheezing, cough, hypoxia and/or laryngeal edema. Individuals having these symptoms may benefit from additional medications/management strategies. Supplemental oxygen, by facemask should be administered to maintain adequate oxygenation. Albuterol, as mentioned previously, in addition to epinephrine can help relieve bronchoconstriction, wheezing, and V-Q mismatching. Rarely, airway oedema prevents endotracheal intubation and a surgical airway (e.g., emergency tracheostomy) is needed.

Treatment of Hypotension

The patient should be placed supine or in Trendelenburg's position, with the lower extremities elevated to maximize perfusion of vital organs. This also helps prevent 'empty ventricle syndrome" in which severe hypotension leads to inadequate cardiac filling and pulseless cardiac activity [23]. In this syndrome, death can occur within seconds. In an evaluation of fatal anaphylaxis, positioning was noted to be a common factor associated with death [1], [24].

Intravenous access should be secured during resuscitation, since large volumes of fluids may be required to treat hypotension caused by increased vascular permeability and vasodilatation, ideally 14 to 16 gauge for most adults. While volume replacement is central to management of hypotension in anaphylaxis, other vasopressors such as dopamine, 2 to 20 mcg per kg per minute, may be required. Continuous noninvasive monitoring of cardiopulmonary status, including blood pressure, heart and respiratory rate and oxygen saturation is required for the duration of the episode [23, 24].

In summary, prompt evaluation, management, and intervention are critical in anaphylaxis. The core of initial management involves removal of the inciting antigen, call for help which may entail summoning a resuscitation team in the hospital setting, call 911 or an equivalent service in the community setting, and rapid administration of epinephrine.

Diagnostic Testing

Anaphylaxis is generally diagnosed clinically, but measurement of serial plasma tryptase is a useful adjunct. Plasma tryptase measured during acute phase can be helpful especially if the person has recurrent episodes and/or when the diagnosis is in doubt.

Tryptase concentrations in the blood may not increase significantly until 30 minutes or more after the onset of symptoms, and peak 1-2 hours after. The half-life of tryptase is short (approximately 2 hours), and concentrations may return to normal within 6-8 hours, so timing of any blood sampling is important.

Serial measurements including 'first' as soon as practically possible after stabilization of patient, 'second' 1-2 hours after onset of symptoms and a 'third' sample at 24 hours are recommended. This approach with serial measurements offers better sensitivity and specificity. Whilst elevated plasma tryptase during an 'acute phase' is diagnostic, a normal value does not exclude the diagnosis. Also, an elevated baseline plasma tryptase indicates underlying mast cell disorder.

Long-Term Management of Individuals with a History of Anaphylaxis

Traditionally physicians are trained to diagnose and treat anaphylaxis as an acute emergency in the health care setting. Equally important however, is the long-term care of a patient who has experienced anaphylaxis. It is crucial to provide a risk assessment for individuals with anaphylaxis and emphasize on education [25]. Appropriate risk assessment involves identifying potential triggers, mechanism and patient-specific risk factors for severity and fatality in those who have previously experienced an acute anaphylactic episode. Important patient-related risk include age, concomitant diseases and concurrent medications as well as other less well-defined factors such as defects in mediatory degradation pathways, fever, acute infections, menses, emotional stress and disruption of routine [26].

The clinical history is extremely important in making the diagnosis of anaphylaxis, determining the triggers and assessing the patient for cofactors that increase the risk for severity.

Previous episode/s should be carefully reviewed, starting with the 24 hour period before the onset of symptoms and paying particular attention to the one to two hours immediately preceding symptom onset. Important information can be obtained from family members, caregivers, friends or other witnesses, emergency medical personnel, and emergency department hospital records. Every effort should be made to identify specific trigger(s), and avoiding recurrence of anaphylaxis.

History

Patient history is crucial in the process of identifying triggers for anaphylaxis. Special attention should be given to the circumstances leading up to the event. Presence of known or suspected triggers (food, medications, stinging insects, etc.,), timing between known or suspected exposures, and development of symptoms, and other details (such as exercise) are important to identify prior to evaluating for allergen triggers.

Testing for Allergen Triggers

In patients with anaphylaxis attributed to an IgE-mediated allergy, sensitization can be confirmed through allergy skin testing and/or measurement of allergen specific IgE levels in serum. Standardized skin testing extracts are commercially available for insect venoms, latex and penicillins, but not for foods, most medications, biting insect saliva [26-27]. In patients with a history of food-induced anaphylaxis, fresh version of the suspected food (e.g.: vegetable, fruits, nuts, etc.,) may be used for skin prick testing.

In vitro testing for allergen specific IgE is relatively less sensitive, and depends on clinical correlation and the availability of specific assays, of which there are over 500 different allergens available for testing with the ImmunoCAP System®, Pharmacia Upjohn Diagnostics, (Uppsala, Sweden), or radio-allergosobent (RAST) technique. Patients with a history of a clinical reaction to a specific food in combination with evidence of IgE sensitization (an elevated specific IgE level to that food and/or a positive skin test to that food) do NOT require a 'food challenge' for confirmation. In such patients, challenges are likely to be positive and can potentially trigger anaphylaxis [28, 29].

Positive skin prick tests (SPT) for food allergens and specific IgE (sIgE) in serum indicate sensitization but do not enable distinction between sensitized but tolerant and clinically allergic patients.

Education

Education is critical in the care of the individuals with an IgE mediated allergy. Anyone with a history of anaphylaxis should be counseled about avoidance measures, identify the signs/symptoms of anaphylaxis, the importance of being prepared and how to manage a reaction if inadvertent exposure occurs.

Food is the most common cause of anaphylaxis in an outpatient setting, and food allergens account for 30% of fatal cases. Reading ingredient labels for all foods is the 'key' to effective avoidance. If a product does not have a label, individuals with a food allergy should avoid consumption.

Studies investigating primary prevention have been inconclusive and there is currently no cure for food allergy. Studies investigating role for oral immunotherapy are underway and early studies have shown some promising results in patients with allergy to peanut, egg and milk.

Venom Immunotherapy is the only specific treatment available for patients with history of anaphylaxis to hymenoptera stings – can significantly reduce frequency and severity of systemic reactions to future stings and has long term efficacy.

A patient with a history of anaphylaxis should be trained in self-management including the use of epinephrine autoinjector and written instructions provided. Two strengths are available: 0.3 mL of 1:1,000 epinephrine for adults, and 0.3 mL of 1:2,000 for children. Training kits containing empty syringes are available for patient education.

Family members and care-givers of young children should be trained to inject epinephrine. The patient also may take an antihistamine at the onset of symptoms. The patient must be told to seek immediate professional help regardless of initial response to self-treatment.

If possible, the patient should avoid taking beta blockers, angiotensin-converting enzyme (ACE) inhibitors, angiotensin-II receptor blockers, and monoamine oxidase inhibitors, because these drugs may interfere with successful treatment of future anaphylactic episodes or with the endogenous compensatory responses to hypotension. Finally, the patient should be advised to wear or carry a medical alert bracelet, necklace, or keychain to alert health care professionals about their allergy/ies.

Deciding which patients should carry an epinephrine autoinjector can be challenging. There are many clear indications, such as: Food Allergy (IgE Mediated), Exercise Induced Anaphylaxis, Food Dependent Exercise Induced Anaphylaxis, Venom Allergy, Systemic Mastocytosis, and Idiopathic Anaphylaxis. There are also individuals who have had anaphylaxis that clearly do not require an epinephrine autoinjector, such as drug allergy.

Finally, there are many other situations that providers may wish to consider prescribing an epinephrine autoinjector that are less clear such as: large local reactions to vespids, and oral allergy syndrome. A good 'rule of thumb' is if the provider and/or patient consider that there is a risk of anaphylaxis, an epinephrine autoinjector should be considered.

The American Academy of Allergy Asthma and Immunology (www.aaaai.org), and the American College of Allergy Asthma and Immunology (www.acaai.org), FARE (www.foodallergy.org) are a few examples of national organizations with information for those affected by anaphylaxis.

Clinical Pearls

- Anaphylaxis is a life threatening condition and can affect the skin, respiratory, gastrointestinal and cardiovascular system.
- Early intervention is key to successful clinical outcome and delay in treatment has been shown to increase risk of death.
- Rapid administration of epinephrine, placing a hypotensive patient on their back (supine) with the feet raised (Trendelenberg's), Oxygen, intravenous fluids and consideration of adjunctive medications (antihistamine/s, corticosteroids, bronchodilators) constitutes standard acute treatment of anaphylaxis.
- Long term management includes identification of trigger/s, appropriate allergen avoidance, provision of written self-management plan and counseling the patient and where relevant family member/s, care givers and in case of children liaison with the school.

Statement of Conflict of Interest

The authors assert that they have no conflict of interests.

References

[1] Pumphrey RS. Lessons for management of anaphylaxis from a study of fatal reactions. *Clinical Exp. Allergy 2000;* 30(8):1144.

[2] Sampson HA.Fatal and near-fatal anaphylactic reactions to food in children and adolescents. *New England Journal of Medicine* 1992; 327(6): 380.

[3] Bock SA.Fatalities due to anaphylactic reactions to foods. *J. Allergy Clin. Immunol.* 2001;107(1): 191.

[4] Brown SG. Cardiovascular aspects of anaphylaxis: implications for treatment and diagnosis. *Curr. Opin. Allergy Clin. Immunol.* 2005; 5(4): 359.

[5] Simons FE. Epinephrine dispensing patterns for an out-of-hospital population: a novel approach to studying the epidemiology of anaphylaxis. *J. Allergy Clin. Immunol.* 2002; 110 (4):1166-1168.

[6] Kemp SF, Lockey RF. Epinephrine: the drug of choice for anaphylaxis. A statement of the World Allergy Organization. *Allergy* 2008; *63*(8): 1061.

[7] Demuth KA, Fitzpatrick A. Epinephrine autoinjector availabilty among children with food allergy. *Allergy Asthma Proc.* 2008; 32:295-300.

[8] .Mehr S, Robinson M, Tang M. Doctor: how to I use my EpiPen? *Pediatr. Allergy Immunol.* 2007; 18:448-452.

[9] Sicherer SH, Forman JA, Noone SA. Use assessment of self-administered epinephrine among food-allergic children and pediatricians. *Pediatrics* 2000; 105:359–362.

[10] Haymore BR, Carr WW. Anaphylaxis and epinephrine prescribing patterns in a military hospital: underutilization of the intramuscular route. *Allergy Asthma Proc.* 2005; 26 (5): 361-5.

[11] Simons KJ, Simons FE. Epinephrine and its use in anaphylaxis: current issues. *Curr. Opin. Allergy Clin Immunol.* 2010;10(4):354.

[12] Simons FE. First-aid treatment of anaphylaxis to food: focus on epinephrine. *J. Allergy Clin. Immunol.* 2004;113(5): 837.

[13] Lieberman P. Use of epinephrine in the treatment of anaphylaxis. *Curr. Opin. Allergy Clin. Immunol.* 2003; 4(4):313-8.

[14] Clark S, Bock SA. Multicenter study of emergency department visits for food allergies. *J. Allergy Clin. Immunol.* 2004; 113(2): 347.

[15] Gaeta TJ, Clark S. National study of US emergency department visits for acute allergic reactions, 1993 to 2004. *Ann. Allergy Asthma Immunol.* 2007;98(4):360.

[16] Banerji A, Long AA Diphenhydramine versus nonsedating antihistamines for acute allergic reactions: a literature review. *Allergy Asthma Proc. 2007*; 28 (4): 418.

[17] Macdougall CF, Cant A How dangerous is food allergy in childhood? The incidence of severe and fatal allergic reactions across the UK and Ireland. *Community child health, public health, and epidemiology 2002;* 86: 236-239.

[18] Sheikh A, Ten B. H1-antihistamines for the treatment of anaphylaxis: Cochrane systematic review. *Allergy 2007;* 62: 830-837.

[19] Alrasbi M, Sheikh A. Comparison of international guidelines for the emergency medical management of anaphylaxis. *Allergy 2007;*62: 838-841.

[20] Tole JW, Lieberman P. Biphasic anaphylaxis: review of incidence, clinical predictors, and observation recommendations. *Immunol. Allergy Clin. North Am. 2007;*27:309-326.

[21] Choo KJ, Simons E. Glucocorticoids for the treatment of anaphylaxis: Cochrane systematic review. *Allergy 2010 ;* 65 (10): 1205-1211.

[22] Thomas M, Crawford I. Best evidence topic report. Glucagon infusion in refractory anaphylactic shock in patients on beta-blockers. *Emerg. Med. J. 2005;* 22 (4): 272.

[23] Soar J, Pumphrey R Emergency treatment of anaphylactic reactions—guidelines for healthcare providers. *Resuscitation* 2008; 77:157-169.

[24] Brown SGA, Mullins Raymond. Anaphylaxis: diagnosis and management. *Med. J. Aust.* 2006;185: 283-289.

[25] Simons FE. Anaphylaxis, killer allergy: long-term management in the community. *Journal of Allergy and Clinical Immunology* 2006; 11 (2): 367.

[26] Simons FE. Anaphylaxis. *J. Allergy Clin. Immunol.* 2010; *125* (2 Supplement 2): S161.

[27] Bilò BM, Ruëff F, Mosbech H, Bonifazi F, Oude Elberink JNG; the EAACI Interest Group on Insect Venom Hypersensitivity. Diagnosis of hymenoptera venom allergy. *Allergy* 2005; 60(11): 1339–1349.

[28] Boyce JA, Assa'ad A. Guidelines for the Diagnosis and Management of Food Allergy in the United States: Summary of the NIAID-Sponsored Expert Panel Report. *J. Allergy Clin. Immunol.* 2010; 126 (6): 1105-1118.

[29] Sicherer SH, Sampson SH. Food allergy. *J. Allergy Clin. Immunol.* 2010; (125) S116-25.

In: Anaphylaxis: Principles and Practice
Editor: M. Thirumala Krishna
ISBN: 978-1-62618-688-0

Chapter V

Food-Induced Anaphylaxis

Harshna Mehta and Scott H. Sicherer*
Allergy and Immunology, Jaffe Food Allergy Institute, Department of Pediatrics, Mount Sinai School of Medicine, New York, NY, US

Abstract

Outside of the hospital setting, foods are the most common trigger of anaphylaxis. Food allergy appears to be increasing in prevalence and there is growing understanding of the underlying pathophysiology. Regarding treatment, education about allergen avoidance is crucial. Most fatal food-induced reactions occur in those with known food allergies. The most common allergens triggering food-induced anaphylaxis are peanut, tree nuts, fish, shellfish, milk and egg. Presence of asthma, being an adolescent or young adult, and delaying treatment with epinephrine are risk factors for fatal food-induced anaphylaxis. Clinical signs and symptoms of food-induced anaphylaxis are similar to those induced by other allergens. Prompt injection of epinephrine is the cornerstone of treatment. Though food allergen avoidance is the current primary therapy, there is ongoing research for novel treatments of food allergy, including allergen specific and non-specific therapies.

Introduction

Foods are the leading cause of anaphylaxis in an outpatient setting and the rate of food-induced anaphylaxis appears to be increasing. [1] Among cases of anaphylaxis presenting to emergency rooms in North America, Europe, Asia and Australia, foods account for one third to one half of cases. [2-4] Food-induced anaphylaxis is defined as a serious allergic reaction that is rapid in onset and can potentially be fatal. [5] Allergic reactions to food can range in

* Correspondence: Scott H. Sicherer, MD scott.sicherer@mssm.edu. Division of Allergy/ Immunology, Mount Sinai Hospital, Box 1198, One Gustave L. Levy Place, New York, New York 10029-6574. Voice: 212 241-5548; FAX: (212) 426-1902.

severity from mild skin or gastrointestinal symptoms to severe multi-organ involvement, with respiratory and/or cardiovascular compromise leading to death. Severe anaphylactic reactions are most frequently caused by peanuts, tree nuts, fish and shellfish, which also tend to be the most persistent food allergies. [3, 6-8] Treatment with epinephrine can be life-saving; however, reports suggest that it is often underutilized and treatment delays are associated with fatalities. [6, 9] Novel therapies and diagnostic tools for food allergy that are currently undergoing research will hopefully aid in the treatment and management of food-induced anaphylaxis in the future.

Food Allergy

Definition

The recent National Institute of Allergy and Infectious Disease (NIAID)-sponsored expert panel report "Guidelines for the Diagnosis and Management of Food Allergy in the United States", defined food allergy as "an adverse health effect arising from a specific immune response that occurs reproducibly on exposure to a given food". [5] This definition includes immune responses that are IgE-mediated causing immediate symptoms, non-IgE mediated (cell mediated reaction with delayed reactions), or a combination of both, and is in agreement with other international guidelines [10].

Prevalence

A number of studies suggest that the prevalence of food allergy is increasing. [11] A recent systematic review of four major electronic databases identifying 12,378 citations estimates food allergy to affect more than 1% to 2% but less than 10% of the population in the United States. [12] A meta-analysis of 51 articles by Rona et al [13], as a part of the EuroPrevall program, estimated rates of self-reported allergy to cow's milk, hen's egg, peanut, fish and shellfish to be 3% to 35%. They also estimated rates of 1% to 10.8% based on 6 studies using oral food challenges. A systematic review of 33 population-based publications (6 studies using oral food challenges) focusing on fruits, vegetables/non peanut legumes, tree nuts, soy and wheat indicated allergy rates from 0.1% to 4.3% for fruits and tree nuts, 0.1% to 1.4% for vegetables and less than 1% for wheat, soy and sesame. [14]

Six million children in the United States are estimated to have food allergy, based on a large population based survey study. [15] Branum et al. [16] from the Center of Disease Control and Prevention reported an increase of 18% in food allergy in children from 1997 to 2007 using data from a cross sectional analysis of several national health surveys. Studies on peanut allergy from the United States, United Kingdom and Canada indicate an increase in prevalence. [17-20] A telephone survey of self-reported peanut allergy across the United States showed a steady increase from 1 in 250 individuals affected in 1997, to 1 in 125 in 2002 to 1 in 70 in 2008. [21] Increased rates of food allergy are likely to result in higher numbers of persons experiencing food-induced anaphylaxis.

Development of Food Allergy

Multiple genetic and environmental factors may influence the development of food allergies. Findings from a twin study found a higher rate of peanut allergy among monozygotic twins (64%) as compared to dizygotic twins (7%)), suggesting that a genetic factor may be involved. [22] Earlier introduction of complementary foods to infants may be protective of allergy to those foods, as suggested by population studies from Israel where infants are fed a peanut snack at an early age and have 10-fold lower incidence of peanut allergy when compared to a culturally similar cohort of Jewish children in London where introduction is delayed. [23] A large, population-based cross sectional study of 2589 infants from Australia reported that introducing cooked egg into the infant's diet at 10-12 months and after 12 months was associated with a higher risk of egg allergy (OR 1.6 [95% CI 1.0-2.6]) and (OR 3.4 [95% CI 1.8-6.5]) when compared to introduction at 4 to 6 months of age. [24] However, the influence of time of introduction may vary for different foods. Katz et al. [25] reported, a prospective telephone study of 13,019 infants showed that introduction of milk within the first 2 weeks may offer protection; however introduction between 4 and 6 months was associated with a higher risk of developing food allergy. Determinants of food allergy are likely to be multifactorial. For example, interruption of the gastrointestinal barrier function or digestion may increase the risk. Increased food sensitization was reported in 25% of 152 patients placed on antacid medication after 3 months. [26] The allergenicity of certain food proteins, such as egg ovomucoid has been shown to be decreased due to gastric digestion. [27]

Pathophysiology of Food Allergy

Food-induced anaphylaxis is considered to be IgE dependent and triggered by allergens binding to allergen-specific IgE. [28] Once sufficient food allergen crosses the oral or gastrointestinal mucosal barrier (or rarely the respiratory mucosal barrier), it circulates throughout the body, cross links food allergen-specific IgE antibodies bound to circulating basophils and tissue mast cells in the skin, gastrointestinal tract, respiratory tract and/or cardiovascular system. Activation of these cells results in release of a variety of pro-inflammatory mediators. [29] Other adverse reactions such as food protein-induced enterocolitis syndrome and eosinophilic esophagitis may present with symptoms similar to those associated with food-induced anaphylaxis, but occur through different mechanisms.

Food protein-induced enterocolitis syndrome (FPIES) is a non-IgE mediated gastrointestinal food hypersensitivity. Patients can present with chronic symptoms of diarrhea, emesis, lethargy, failure to thrive, become hypotensive and require hospitalization. [30] Therapy involves fluid resuscitation and supportive care. [31] Eosinophilic esophagitis is an inflammatory disorder characterized by eosinophilic inflammation resulting from immune response to foods. [32] Patients, who often also have food allergies, may have food impaction that results in pain and breathing discomfort that may mimic an anaphylactic reaction.

Initial sensitization to foods may not always occur from gastrointestinal exposure. Oral allergy syndrome, also known as pollen-food allergy syndrome is due to cross reactivity seen between pollen and plant derived foods. Cross reactivity occurs when a specific antibody formed in response to a pollen protein reacts with a homologous protein in the food. For example, respiratory sensitization to Bet v1 a birch pollen protein, may lead to local symptoms (oral pruritus) in an allergic patient eating raw apples due to cross reactivity to a homologous protein in apple called Mal d 1.

The symptoms are usually mild and heating the food generally denatures the protein such that the food is tolerated without symptoms. In a review of several studies which included 1361 subjects it was reported that 8.7 % experienced symptoms outside of the gastrointestinal tract when eating raw forms, 3% had systemic symptoms without oral involvement and 1.7% had anaphylaxis [33].

Epidemiology of Food Induced Anaphylaxis

With the apparent recent increase in prevalence of food allergy, the incidence of food-induced anaphylaxis has also increased. [34-36]. Clark et al. [37] reported the natural burden of food-related acute allergic reactions treated in the emergency department in the United States by using data from 2 large emergency department based cohort studies and the National Hospital Ambulatory Medical Care Survey. Overall, from 2001 to 2005 there were approximately 203, 000 emergency room visits for food-related reactions each year, averaging an emergency department visit occurring for food related reaction every 3 minutes. Visits to the emergency department for probable anaphylactic reactions were estimated to be 90,000 per year from 2001 to 2005.

These results are higher than those reported previously. In 1999, results from Yocum et al. [38] could be extrapolated to estimate 30,000 food-induced anaphylactic reactions treated in emergency departments. Using symptom codes in the National Electronic Injury Surveillance System during August and September 2003, Ross et al. [39] estimated 125,000 visits to the emergency department for food-related allergic reactions and 14,000 for food-induced anaphylaxis annually.

Though the exact prevalence of food-induced anaphylaxis has been difficult to determine, food appears to be the most common cause of anaphylaxis in an outpatient setting. [1-4] A population-based study of the incidence and causes of anaphylaxis in Rochester, Minnesota between 1990 and 2000 showed that allergic reactions to food continue to be the most common cause of anaphylaxis, accounting for 33% of the cases. [35]

In the pediatric population, food allergens are the most common cause of outpatient anaphylaxis, whereas in adults the primary culprits are drugs and insect venom. [8] Branum and Lukacs reported 25,000 annual visits for food allergy to hospital outpatient departments, physician offices and emergency department among children < 18years of age. [40] In a recent study from Clark et al. [37], children accounted for 38% of all food related allergic reactions. In a review, de Silva et al. [41] reported food was the most common trigger for anaphylaxis in the 117 pediatric patients seen from a hospital in Melbourne, Australia, with one death of a peanut allergic 7 year old.

Both sexes are equally affected, although studies have reported that in Australia females have higher rates and in Hong Kong males have higher rates of food-induced anaphylaxis. [2, 4] The most common location for reactions to occur is in the home. [42, 43]

Fatal Food-Induced Anaphylaxis

Food allergy deaths appear to be rare and incidence rates are difficult to determine. In 2007 Pumphrey and Gowland reported 48 cases of fatal food induced anaphylaxis in the United Kingdom from 1999 to 2006. [44] From the Allergy Vigilance Network in France, Moneret et al identified 107 cases of severe anaphylaxis and 2 fatalities. [45] More recently Liew et al [34] reported an increase of 350% in hospital admissions based on retrospective review of national databases in Australia from 1997 to 2005, but found no increase in fatalities. Fatality rates were extrapolated to be 0.64 per million inhabitants a year and 6 % were food related.

Risk Factors for Fatal Food Induced Anaphylaxis

An obvious but major risk factor for fatal food-induced anaphylaxis is the presence of a food allergy. In an analysis of 32 fatal cases of food induced anaphylaxis in the United States, Bock et al reported that all but one individual was known to have food allergy with a prior reaction to the food that triggered the fatal reaction. [6] Indeed, the majority of victims of fatal or near fatal anaphylaxis are aware of their food allergy. [6-8, 46, 47] The severity of a previous reaction cannot predict the nature of a subsequent reaction; therefore NIH guidelines encourage clinicians to prescribe epinephrine auto injectors for all patients with suspected food allergy to foods that may trigger severe reactions, those with prior history of anaphylaxis as well as patients with food allergy and asthma. [5] This advice reflects observations made in a number of studies of fatal anaphylaxis. Bock et al. [6] reported that the majority of victims were young adults, 96% had a history of asthma, only 10% had epinephrine available, and peanut and tree nuts were the most common food allergens responsible. A follow up publication of 31 fatalities from 2001 to 2006 reported similar results with peanuts and tree nuts continuing to be the most common culprits and a majority of victims having a history of asthma. [7] Lack of epinephrine remained a substantial problem with only 4 individuals appearing to have injected epinephrine in a timely manner. In a study of 202 cases of fatal anaphylaxis, Pumphrey et al. [8] reported that 45 were food related and another 18 were thought to possibly be due to food. Most victims were young adults with asthma and had a prior history of reacting to the responsible allergen usually with a milder reaction. Risk taking behaviors, increasing independence, susceptibility to peer pressure and ingesting risky foods at social events may be contributing factors for young adults being more affected. [48] More than 50% of 176 adolescents and young adults reported purposefully ingesting a potentially unsafe food. [48] Summers et al. [49] demonstrated that that severity of co-existing atopic diseases predicted which patients were at higher risk to develop a life threatening allergic reaction due to peanuts and tree nuts.

Factors such as medications, exercise and alcohol can also affect the probability and/or severity of potential reactions by increasing the allergen uptake (i.e. exercise, alcohol, drugs that increase gastric pH or non-steroidal anti-inflammatory drug use) or by enhancing the inflammatory response (i.e., febrile illness, asthma exacerbation). [50] A retrospective analysis from Japan showed that NSAIDS enhanced immediate reactions due to food allergy in 9 out of 47 cases evaluated. [51] Aspirin, alcohol, angiotensin converting enzyme inhibitors, monoamine oxidase inhibitors, tricyclic antidepressants, and infection may increase the severity of anaphylactic reactions or decrease the efficiency of epinephrine. [8, 52] Please refer to table 1 for major risk factors for food-induced anaphylaxis.

Food Allergens

Any food that is intended for human consumption can cause a severe allergic reaction. However, the most common causes of these reactions are peanuts, tree nuts, milk, egg, shellfish, fish, wheat, soy and seeds. Jenkins et al determined that allergenicity of protein decreases as function of its relatedness to human homologs. [53] Proteins with sequence identity greater than 63% to human homologs were less likely to be allergenic.

Table 1. Risk Factors for food-induced anaphylaxis

Presence of asthma
Allergy to peanut, tree nuts, shellfish, fish or milk
Young adults
History of anaphylaxis Lack/delay of epinephrine administration Medications: *NSAIDS, angiotensin converting enzyme inhibitors, monoamine oxidase inhibitors, tricyclic antidepressants* Exercise Alcohol Illness Presence of other atopic disease

Major food allergens share similar properties, such as being water soluble glycoprotein, 10-70 kd in size and relatively stable to heat, acid and proteases. Preparation of the food can also affect the allergenicity.

Peanut/Tree Nuts

Peanuts and tree nuts are the most common food allergens to cause fatal anaphylactic reactions and visits to the emergency room, particularly in the United States, Germany, Australia and the United Kingdom, but these are less common triggers in China, Spain or Italy. [6, 34, 54-57] The prevalence of anaphylaxis due to nuts has been estimated to be 0.25% to 0.95% in the United Kingdom and United States pediatric population. [17, 58, 59]

Food-induced fatality case series from the United States and United Kingdom report peanuts and tree nuts as being the most common food allergen associated with death. [6-8, 60] The ubiquitous nature of tree nuts may be a contributing factor in that commercially prepared foods accounted for 68% of the reactions. [8] Tree nuts, in comparison to other food allergens, cause particularly severe reactions with multi-systemic or respiratory symptoms in up to 81% of cases [58].

Peanut proteins have been isolated and characterized, revealing 11 major antigens, Ara h 1 - Ara h 11, with different allergenic potential that can be used for improved allergy testing (component testing) and 'risk-stratification' of patients. The dominant allergens are Ara h 1-3 which are vicilin, conglutin and glycinin seed storage proteins respectively. Studies suggest that Ara h 2 is strongly associated with clinical reactivity [61] and in the United States and United Kingdom, more than 90% of peanut allergic patients demonstrate specific IgE to Ara h 1 and Ara h2. [62, 63] Ara h 1 and 2 have several physicochemical properties that make them particularly resistant to heat and digestive enzymes. [64]

The Maillard reaction, a carmelization reaction that occurs during high temperature heating/roasting, increases the stability and allergenicity of some of the peanut proteins. [65, 66] It is hypothesized that the lower prevalence rates of peanut allergy in China may be due to the preparation method which includes boiling and frying, as opposed to primarily roasting in the United States.

Another theory suggests that emulsification also increases allergenicity through an adjuvant effect. [64] The presence of carbohydrates can also affect the allergenicity. Whereas glycosylated Ara h 1 has been shown to act as a Th2 adjuvant, the deglycosylated form did not possess the same effect. [67] In contrast Ara h 5, 8 and 9 are proteins that are associated with pollen-food allergy syndrome or fruit allergies. Arah 8 is cross reactive with Bet v 1 and Ara h 9 is non-specific lipid transfer protein (LTP) similar to Pru p 3 (a peach allergen) [68, 69] and is more common in individuals with concomitant birch pollen or peach sensitization particularly in northern and southern Europe (however, LTP has been associated with severe reactions as well. [25, 70-72]

The presence of IgE antibodies recognizing a larger diversity of binding sites on proteins (epitopes) also appears to be related to increasing severity of reactions as demonstrated in a retrospective study of peanut allergic patients. [73] Higher diversity of IgE binding to various peanut epitopes on peanut allergens Ara h1, Ara h 2 and Ara h 3 was found in patients with a history of more severe allergic reactions to peanut. [73] The correlation between IgE sequential epitope diversity and clinical sensitivity was further explored by Flinterman et al [74]. The clinical reactivity of 24 peanut allergic children was determined prospectively by means of double-blind, placebo-controlled peanut challenges. A positive correlation ($r = 0.6$) between IgE epitope diversity and clinical reactivity was confirmed.

Though in the past peanut allergy was thought to uniformly persist, several large studies have demonstrated otherwise. [75, 76] Hourihane et al. [75] showed that 18% of children had resolution of their peanut allergy at a median age of 5 years in a cohort of 120 patients. Skolnick et al. [77] showed similar results with 21.5% resolution rate in 223 peanut allergic patients.

Patients sensitized to peanut or tree nut are also commonly sensitized other nuts. Sicherer et al. [78] demonstrated that 92% of 111 patients with peanut allergy, tree nut allergy or both had an IgE antibody to more than 1 tree nut and 37% of 54 had experienced convincing reactions to more than one nut. Clinical reactions to tree nuts can be severe, potentially fatal, and can occur from the first exposure to a nut [79].

A commonly reported tree nut allergy is cashew, and one-third of these patients will also react to pistachio due to cross reactivity. Hazel nut allergic patients sensitized to Cor a 8 (LTP) and Cor a 9 (11s globulin) have had severe reactions. If the test reactivity to a tree nut is due to pollen cross reactivity, ingestion reactions are typically mild or absent. [80] Some nuts have homologous proteins and cause cross reactions, for example, pistachio and cashew, whereas others, though homologous, will rarely cause reactions in the same patient, e.g., coconut and walnut.

Fish and Shellfish

Seafood allergy is the most common allergy in adults and among the six most prevalent food allergies in young children. [81] Turner et al. [82] showed that seafood is a common cause of anaphylaxis with a rate of 20% in sensitized patients in a retrospective study of 167 children. Rate of fish allergy was lower for children (0.2%) than for adults (0.5%) as determined by a telephone survey in the United States. [83] The major allergen responsible for cross reactivity among fish is parvalbumin, which is resistant to thermal and enzymatic degradation. Although canned fish is cooked for 7 hours under pressure (making it less allergenic) anaphylaxis has been reported.

Based on a telephone survey in the United States, shellfish anaphylaxis has a prevalence of 0.44%. [83] Shellfish such as shrimp and prawn are the most common types implicated. Tropomyosin is the major shellfish allergen responsible for cross reactivity between crustaceans, and homologous proteins are also present in insects (cockroach), house dust mite and different classes of molluscs.

Cross reactivity between shellfish and fish has not been reported, so affected individuals usually do not need to avoid fish if they are shellfish allergic or *vice versa*. However, patients should be cautioned about risk of cross contamination (see below) between fish and shellfish. Importantly, presence of seafood allergy is not related to reactions to intravenous contrast, a common misconception [84].

Milk

In children, milk appears to be one of the most common causes of anaphylaxis worldwide. [47, 57, 85, 86] Milk is an increasingly recognized cause of fatal or near fatal reactions. [6-8, 60] Earlier reports indicated that most children with an IgE mediated cow's milk allergy became tolerant by the age of 3. [87] However, a more recent study from a referral center indicates that cow's milk allergy may be more persistent, with only 64% of children developing tolerance by 12 years of age. [88] Casein and whey are the main milk allergens that cause reactions and account for 80% and 20% of the total milk protein respectively. [89] Phylogenetically related mammals produce homologous milk proteins, therefore cow's milk allergic patients should be advised to avoid most mammalian milks (e.g., sheep, goat).

Egg

Fatal reactions due to egg, though rare, have been reported. [90] Egg allergy is generally considered to have a good prognosis with most children eventually showing tolerance. A prospective study in a cohort of 58 children showed that 50% developed tolerance by 4 ½ years of age. [91] More recently, a large retrospective analysis of 850 patients with an IgE mediated egg allergy presenting to a referral center suggested that resolution may occur in late childhood and adolescence. Their results showed that only 68% of patients were tolerant at 16 years of age. [92] Anaphylaxis to egg, particularly in individuals with asthma, has been frequently reported. [9, 39, 93] A German study [94] reported that egg accounted for 7% of severe anaphylactic reactions in infants and children. Ingestion of raw or undercooked egg may trigger more severe clinical reactions than well cooked version. [95]

Five major allergenic proteins from hen's egg have been identified and are designated Gal d 1 to Gal d 5. Egg white contains several allergenic proteins such as ovomucoid (Gal d 1), ovalbumin (Gal d 2), ovotransferrin (Gal d 3), and lysozyme (Gal d 4) ovomucin. Ovomucoid (OVM) is the immunodominant allergen in egg, although ovalbumin (OVA) is the most abundant in hen's egg white. Bernhisel-Broadbent et al [96] demonstrated that children with persistent egg allergy have higher levels of IgE antibodies reacting against ovomucoid and ovalbumin than those with transient allergy. Jarvinen et al. [97] reported IgE antibodies directed at the four major sequential epitopes of ovomucoid in all seven subjects with persistent egg allergy compared with none in the 11 children with transient allergy. Ingestion and tolerance of baked egg appears to accelerate the development of tolerance to raw egg and similarly to oral immunotherapy. [98]

Soy

A Swedish study [99] of food related anaphylaxis reported that 4 of 6 fatalities were due to soy, suggesting that it may often be underestimated as a cause of anaphylaxis, although this experience has not been reported elsewhere. As many as 28 different soy proteins have been recognized as being allergenic but only a few are considered "major" allergens defined as those to which more than 50% of the tested population reacted. The Internal Union of Immunological Societies Allergen Sub Committee have recognized the birch pollen related allergens (Gly m 3 and Gly m 4), and soybean hull proteins (Gly m 1 and Gly m2). Holzhauser et al. [100] were able to demonstrate that the presence of IgE antibodies to Gly m 5 and Gly m 6 is a predictor for severe allergic reactions. Most individuals with soy allergy will eventually become tolerant. A retrospective study describing the natural history of 133 of soy allergic patients by Savage et al found that 50% of children outgrew their allergy by age of 7 years and 69% by 10 years of age. [101] Soy allergy may develop due to sensitization to birch pollen and resulting cross reactivity. A study [102] of 273 infants from the German Multi-Centre Allergy group revealed soy sensitization was rare, and it was more frequently found at school age due to cross reacting pollen with initial sensitization *via* inhalation. Soy proteins can elicit oropharyngeal or systemic reactions in patients sensitized to the major birch pollen Bet v1 due to cross reactivity to Gly m4, a pathogenesis related protein (PR-10).

Delayed Anaphylaxis to Meat

One of the first reports of a carbohydrate (galactose α-1,3 galactose, alpha-gal) as a potential food allergen causing a delayed hypersensitivity reaction to red meats such as beef, pork and lamb was published by Commins et al. [103] Commins et al. identified 24 patients from Southeastern United States with similar histories of delayed anaphylaxis, angioedema or urticaria, each of whom had detectable IgE antibodies to alpha gal; however they had a wheal response of less than 4 mm to the causal food. Patients consistently reported episodes of allergic reactions and anaphylaxis associated with having eaten beef, pork, or lamb 3 to 6 hours earlier. In 2011 the first cases from Europe of delayed anaphylaxis to meat with sensitization to α gal were reported. [104] Additional studies [105] are needed to explore the mechanism and mode of sensitization in these patients, but sensitization *via* tick bites has been suggested.

Additives

Though very rare, anaphylaxis to additives such as annatto, carmine, erthrito, guar gum and psyllium have been reported; they are primarily protein-bearing additives derived from plant, insect and animal products. [106-111]

Clinical Features of Food-Induced Anaphylaxis

Clinical signs and symptoms of food-induced anaphylaxis are similar to those induced by other allergens. Symptoms include but are not limited to pruritus, flushing, urticaria, angioedema, vomiting (large amounts of stringy mucus), diarrhea, abdominal pain, a feeling of impending doom, respiratory difficulty, wheezing, hypotension, syncope and shock. Cutaneous symptoms are common and appear in 80% of food-induced cases. A study of fatal and near-fatal reactions reported that all patients with near-fatal reactions developed cutaneous symptoms whereas only one patient with fatal anaphylaxis had skin rashes/hives, possibly leading to a delay in diagnosis and treatment. [9] Though cardiovascular symptoms are not as common in food-induced anaphylaxis, an eleven year retrospective study reported 39% of food-induced anaphylactic reactions had cardiovascular involvement. [112] Hypotension can manifest with nausea, diaphoresis, dyspnea, hypoxia, seizures and collapse. Within 10 minutes, a decrease in circulating blood volume of up to 35% can occur due to vasodilation and fluid extravasation, so aggressive fluid resuscitation is recommended. [113] Additional recommendations include supine positioning and elevation of legs. Coming to an upright posture has been rarely reported to result in sudden fatalities in cases of anaphylaxis. [114] The suggested mechanism for this is the incapacity of sufficient blood to return to the vena cava and the right side of the heart due to vasodilation of the veins and capillaries during anaphylactic shock. Once the vena cava is empty, epinephrine cannot circulate and reverse the shock.

The onset of symptoms can vary from immediately to a few hours following ingestion of the food allergen. A slower onset of symptoms often correlates with a less severe reaction and a majority of reactions occur within 1 hour of exposure. [3] Food-induced fatalities commonly associated with peanut or tree nut ingestion have been reported to occur within 30 minutes to 2 hours of exposure. Usually, fatal food-induced anaphylaxis reactions occur within 25-35 minutes of ingesting the eliciting food allergen, whereas fatal anaphylaxis due to medication or insect venom occurs with 5 to 12 minutes. [8]

Most anaphylactic reactions are monophasic with complete resolution within 2 hours of appropriate treatment. Biphasic reactions occur when there is a reoccurrence of symptoms 2 to 72 hours after complete resolution of initial symptoms. The reported rate of biphasic reactions in food induced anaphylaxis varies by study. Biphasic reactions were reported to occur in 25% of fatal or near fatal food reactions. [115] However, in a retrospective review of 1273 oral food challenges offered at a tertiary center, only one patient was found to have a biphasic reaction with symptoms reoccurring one hour after resolution with epinephrine, [116] it is unclear if this is related to the gradual feeding of a food allergen over a prolonged period of time during a supervised food challenge, compared to ingestions occurring more rapidly and with larger doses by accident or during meals. Based upon various studies of the time course for biphasic reactions, recommendations range from 4 hours to 24 hours for observation of patients in a medical setting following food-induced anaphylaxis. [9, 117, 118] It is unclear why food allergic individuals on a number of occasions will manifest only mild symptoms whereas at other times will have a life threatening reaction.

In addition to medications, exercise, alcohol, illness and the presence of atopic disease - other cofactors that may potentially influence the onset and severity of symptoms include the following: [6, 8, 119].

1. The quantity of food allergen ingested; the larger the dose, the more rapid and pronounced the onset of symptoms.
2. The composition of food containing the allergen: fatty foods tend to slow absorptions rate and delay onset/prolong onset of symptoms

The presentation of food-induced anaphylaxis can overlap with other illnesses. Table 2 shows examples of non-allergic adverse reactions to food.

Table 2. Examples of Non Allergenic Adverse Reactions to Food

Metabolic
Lactose Intolerance
Galactosemia
Alcohol Intolerance
Pharmacologic
Tyramine: present in aged cheeses which trigger migraines
Caffeine: coffee, tea, energy drinks causing jitters and dysrhythmia
Histamine like substances: fish, wine, strawberry causing flushing
Sodium metabisulfite: triggering wheeze
Food Poisoning
Scombroid: spoiled dark meat fish such as tuna and mackerel mimicking anaphylaxis
Psychologic
Food Aversion
Eating Disorder: anorexia nervosa
Neurologic
Auriculotemporal syndrome: manifested by facial flush from tart foods
Gustatory rhinitis: rhinorrhea from hot or spicy foods

When the clinical history is not convincing, it is important to evaluate for other potential causes and diseases that may mimic food induced anaphylaxis. Adverse reactions to foods that are not food allergies should be addressed when considering the diagnosis of food allergy.

Exercise

Exercise induced anaphylaxis (a detailed discussion is present in chapter - 6) is a rare, potentially fatal, reaction that is associated with physical activity. This reaction may occur independently or may occur only after ingestion of a food allergen, a disorder known as food-dependent, exercise-induced anaphylaxis (FDEIA). In FDEIA, both exercise and the food allergen are independently tolerated. There are very limited data on the prevalence of FDEIA. Females are more commonly affected and the majority of cases are of patients less than 30 years of age.

The most common specific food allergen to induce FDEIA is wheat, in particular the wheat protein omega-5- gliadin, followed by other grains, nuts and seafood. [120] Certain characteristics of food proteins such as resistance to digestion during exercise, abundance of protein, and multiple linear epitopes may make some food proteins more likely to cause FDEIA. [121, 122] The severity of FDEIA reactions to the same food is not stereotypical and there is both inter- and intra-individual variability with respect to the dose of allergen required to induce FDEIA. [123]

Various physical activities including high and low aerobic sports have been associated with FDEIA. Symptoms usually begin within 30 minutes of the start of exercise but also have occurred during all phases of exercise. The pathophysiology of FDEIA is not well understood and remains unclear as to which exercise specific or combination of factors up regulates immune responses and leads to a transient loss of tolerance. Enzyme activity, epitope recognition, altered gastrointestinal permeability and autonomic aberrations are being researched as potential etiologic factors.

Diagnosis is made by convincing clinical history. Currently there is no established protocol for exercise challenge to evaluate patients for FDEIA as many studies have reported variable rates of success in eliciting symptoms. In a literature review of 234 cases of FDEIA, food/exercise challenges failed to reproduce symptoms in 36%. [114] The management of FDEIA is focused on prevention. It is recommended that patients avoid the food allergen for up to 4 hours prior to undertaking a physical activity. The simultaneous intake of alcohol and or salicylates may facilitate the onset of FDEIA. [124-126]. The presence of the following factors may trigger the reaction although exercise remains the inciting factor:

1. NSAIDS
2. Alcohol
3. Premenstrual or ovulatory phase of the menstrual cycle
4. Extremes of temperature
5. Seasonal pollen exposure in pollen sensitized patients

Diagnostic Testing

Anaphylaxis is diagnosed by obtaining a thorough history and physical examination. A comprehensive history should include the details about the possible food trigger, quantity ingested, time of onset of reaction, clinical features of the reaction, presence of modifying factors, and reaction consistency. Identification and diagnosis of the eliciting food allergen is an essential initial step in preventing further episodes. Skin prick testing [SPT] and food specific IgE by serum immunoassay are utilized to assess IgE-mediated food allergies. Negative SPT responses have a 90% negative predictive accuracy. A positive test, however does not prove that the food is the trigger unless it is combined with a recent or convincing history of a food induced reaction. [81] Increasing wheal size is positively correlated with possibility of clinical allergy. [127, 128] Serum tests for food specific IgE antibodies can be important particularly when there is persistent dermatographism in the few weeks after anaphylactic shock, severe eczema or when the patient is on an antihistamine. The presence of serum food-specific IgE or a positive SPT alone reflects allergic sensitization and not necessarily clinical allergy. [5] Increasing wheal diameter and higher concentrations of food specific IgE levels correlate with the increasing likelihood of a reaction, however these parameters do not correlate well with severity [81] When the history and serum food-specific IgE testing have not confirmed an allergy, an oral food challenge (OFC) is required to confirm the diagnosis. An OFC is performed by gradually feeding increasing amounts of the suspected food allergen under a controlled medical setting. A double-blind, placebo-controlled OFC is however considered the 'gold standard' for diagnosis of a food allergy. [129]

Currently, there is no 'gold standard' laboratory test to evaluate for anaphylaxis. Lin et al showed that in a study of 97 emergency room patients with anaphylaxis, 42% had increased plasma histamine and 21% had increased tryptase. [130]

Serum histamine is transiently elevated after the onset of a reaction so it can be easily missed. Serum tryptase is not generally increased in food induced anaphylaxis and therefore would be a poor marker. [9, 131] In a study by Sampson et al [9], the majority of patients with fatal anaphylaxis and near fatal anaphylaxis did not have detectable increases in tryptase. Sampson and Jolie also failed to demonstrate elevated tryptase in patients with anaphylaxis undergoing food challenges even though the samples were obtained at the ideal time. [132] Detection of greater epitope diversity by microarray immunoassay shows promise in the diagnosis of food allergy as it is correlated with reaction severity. [104] However, its role in diagnosis of potential for food-induced anaphylaxis remains to be determined. [73] Platelet activating factor (PAF) is currently being investigated as a potential biomarker for anaphylaxis. Vadas et al. [133] reported a direct correlation of serum PAF and an indirect correlation of PAF acetylhydrolase activity with the severity of anaphylaxis.

Treatment

Anaphylaxis should be treated the same regardless of the cause and a more detailed discussion is presented in chapter 4. We will briefly review medical management of food induced anaphylaxis and focus on avoidance.

Epinephrine

The treatment for food-induced anaphylaxis is the same as it is for anaphylaxis due to other allergens: intramuscular epinephrine (0.01ml/kg aqueous epinephrine 1:1000, up to 0.5 mL) into the lateral thigh. [134] During severe episodes, intravenous epinephrine has been used. Vasoconstrictors can be used in extremely severe cases refractory to epinephrine and fluids. [135]

Though epinephrine is well recognized as first line treatment it is not always utilized and administered in a timely manner. In a follow up report from Bock et al. [6] it was reported that of the 31 deaths due to food anaphylaxis between 2001 to 2006, only 4 individuals appeared to have had epinephrine administered in a timely manner. A study in Hong Kong demonstrated that 67% cases of anaphylaxis treated in the emergency room were given epinephrine. [4] A similar study based in Italy showed that only 15% of anaphylactic cases admitted to the hospital were given epinephrine. [112] In a chart review of patients presenting to 21 North American emergency departments for food allergy, Clark et al., [136] reported that 22% of anaphylaxis cases were treated with epinephrine.

These studies clearly show that there is underutilization of epinephrine in food related anaphylactic reactions. Additionally, there may be differences in the treatment of children and adults. In an Australian study, 57% of adults with anaphylaxis received epinephrine as opposed to only 26.3% of children. [137] In the United Kingdom it was shown that 11% of children and 32% of adults used available epinephrine at the time of their food related reaction. [42]

All patients with a serious food reaction should be discharged with an epinephrine auto-injector; however, according to Clark et al. [136] only 16% of patients who presented to the emergency department were discharged with a prescription for epinephrine and only 12% were referred for an allergy evaluation. Other studies have also investigated the frequency of epinephrine prescriptions given by the emergency room staff for anaphylaxis management and found rates to be 0 % to 38%. [2, 138, 139] Gold and Sainsbury [140] reported that in 71% of patients experiencing anaphylactic reactions, an auto-injector was not used as first line treatment. Of the 32 occasions when the injection was not given, 47% of patients had admission to the hospital compared to 15% when the injection was administered. [140] The importance of timely administration of epinephrine and management of food-induced anaphylactic patients in the emergency department and in the outpatient setting cannot be over emphasized. Self-injectable epinephrine (2 doses) should be prescribed to any patient diagnosed with a potentially serious food allergy particularly those at high risk for severe reactions such as individuals with asthma irrespective of severity or to individuals with a history of previous reactions involving the cardiovascular or respiratory system. [5] In addition, patients should receive a plan for monitoring for auto-injector expiration dates, an anaphylaxis emergency action plan, plan for further evaluation, and printed information about anaphylaxis and its treatment. [5] Children (age appropriate) and care givers should be taught how and when to administer epinephrine. Sicherer et al. [141] demonstrated that although 86% of food allergic patients carry self-injectable epinephrine at all times, only 71% had the device during the study visit and only one third were to correctly demonstrate its use. Interestingly, less than half of the pediatricians in that study were able to correctly demonstrate the use of epinephrine auto-injectors. Studies based on retrospective reviews convincingly show that lack of prompt treatment with epinephrine is one of the major risk factors for fatalities in food related reactions. [6] However, despite having received management advice and having epinephrine present, anaphylactic reactions are often not appropriately treated. In a large, prospective multi-center study evaluating reactions in children with a certain or likely diagnosis of food allergies who have received avoidance advice, of 134 severe reactions, only 40 were treated with epinephrine. [142] The most common reason for not injecting was not recognizing the reaction, followed by unavailability of epinephrine, too afraid, waiting for more symptoms and uncertainty about whether it was needed. Caretakers admitted retrospectively that epinephrine was warranted. These studies underscore the need for clinicians to educate patients about the indications and technique of use for self-injectors, and the safety of epinephrine.

Antihistamines

H1 histamine receptor antagonists are often used during the management of food-induced anaphylaxis. Though they can decrease nasal and cutaneous symptoms (urticaria, pruritus, flushing), they do not prevent or treat respiratory, gastrointestinal and cardiovascular manifestations of anaphylaxis. Antihistamines are not considered first line therapy during an anaphylactic food related reaction. [46] They may however be used as adjunctive therapy in conjunction with epinephrine. It is advised for patients to take an H1 antihistamine immediately if there is an accidental ingestion of known food allergen.

Combination of H1 and H2 antihistamines have been shown to more effective than either alone [143]. The evidence to support H2 antagonist in treatment of anaphylaxis due to food is also limited.

Corticosteroids

Many health care professionals empirically use corticosteroids in patients with food-allergic reactions; however, studies are contradictory regarding their role. [117] These medications are often prescribed for their anti-inflammatory activity and a notion that they may be helpful for protracted or biphasic reactions but the evidence is lacking. [144, 145] Prospective, randomized double- blinded placebo controlled studies are needed to further evaluate the role of steroids in food-induced anaphylaxis.

Supplemental Measures

Beta adrenergic agents and supplemental oxygen are recommended for patients with respiratory symptoms. Shock with symptoms of severe hypotension can be refractory to epinephrine, therefore aggressive fluid resuscitation or intravenous vasopressors may be necessary. Glucagon can be used for patients on beta blockers if other treatments are ineffective.

Avoidance

Currently, prevention of food-induced anaphylaxis is based on avoidance. This underscores the importance of education about identification of food allergens by reading labels, understanding how to avoid cross contact during food preparation, and communicating effectively with persons who are providing meals such as relatives and restaurant personnel. Patients should also be instructed to wear medical jewelry that easily identify themselves as individuals with potential for food induced anaphylaxis [146].

Label Reading

By using the United Kingdom fatal anaphylaxis register, Pumphrey et al [8] were able to demonstrate that over two-thirds of those dying from sting reaction and over four-fifths dying from drug anaphylaxis had no previous indication of allergy. However, patients with food related fatalities had a history of reactions to that food allergen. This demonstrates the importance of correctly identifying all the ingredients present in foods consumed by allergic individuals. [147] On 01 January, 2006 the Food Allergen Labeling and Consumer Protection Act of 2004 went into effect in the US requiring that packaging labels clearly identify ingredients such as milk, egg, peanut, tree nut, shellfish, wheat and soy. However this policy only applies to the 8 major allergens, sesame for example can be listed using ambiguous term and does not need to be included in the "contains." statement. Similar labeling laws are also in effect for Canada, Europe, New Zealand and Australia. The European Union enacted legislation in 2005 requiring that common allergens such as milk, egg, fish, crustacean shellfish, peanuts, soybean, tree nuts, gluten, celery, mustard and sesame seeds be listed if present in any amount and any ingredients that comprise 5 percent or more must be listed. [148, 149] Advisory wording such as "may contain", "processed in a facility with", "manufactured on shared equipment with" and others have become commonly used by manufacturing companies. A study of over 600 subjects who shop for food allergic individuals showed that they were more likely to purchase products that were labeled "made in a facility that may contain" rather than "may contain peanut" when shopping for a peanut allergic patient. [150] However, assays of over 179 products with such labeling for peanut disclosed that 7% contained detectable peanut protein regardless of the advisory wording. Another study examining milk products revealed 34 of 81 of products with advisory labeling had milk detectable milk. [151] Based on these studies, it appears that sensitive patients should be advised to avoid all foods that describe the allergen in an advisory label because it is impossible to determine the actual risk and serious reactions from cross contact have been reported. [152] Regardless of appropriate labeling, Sampson et al demonstrated that among 174 adolescents with food allergy, 42% were willing to eat food labeled as "may contain." [48]

Despite receiving avoidance advice, 72% of participants in a multicenter observational study of 512 children experienced a reaction. [153] Most of accidental reactions that occurred in patients were due to unintentional ingestions due to forgetfulness or lack of attention (64.9%), label reading error (15.8%), cross contamination (15.1%), error in preparation (4.1%) and manufacturer labeling error (0.1%). These findings emphasize the need for supervision, vigilance with checking ingredients lists, education about label reading and avoiding allergens in meal preparation and restaurants. In the same study it was reported that parents were most often the providers of the food, followed by the patients, and then various relatives. [153] These results underscore the need to educate all caregivers. Patients should also be made aware that alcoholic beverages may contain allergens such as eggs, milk and seafood which is not subject to labeling laws in the United States or in the European Union. [148]

Food allergic individuals should receive guidance for managing their food allergies in the home and outside of it, such as in schools and restaurants. In the home of individuals with food allergies, families may decide to remove the food allergen or, if left in the home, take the necessary precautions to avoid cross contact. Cross contact occurs when an allergen is introduced unintentionally to an otherwise safe food. For example, cross contact could occur from using a utensil in peanut butter and then using the same utensil in jelly, or using a fish fryer to cook otherwise safe potatoes, or chopping nuts on a cutting board and then using the same board to chop otherwise safe lettuce. All dishware and utensils should be thoroughly cleaned if they are in contact with an allergen. All family members should be educated on cross contact. When eating outside of the home, patients should take precautions and discuss issues of hidden ingredients, nature of allergy and cross contamination of cookware and serving utensils with restaurant staff. Establishments such as Ice cream parlors, bakeries and Asian restaurants are particularly high risk for peanut and tree nut allergic individuals. [154] In a telephone survey of 100 employees in the food industry in the New York City area it was found that only 22% were able to provide correct answers to 5 true or false food allergy questions. [155] Inaccurate beliefs such as removal of allergen from a plate, only ingesting small amounts of an allergen and frying the allergen would eliminate the risk of a reaction were discovered. Despite these results, more than 90% rated themselves as being "comfortable" in providing safe meals to food allergic customers. Therefore, patients should review the nature of allergy, cross contact risks and potential hidden ingredients with all personnel that will handle their food to minimize the possibility of a reaction.

School should be notified about a child's potentially life threatening allergy. Allergic reactions induced by food at school are common, but preparation for managing them is usually inadequate. [156-158] In a telephone survey of 80 schools and parents of the 132 food allergic children, 39% of schools reported at least one food allergic reaction during the prior two years. In the same period, 58% of food allergic children experienced a reaction at school and of those 30% did not have an action plan or medication available at the school at the time of the reaction. [156] An expert panel recommends that all patients with food allergies at risk of anaphylaxis should leave the hospital or physician's office with a written action plan (figure 1: emergency action plan) clearly indicating the food allergies, the dose of epinephrine to be used, symptoms that should induce epinephrine use, emergency contact information and, if applicable, a photo of the child. [5] The emergency plan should be reviewed with all caregivers (parents, relatives, school staff, camp staff, etc.). Self-injectable epinephrine should be available to use at school: carried by the child if age appropriate otherwise kept with a supervising adult and kept in a health office. [159] Based on a survey study of members of the American Academy of Pediatrics Section on Allergy and Immunology it was reported that most allergists transition the responsibilities of anaphylaxis recognition and management from parents or caregivers to children by age 12 to 14 years and begin the gradual teachings of these responsibilities when patients are younger. [160]

Class projects where food is involved or special events can be problematic since 79% of peanut and tree nut reactions that occurred in the school setting were during these times. [78] Schools and camps should be proactive in planning on how to manage food allergies and reactions that may occur. [159, 161, 162] Craft projects with allergens should be curtailed. Standard cleaning and lack of visible contamination should suffice for most children with peanut allergy [159].

The route of exposure is important in determining the risk and severity of allergic reaction. Ingestion is the cause of most food allergic reactions whereas cutaneous and inhalation exposure cause milder symptoms. One study applied 1 gram of peanut butter for 15 minutes to the skin of 281 skin prick peanut positive children. The results revealed that though contact urticaria was common among peanut allergic children, no systemic reactions occurred. [163] In a double-blind, placebo-controlled study, 30 children with a positive history for a severe allergic reaction to peanut ingestion smelled peanut butter. No child experienced symptoms, except one child during exposure to placebo [164].

Food Allergy Action Plan

Emergency Care Plan

Place Student's Picture Here

Name: ________________________ **D.O.B.:** __/__/__

Allergy to: ________________________

Weight: ______ lbs. **Asthma:** ☐ Yes (higher risk for a severe reaction) ☐ No

Extremely reactive to the following foods: ________________________

THEREFORE:

☐ If checked, give epinephrine immediately for ANY symptoms if theallergen was *likely* eaten.

☐ If checked, give epinephrine immediately if theallergen was *definitely* eaten, even if no symptoms are noted.

Any SEVERE SYMPTOMS after suspected or known ingestion:

One or more of the following:

LUNG: Short of breath, wheeze, repetitive cough
HEART: Pale, blue, faint, weak pulse, dizzy, confused
THROAT: Tight, hoarse, trouble breathing/swallowing
MOUTH: Obstructive swelling (tongue and/or lips)
SKIN: Many hives over body

Or **combination** of symptoms from different body areas:

SKIN: Hives, itchy rashes, swelling (e.g., eyes, lips)
GUT: Vomiting, diarrhea, crampy pain

1. **INJECT EPINEPHRINE IMMEDIATELY**
2. Call 911
3. Begin monitoring (see box below)
4. Give additional medications:*
   -Antihistamine
   -Inhaler ([bronchodilator) if asthma

*Antihistamines & inhalers/bronchodilators are not to be depended upon to treat a severe reaction (anaphylaxis). USE EPINEPHRINE.

MILD SYMPTOMS ONLY:

MOUTH: Itchy mouth
SKIN: A few hives around mouth/face, mild itch
GUT: Mild nausea/discomfort

1. **GIVE ANTIHISTAMINE**
2. Stay with student; alert healthcare professionals and parent
3. If symptoms progress (see above), USE EPINEPHRINE
4. Begin monitoring (see box below)

Medications/Doses

Epinephrine (brand and dose): ________________________

Antihistamine (brand and dose): ________________________

Other (e.g., inhaler-bronchodilator if asthmatic): ________________________

Monitoring

Stay with student; alert healthcare professionals and parent. Tell rescue squad epinephrine was given; request an ambulance with epinephrine. Note time when epinephrine was administered. A second dose of epinephrine can be given 5 minutes or more after the first if symptoms persist or recur. For a severe reaction, consider keeping student lying on back with legs raised.Treat student even if parents cannot be reached. See back/attached for auto-injection technique.

Parent/Guardian Signature ____ Date ____ Physician/Healthcare Provider Signature ____ Date ____

EPIPEN Auto-Injector and EPIPEN Jr Auto-Injector Directions

- First, remove the EPIPEN Auto-Injector from the plastic carrying case
- Pull off the blue safety release cap

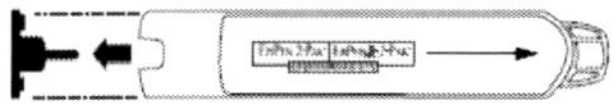

- Hold orange tip near outer thigh (always apply to thigh)

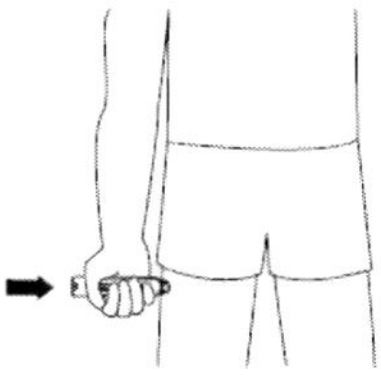

- Swing and firmly push orange tip against outer thigh. Hold on thigh for approximately 10 seconds. Remove the EPIPEN Auto-Injector and massage the area for 10 more seconds

DEY® and the Dey logo, EpiPen®, EpiPen 2-Pak®, and EpiPen Jr 2-Pak® are registered trademarks of Dey Pharma, L.P.

Adrenaclick™ 0.3 mg and Adrenaclick™ 0.15 mg Directions

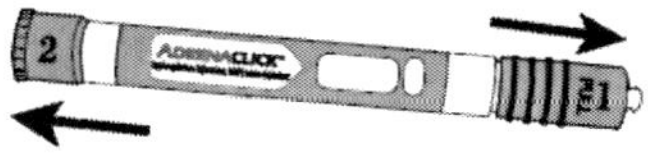

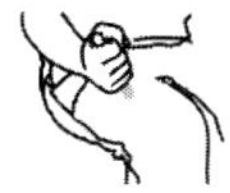

Remove GREY caps labeled "1" and "2."

Place RED rounded tip against outer thigh, press down hard until needle penetrates. Hold for 10 seconds, then remove.

A food allergy response kit should contain at least two doses of epinephrine, other medications as noted by the student's physician, and a copy of this Food Allergy Action Plan.

A kit must accompany the student if he/she is off school grounds (i.e., field trip).

Contacts

Call 911 (Rescue squad: (___) _____-_________) Doctor: _______________ Phone: (___) _____-________

Parent/Guardian: ____ Phone: (___) _____-________

Other Emergency Contacts

Name/Relationship: ____ Phone: (___) _____-________

Name/Relationship: ____ Phone: (___) _____-________

Form provided ©2011, The Food & Anaphylaxis Network. Used with permission.

Figure 1. Emergency Action Plan.

Contact between airborne volatile organic compounds which are continuously given off by foods and the nasal mucosa results in smelling whereas during aerosolization actual food proteins become airborne. Inhalation contact with aerosolized food has been shown to induce asthmatic symptoms in highly sensitive individuals [165, 166], therefore situation where food protein is becoming aerosolized (cooking or processing) should be avoided.

Another route through which systemic reactions can occur is via kissing, particularly passionate kissing. Studies report that 5% to 16 % of reactions have occurred due to kissing. [167, 168] In a study of 36 individuals, 30 had detectable Ara h1 at 5 minutes after ingesting 2 tablespoons of peanut butter, and 87% of the 30 had undetectable protein levels after 1 hour without interventions. Interventions such as brushing teeth, rinsing, waiting then brushing and waiting then chewing gum did not consistently result in undetectable levels, but waiting several hours and consuming a peanut-free meal resulted in no detectable peanut protein. [169]

Strategies for minimizing risks at school may include:

- Increased supervision
- No food trading

- Wearing medical identification jewelry
- No food in classrooms
- No home-made food allowed for class celebrations or parties
- Designating the parent of the allergic student to be responsible for selecting food for class celebrations
- Celebration of birthdays or special events with books or music instead of food
- Designated peanut/ nut safe tables in the cafeteria
- Education of all students and implementation of student focused allergy programs

Other Settings

Avoidance advice and emergency management preparedness at camps is very similar to that provided for school. Studies based on self-reported reactions to peanut on commercial airlines indicate there is a potential risk present; however, the degree of risk is difficult to ascertain [170]. The safe option would be for patients to carry on their own meal and for parents to clean tray tables and inspect the sitting area for residual foods.

Future Therapies for Food Induced Anaphylaxis

Food allergies seriously affect the quality of life of food allergic patients. [171] Novel therapies are currently being investigated to lead to oral tolerance or increase the threshold dose for desensitization to food allergen. Approaches that are being pursued are allergen and non-allergen specific. Allergen specific therapies include immunotherapy with native food allergens and mutated proteins with decreased binding capacity to generate maximum immune response. Examples of nonspecific approaches include Chinese herbal medication and monoclonal anti-IgE antibodies. Table 3 provides a summary of novel therapies being invested for food allergy.

Allergen Specific Immunotherapy

Subcutaneous Peanut Therapy

For over 100 years subcutaneous immunotherapy has been used to treat environmental allergies and is currently used to effectively treat environmental and venom allergies. [172] Early attempts at immunotherapy using native peanut allergens resulted in modest clinical improvement, but was associated with significant adverse effects, including anaphylaxis. [173-175] Due to these pitfalls, alternative routes of administration attempting to avoid serious adverse effects have been investigated.

Food Oral Immunotherapy (OIT)

There are a number of studies exploring oral immunotherapy, where a food allergen is ingested in gradually increasing doses over months. One of the earliest reports of successful oral immunotherapy (OIT) was in 1908 when a boy was treated for egg induced anaphylaxis. [176] Currently, OIT to food represents one of the most active areas of research in the field of food allergy.

Table 3. Future Therapies

Therapy	Mechanism	Benefits	Observations
Subcutaneous immunotherapy	Antigen presentation in non-mucosal site results in Th1 skewing	Proven for venom and aeroallergens, Might benefit oral allergy syndrome	Primarily avoided for risk of anaphylaxis
Sublingual/OIT	Antigen presentation to mucosal site provides desensitization and might induce tolerance	Natural foods, reduced risk of systemic reactions compared with subcutaneous IT	Increasing evidence for desensitization and relative safety; unclear effect on tolerance
EPIT	Antigen presentation by Langerhans cells leading to tolerance	Low doses of natural protein, reduced risk of systemic reactions	Clinical trials ongoing
Modified Protein Vaccine	Reduced IgE activation by mutation of IgE binding epitope	Safer form of IT compared with native protein IT	Murine models show promise, human studies needed
Peptide Vaccine	Peptides are less likely to cross link IgE, avoiding mast cell activation	No requirement for IgE epitope mapping/mutation	Limited
Anti IgE antibodies	Targeting towards Fc portion of antibody can inactivate IgE with reduced risk for activating mast cells	Not food specific. Some response in eosinophilic gastroenteropathy	Preliminary study showed improved threshold over but did not show protection
Plasmid DNA coded vaccines	Endogenous production of allergen might result in tolerance	Possible 1 time dose treatment	Murine models reveal strain specific response
Conjugation of immune stimulatory sequences	Enhance Th2 response by activating innate immune receptors	Increased efficacy, possible improved safety	Preclinical studies
Modified Protein Vaccine	Reduced IgE activation by mutation of IgE binding epitope	Safer form of IT compared with native protein IT	Murine models show promise, human studies needed
Chinese herbal medicine	Mechanisms unknown	Not food specific	Murine models show efficacy. Human studies underway
Probiotics	Improve defective skin barrier in atopic dermatitis therefore decrease sensitization	Murine model has shown decrease systemic reactions	Lack of support from human studies
Trichurissuis Ova Therapy	Stimulation of IL-10	Not food specific.	Murine models show anaphylaxis protection. Unclear role in humans
Toll receptor agonist	Th1 skewing		Murine models show anaphylaxis protection

Studies have demonstrated desensitization (an increased threshold during treatment), however few studies have demonstrated tolerance (permanent loss of reactivity independent of treatment dosing). [174, 177, 178] The more recent and larger studies have focused on oral immunotherapy for milk and egg. [179-182]

Success rates vary and failures appear more commonly in patients with higher food specific IgE, although Longo et al reported 90% success rate in 30 children with severe milk allergy. [183] Adverse reactions during treatment have been reported, particularly during exercise or illness and early during OIT. [182] Skripak et al [184] published the first double-blind, placebo-controlled milk OIT study with 20 subjects in the active arm who achieved a 50 to 100 fold increase in the threshold dose needed for reactivity. Most patients were successfully desensitized, however it is unclear if tolerance, as described earlier, was achieved as participants continued daily consumption of milk without a period of abstinence. Staden et al [182] reported that only 36% of subjects of a milk and egg OIT trial demonstrated tolerance when challenged two month post treatment. This percentage exactly matched tolerance achieved by the control untreated group. Most recently Burks et al [178] published results from a large double blind randomized placebo controlled study with 55 egg allergic children who received immunotherapy or placebo.

After 10 months of therapy none of children on placebo and 55% of treatment group passed an OFC and were considered desensitized and after 22 months 75% of the active arm were desensitized. Children who passed the OFC at 22 months discontinued oral immunotherapy and avoided all egg consumption for 4 to 6 weeks. In the oral immunotherapy group 28% passed OFC at 24, 30 and 36 months while on a diet with ad libitum egg consumption suggesting that tolerance was achieved. Most reactions that occurred were mild with less than 1% scored as moderate. These results seem encouraging however adverse reactions are variable therefore more studies are required to further assess safety and efficacy of OIT.

Sublingual Immunotherapy (SLIT)

Another modality for immunotherapy is *via* the sublingual route where a food allergic individual may be gradually exposed to a native food protein allowing for immune processing while avoiding acute allergic reaction triggered by larger exposures. Sublingual immunotherapy treating a 29 year old woman with kiwi induced anaphylaxis was one of the first successful reports. [185] Enrique et al [186, 187] have also demonstrated success with hazel nut SLIT.

In a placebo controlled double blind study for hazel nut allergy confirmed by double-blind, placebo-controlled food challenge, 50% of treated subjects tolerated the highest dose (20 grams) of hazelnut compared with 9% in the placebo group. Systemic reactions occurred in 0.2% of the total doses during the escalation phase and were treated with oral antihistamines.

Results from a controlled trial of peanut SLIT showed promise, although with less robust response compared to OIT. Eighteen children completed twelve months of peanut SLIT dosing and the subjects achieved clinical desensitization, being able to ingest 1,710 gram of peanut protein. Long term study follow up is required to assess tolerance. [188] Keet et al [177] demonstrated OIT was more efficacious for desensitization to cow's milk than SLIT.

Thirty subjects with cow's milk allergy were enrolled in a three arm clinical trial of SLIT, SLIT/OIT and OIT alone. Though more subjects were desensitized with OIT, it was associated with more systemic side effects. Numerous studies suggest beneficial effects of OIT and SLIT, though the latter has less severe adverse reactions. These treatments needed further investigation regarding optimal doses, duration, degree/length of protection, applicability to various types and severity of food allergies, efficacy for different ages, and need for patient protection at home. [189, 190]

Epicutaneous Immunotherapy (EPIT)

Allergen delivery through an epicutaneous route delivers the food allergen in small doses by placing an allergen containing patch on the skin. Dupont et al. [135] showed a trend toward increased threshold doses in EPIT treated milk allergic children. Side effects included local pruritus and eczema at the site of EPIT patch. The only systemic reaction reported was in one child with repeated episodes of diarrhea after the EPIT. Currently, EPIT is undergoing further evaluation in several studies for food allergy.

Heated Milk and Egg Diet

Clinical studies are investigating the role of baked milk and egg as a form of immunotherapy since 70-80% of milk and egg allergic patients can tolerate baked forms of these foods. Regular ingestion of these extensively heated milk and egg products has resulted in decreased skin test wheal diameters, and increased IgG4 levels and appears to accelerate the development of tolerance of unheated milk and egg. [71]

In a prospective study of 65 baked milk tolerant patients who incorporated baked milk into their diet, 60% were able to tolerate unheated milk. [191] In retrospective comparison they were 16 times more likely to become unheated milk tolerant when compared to children who were strictly avoiding milk ($P<0.001$). Similarly, Nowak-Wegrzyn et al [192] showed in a prospective study that that baked egg tolerant children who incorporated baked egg into the diet were 14.6 times (95% confidence interval, 5.8-36.4; $P<0.0001$) more likely to develop egg tolerance when compared to children who strictly avoided egg. Clinical studies are ongoing to determine the safety and efficacy of this approach.

Immunotherapy with Modified Recombinant Engineered Food Proteins

Site directed mutagenesis can be used to create proteins with modified IgE antibody binding sites, decreasing IgE binding and reducing the risk of an allergic reaction to the therapy. Bacterial adjuvants can be combined with modified food allergens to enhance the Th1 skewing effect and decrease the Th2 response. Initial studies with peanut anaphylactic murine models suggested protection after treatment with a subcutaneous recombinant modified major peanut allergen and a bacterial adjuvant. [193] Subsequent murine studies using a non-pathogenic bacterial adjuvant and modified peanut protein delivered *via* rectal route have supported these findings. [194] A phase 1 clinical safety study is underway.

Allergen Nonspecific Therapy

Humanized Monoclonal Anti-IgE

Humanized monoclonal murine anti IgE IgG1 antibodies prevent IgE from binding to high affinity receptors expressed on the surface of mast cells and basophils and low affinity receptors expressed on the surface of B cells, dendritic cells, and intestinal epithelial cells. There is also decreased activation and release of histamine and other mediators due to decrease in free IgE molecules caused by anti IgE therapy. [195]

In a multicenter clinical trial, 84 peanut allergic patients received humanized monoclonal anti IgE murine IgG1 antibody in three different doses. [196] All 3 groups had a trend in increase of threshold, however the increase was statistically significant in the group that received the highest dose. In this group the threshold dose increased from ½ peanut to almost 9 peanuts. The occurrence of 2 severe peanut allergic reactions during initial screening food challenges terminated a controlled trial of omalizumab, an anti-IgE preparation approved for asthma treatment. [197]

Traditional Chinese Medication (TCM)

TCM has been used for many centuries for various ailments. Initial studies in peanut allergic murine models with Food Allergy Herbal Formula 1 (FAHF-1), an 11 herb mixture demonstrated protection against peanut induced anaphylaxis. [198] Subsequent murine studies with a more simplified formula FAFH-2 containing 9 herbs demonstrated similar results. [199] A phase 1 study with 19 subjects with peanut and tree nut allergy recently demonstrated that FAFH 2 is safe and well tolerated. [200] Currently, a phase II safety and efficacy trial is enrolling 12 to 45 years of age subjects with peanut, tree nut, sesame, fish or shellfish allergy.

Other Approaches

Alternative approaches being investigated for their potential utility in the treatment of food allergies include probiotics, toll like receptor agonists and trichuris suis ova therapy. Recently probiotics such as Lactobacillus and Bifodobacterium have gained popularity due to their role in improvement of intestinal microbial balance. However the benefit of this therapy has not been demonstrated in food allergy. In a double-blind, randomized, placebo controlled trial in 119 patients with cow's milk allergy treated with probiotics for 12 months, no benefit was observed. [201]

Toll like receptor 9 (TLR9) agonists induce Th1 immune response and in a murine model it was demonstrated that administration of a synthetic TLR9 agonist resulted in protection from peanut induced anaphylaxis. [202] The role of helminthic infections is also being explored in food allergy as observational studies suggest that they may be beneficial in other allergic diseases such as asthma and atopy. [129-131 [203]] Murine models suggest protection against IgE sensitization and anaphylaxis. [204, 205] However the role of T suis in humans is unclear as a more recent randomized double blinded study of T suis ova therapy by Bager et al [206] in adults with allergic rhinitis failed to show improvement in symptoms.

Clinical Cases

Case 1: An 8 year old male with a known diagnosis of cashew nut allergy develops vomiting and generalized urticaria minutes after ingesting chicken and broccoli from a local Chinese restaurant. Upon arrival to the emergency department he becomes hypotensive. He is treated with epinephrine, Benadryl and his symptoms resolve. He is observed for 4 hours and discharged home with his parents.

Comments: The clinical symptoms and time of onset clearly indicate a food induced anaphylactic reaction most likely due to cross contamination at the restaurant. Establishments such as Ice cream parlors, bakeries and Asian restaurants are particularly high risk for peanut and tree nut allergic individuals. [154] First line treatment for food induced anaphylaxis should be epinephrine. Once epinephrine is injected, vitals should be monitored and patient observed. This patient was discharged home after being appropriately treated for food induced anaphylaxis however his discharge plan was lacking. Self-injectable epinephrine (2 doses) should be prescribed to any patient diagnosed with a potentially serious food allergy particularly those at high risk for severe reactions such as individuals with a history of previous reactions involving the cardiovascular or respiratory system which this patient clearly had. [5] In addition, patients should receive a plan for monitoring for auto-injector expiration dates, an anaphylaxis emergency action plan, plan for further evaluation, and printed information about anaphylaxis and its treatment. [5] Children (age appropriate) and care givers should be taught how and when to administer epinephrine.

Case 2: A 25 year old male with mild asthma, atopic dermatitis, peanut and apple allergy presents for his annual follow up. His previous reaction history consists of having repetitive coughing and vomiting when he was 17 years old after ingesting a sandwich containing peanut butter. One year ago he required his albuterol inhaler after ingesting a chocolate candy. His physical examination is normal and his serum specific peanut IgE is 2.78 kU/L. He is advised to continue to avoid peanut, prescribed a self-injectable epinephrine, given an emergency action plan, and written information about anaphylaxis.

Comments: Despite this patient's low serum specific peanut IgE, his clinical history clearly indicates that he continues to have a peanut allergy as evidenced by his most recent reaction most likely due to cross contamination. In addition to the recommendations he has already received he should also be instructed to wear medical jewelry that easily identifies himself as an individual with potential for food induced anaphylaxis. [146] He also has significant risk factors for fatal food induced anaphylaxis such as presence of a peanut and tree allergy, age (young adults or children), asthma and history of severe reaction in the past.

Case 3: A 36 year old woman with no history of food allergies presents with edema of the lips and palate, vomiting and wheezing which developed while she was running. Two hours prior to this she had eaten a bagel with cream cheese, though she regularly eats this without reactions. She is treated with IM epinephrine and her symptoms resolve. She is prescribed self-injectable epinephrine and recommended that she keep a separation of wheat ingestion up to 4 hours prior to undertaking a physical activity.

Comments: This disorder is known as food-dependent, exercise-induced anaphylaxis (FDEIA). In FDEIA, both exercise and the food allergen are independently tolerated. There are very limited data on the prevalence of FDEIA. Females are more commonly affected and the majority of cases are of patients less than 30 years of age. The most common specific food allergen to induce FDEIA is wheat, in particular the wheat protein omega-5-gliadin, followed by other grains, nuts and seafood [120]. The management of FDEIA is focused on prevention. It is recommended that patients keep a separation of known food allergen for up to 4 hours prior to undertaking a physical activity.

Conclusion

Food induced anaphylaxis is an immediate systemic reaction caused by a rapid IgE mediated immune response triggered by a food allergen. The incidence of food Induced anaphylaxis appears to be increasing and it is currently the leading cause of anaphylaxis presenting to emergency departments. Early recognition, diagnosis and treatment with epinephrine can be lifesaving. Ongoing research in potential novel treatments of food allergy seems promising, but avoidance of the trigger allergen is the key to current therapy.

Clinical Pearls

- Food allergies are adverse immune reactions to food proteins that can lead to mild or severe anaphylactic reactions. Any food can trigger an allergic response but milk, peanut, tree nuts, fish, shellfish, soy and wheat are the major food allergens in Westernized countries.
- Clinical features of food-induced anaphylaxis encompass a variety of symptoms involving the respiratory, gastrointestinal, cutaneous, and cardiovascular systems. The majority of reactions commence within an hour of ingestion and fatal reactions have occurred within 25-35 minutes.
- Risk factors for food related fatalities appear to include the age group of adolescents and young adults, individuals with known history of food allergy particularly to peanut or tree nuts, prior history of anaphylaxis and individuals with asthma.
- Food-induced anaphylaxis is diagnosed clinically and there are no laboratory tests available for the diagnosis.
- Epinephrine is first line treatment for food-induced anaphylaxis. Patients with food allergies at risk of anaphylaxis should receive a written action plan clearly indicating the food allergies, the dose of epinephrine to be used and symptoms that warrant injection of epinephrine. Patients should receive education about recognizing and treating an allergic or anaphylactic reaction.

- Food allergic individuals should be educated about the importance of allergen avoidance by label reading, care in obtaining food in restaurants and understanding and managing risks of cross contamination.

Conflict of Interest

Dr. Sicherer is a consultant for the Food Allergy Initiative and Novartis, medical advisor to the Food Allergy and Anaphylaxis Network, receives grant support from the National Institute of Allergy and Infectious Diseases, and receives royalties from UpToDate. Dr. Mehta has nothing to disclose.

References

[1] Simons FE, Sampson HA. Anaphylaxis epidemic: fact or fiction? *The Journal of Allergy and Clinical Immunology*. 2008 Dec; 122(6):1166-8.

[2] Brown AF, McKinnon D, Chu K. Emergency department anaphylaxis: A review of 142 patients in a single year. *The Journal of Allergy and Clinical Immunology* 2001 Nov; 108(5):861-6.

[3] Sampson HA. Anaphylaxis and emergency treatment. *Pediatrics*. [Review]. 2003 Jun; 111(6 Pt 3):1601-8.

[4] Smit DV, Cameron PA, Rainer TH. Anaphylaxis presentations to an emergency department in Hong Kong: incidence and predictors of biphasic reactions. *The Journal of Emergency Medicine* 2005 May; 28(4): 381-8.

[5] Boyce JA, Assa'ad A, Burks AW, Jones SM, Sampson HA, Wood RA, et al. Guidelines for the diagnosis and management of food allergy in the United States: report of the NIAID-sponsored expert panel. *The Journal of Allergy and Clinical Immunology*. 2010 Dec; 126(6 Suppl):S1-58.

[6] Bock SA, Munoz-Furlong A, Sampson HA. Fatalities due to anaphylactic reactions to foods. *The Journal of Allergy and Clinical Immunology* 2001 Jan; 107(1):191-3.

[7] Bock SA, Munoz-Furlong A, Sampson HA. Further fatalities caused by anaphylactic reactions to food, 2001-2006. *The Journal of Allergy and Clinical Immunology* [Letter]. 2007 Apr; 119(4):1016-8.

[8] Pumphrey R. Anaphylaxis: can we tell who is at risk of a fatal reaction? *Current Opinion in Allergy and Clinical Immunology*. [Research Support, Non-U.S. Gov't Review]. 2004 Aug; 4(4):285-90.

[9] Sampson HA, Mendelson L, Rosen JP. Fatal and near-fatal anaphylactic reactions to food in children and adolescents. *The New England Journal of Medicine*. [Research Support, U.S. Gov't, P.H.S.]. 1992 Aug 6; 327(6):380-4.

[10] Burks AW, Tang M, Sicherer S, Muraro A, Eigenmann PA, Ebisawa M, et al. ICON: food allergy. *The Journal of Allergy and Clinical Immunology*. [Review]. 2012 Apr; 129(4):906-20.

[11] Sicherer SH. Epidemiology of food allergy. *The Journal of Allergy and Clinical Immunology*. [Research Support, Non-U.S. Gov't Review]. 2011 Mar; 127(3): 594-602.

[12] Chafen JJ, Newberry SJ, Riedl MA, Bravata DM, Maglione M, Suttorp MJ, et al. Diagnosing and managing common food allergies: a systematic review. JAMA: *The Journal of the American Medical Association*. [Research Support, N.I.H., Extramural Review]. 2010 May 12; 303(18):1848-56.

[13] Rona RJ, Keil T, Summers C, Gislason D, Zuidmeer L, Sodergren E, et al. The prevalence of food allergy: a meta-analysis. *The Journal of Allergy and Clinical Immunology* [Meta-Analysis Research Support, Non-U.S. Gov't]. 2007 Sep; 120(3):638-46.

[14] Zuidmeer L, Goldhahn K, Rona RJ, Gislason D, Madsen C, Summers C, et al. The prevalence of plant food allergies: a systematic review. *The Journal of Allergy and Clinical Immunology* [Meta-Analysis Research Support, Non-U.S. Gov't]. 2008 May; 121(5):1210-8 e4.

[15] Gupta RS, Springston EE, Kim JS, Smith B, Pongracic JA, Wang X, et al. Food allergy knowledge, attitudes, and beliefs of primary care physicians. *Pediatrics*. [Comparative Study]. 2010 Jan;125(1):126-32.

[16] Branum AM, Lukacs SL. Food allergy among U.S. children: trends in prevalence and hospitalizations. *NCHS data brief* 2008 Oct (10):1-8.

[17] Sicherer SH, Munoz-Furlong A, Sampson HA. Prevalence of peanut and tree nut allergy in the United States determined by means of a random digit dial telephone survey: a 5-year follow-up study. *The Journal of Allergy and Clinical Immunology*. [Research Support, Non-U.S. Gov't Research Support, U.S. Gov't, P.H.S.]. 2003 Dec; 112(6):1203-7.

[18] Grundy J, Matthews S, Bateman B, Dean T, Arshad SH. Rising prevalence of allergy to peanut in children: Data from 2 sequential cohorts. *The Journal of Allergy and Clinical Immunology*. [Research Support, Non-U.S. Gov't]. 2002 Nov; 110(5):784-9.

[19] Venter C, Hasan Arshad S, Grundy J, Pereira B, Bernie Clayton C, Voigt K, et al. Time trends in the prevalence of peanut allergy: three cohorts of children from the same geographical location in the UK. *Allergy* 2010 Jan; 65(1):103-8.

[20] Ben-Shoshan M, Kagan RS, Alizadehfar R, Joseph L, Turnbull E, St Pierre Y, et al. Is the prevalence of peanut allergy increasing? A 5-year follow-up study in children in Montreal. *The Journal of Allergy and Clinical*. [Research Support, Non-U.S. Gov't]. 2009 Apr; 123(4): 783-8.

[21] Sicherer SH, Munoz-Furlong A, Godbold JH, Sampson HA. US prevalence of self-reported peanut, tree nut, and sesame allergy: 11-year follow-up. *The Journal of Allergy and Clinical Immunology*. [Comparative Study Research Support, N.I.H., Extramural Research Support, Non-U.S. Gov't]. 2010 Jun; 125(6): 1322-6.

[22] Sicherer SH, Furlong TJ, Maes HH, Desnick RJ, Sampson HA, Gelb BD. Genetics of peanut allergy: a twin study. *The Journal of Allergy and Clinical Immunology*. 2000 Jul; 106(1 Pt 1):53-6.

[23] Du Toit G, Katz Y, Sasieni P, Mesher D, Maleki SJ, Fisher HR, et al. Early consumption of peanuts in infancy is associated with a low prevalence of peanut allergy. *The Journal of Allergy and Clinical Immunology*. 2008 Nov; 122(5): 984-91.

[24] Koplin JJ, Osborne NJ, Wake M, Martin PE, Gurrin LC, Robinson MN, et al. Can early introduction of egg prevent egg allergy in infants? A population-based study. *The*

Journal of Allergy and Clinical Immunology. [Research Support, Non-U.S. Gov't]. 2010 Oct; 126(4):807-13.

[25] Katz Y, Rajuan N, Goldberg MR, Eisenberg E, Heyman E, Cohen A, et al. Early exposure to cow's milk protein is protective against IgE-mediated cow's milk protein allergy. *The Journal of Allergy and Clinical Immunology*. [Research Support, Non-U.S. Gov't]. 2010 Jul; 126(1):77-82 e1.

[26] Untersmayr E, Bakos N, Scholl I, Kundi M, Roth-Walter F, Szalai K, et al. Anti-ulcer drugs promote IgE formation toward dietary antigens in adult patients. *FASEB J* 2005 Apr; 19(6):656-8.

[27] Takagi K, Teshima R, Okunuki H, Itoh S, Kawasaki N, Kawanishi T, et al. Kinetic analysis of pepsin digestion of chicken egg white ovomucoid and allergenic potential of pepsin fragments. *International Archives of Allergy and Immunology*. 2005 Jan; 136(1):23-32.

[28] Lemon-Mule H, Nowak-Wegrzyn A, Berin C, Knight AK. Pathophysiology of food-induced anaphylaxis. *Current Allergy and Asthma Reports*. [Review]. 2008 May; 8(3):201-8.

[29] Sampson HA, Munoz-Furlong A, Bock SA, Schmitt C, Bass R, Chowdhury BA, et al. Symposium on the definition and management of anaphylaxis: summary report. *The Journal of Allergy and Clinical Immunology*. 2005 Mar; 115(3): 584-91.

[30] Nowak-Wegrzyn A, Muraro A. Food protein-induced enterocolitis syndrome. *Current Opinion in Allergy and Clinical Immunology*. [Review]. 2009 Aug; 9(4):371-7.

[31] Sicherer SH. Food protein-induced enterocolitis syndrome: case presentations and management lessons. *The Journal of Allergy and Clinical Immunology*. [Case Reports]. 2005 Jan; 115(1):149-56.

[32] Liacouras CA, Furuta GT, Hirano I, Atkins D, Attwood SE, Bonis PA, et al. Eosinophilic esophagitis: updated consensus recommendations for children and adults. *The Journal of Allergy and Clinical Immunology*. [Research Support, N.I.H., Extramural Research Support, Non-U.S. Gov't Review]. 2011 Jul; 128(1):3-20 e6; quiz 1-2.

[33] Ortolani C, Pastorello EA, Farioli L, Ispano M, Pravettoni V, Berti C, et al. IgE-mediated allergy from vegetable allergens. *Annals of Allergy*. [Meta-Analysis]. 1993 Nov; 71(5):470-6.

[34] Liew WK, Williamson E, Tang ML. Anaphylaxis fatalities and admissions in Australia. *The Journal of Allergy and Clinical Immunology*. 2009 Feb; 123(2): 434-42.

[35] Decker WW, Campbell RL, Manivannan V, Luke A, St Sauver JL, Weaver A, et al. The etiology and incidence of anaphylaxis in Rochester, Minnesota: a report from the Rochester Epidemiology Project. *The Journal of Allergy and Clinical Immunology*. [Research Support, Non-U.S. Gov't]. 2008 Dec; 122(6):1161-5.

[36] Gupta R, Sheikh A, Strachan DP, Anderson HR. Burden of allergic disease in the UK: secondary analyses of national databases. *Clinical and Experimental Allergy*. [Research Support, Non-U.S. Gov't]. 2004 Apr; 34(4):520-6.

[37] Clark S, Espinola J, Rudders SA, Banerji A, Camargo CA, Jr. Frequency of US emergency department visits for food-related acute allergic reactions. *The Journal of Allergy and Clinical Immunology*. [Letter Research Support, Non-U.S. Gov't]. 2011 Mar; 127(3):682-3.

[38] Yocum MW, Butterfield JH, Klein JS, Volcheck GW, Schroeder DR, Silverstein MD. Epidemiology of anaphylaxis in Olmsted County: A population-based study. *The Journal of Allergy and Clinical Immunology.* [Research Support, Non-U.S. Gov't Research Support, U.S. Gov't, P.H.S.]. 1999 Aug; 104(2 Pt 1):452-6.

[39] Ross MP, Ferguson M, Street D, Klontz K, Schroeder T, Luccioli S. Analysis of food-allergic and anaphylactic events in the National Electronic Injury Surveillance System. *The Journal of Allergy and Clinical Immunology* 2008 Jan; 121(1):166-71.

[40] Branum AM, Lukacs SL. Food allergy among children in the United States. *Pediatrics* 2009 Dec; 124(6):1549-55.

[41] de Silva IL, Mehr SS, Tey D, Tang ML. Paediatric anaphylaxis: a 5 year retrospective review. *Allergy* 2008 Aug; 63(8):1071-6.

[42] Uguz A, Lack G, Pumphrey R, Ewan P, Warner J, Dick J, et al. Allergic reactions in the community: a questionnaire survey of members of the anaphylaxis campaign. *Clinical and Experimental Allergy.* [Research Support, Non-U.S. Gov't]. 2005 Jun; 35(6):746-50.

[43] Clark S, Bock SA, Gaeta TJ, Brenner BE, Cydulka RK, Camargo CA. Multicenter study of emergency department visits for food allergies. *The Journal of Allergy and Clinical Immunology.* 2004 Feb; 113(2):347-52.

[44] Pumphrey RS, Gowland MH. Further fatal allergic reactions to food in the United Kingdom, 1999-2006. *The Journal of Allergy and Clinical Immunology.* 2007 Apr; 119(4):1018-9.

[45] Moneret-Vautrin DA, Kanny G, Morisset M, Rance F, Fardeau MF, Beaudouin E. Severe food anaphylaxis: 107 cases registered in 2002 by the Allergy Vigilance Network. *European Annals of Allergy and Clinical Immunology.* 2004 Feb; 36(2): 46-51.

[46] Neugut AI, Ghatak AT, Miller RL. Anaphylaxis in the United States: an investigation into its epidemiology. *Archives of Internal Medicine.* [Research Support, Non-U.S. Gov't Review]. 2001 Jan 8; 161(1): 15-21.

[47] Silva R, Gomes E, Cunha L, Falcao H. Anaphylaxis in children: a nine years retrospective study (2001-2009). *Allergol. Immunopathol.* (Madr) 2012 Jan-Feb; 40(1):31-6.

[48] Sampson MA, Munoz-Furlong A, Sicherer SH. Risk-taking and coping strategies of adolescents and young adults with food allergy. *The Journal of Allergy and Clinical Immunology.* [Research Support, Non-U.S. Gov't]. 2006 Jun; 117(6): 1440-5.

[49] Summers CW, Pumphrey RS, Woods CN, McDowell G, Pemberton PW, Arkwright PD. Factors predicting anaphylaxis to peanuts and tree nuts in patients referred to a specialist center. *The Journal of Allergy and Clinical Immunology.* [Research Support, Non-U.S. Gov't]. 2008 Mar; 121(3): 632-8 e2.

[50] Cianferoni A, Muraro A. Food-induced anaphylaxis. *Immunology and Allergy Clinics of North America.* [Research Support, N.I.H., Extramural]. 2012 Feb; 32(1):165-95.

[51] Izumi K, Aihara M, Ikezawa Z. [Effects of non steroidal antiinflammatory drugs (NSAIDs) on immediate-type food allergy analysis of Japanese cases from 1998 to 2009]. *Arerugi = [Allergy].* [Research Support, Non-U.S. Gov't]. 2009 Dec; 58(12):1629-39.

[52] Miller MM. Beta-blockers and anaphylaxis: are the risks overstated? *The Journal of Allergy and Clinical Immunology.* [Comment Guideline Letter Practice Guideline]. 2005 Oct; 116(4):931-3; author reply 3-6.

[53] Jenkins JA, Breiteneder H, Mills EN. Evolutionary distance from human homologs reflects allergenicity of animal food proteins. *The Journal of Allergy and Clinical Immunology.* [Comparative Study]. 2007 Dec; 120(6): 1399-405.

[54] Rudders SA, Banerji A, Vassallo MF, Clark S, Camargo CA, Jr. Trends in pediatric emergency department visits for food-induced anaphylaxis. *The Journal of Allergy and Clinical Immunology.* [Letter Research Support, N.I.H., Extramural Research Support, Non-U.S. Gov't Review]. 2010 Aug; 126(2):385-8.

[55] Bock SA. The incidence of severe adverse reactions to food in Colorado. *The Journal of Allergy and Clinical Immunology* 1992 Oct; 90 (4 Pt 1): 683-5.

[56] Hompes S, Kohli A, Nemat K, Scherer K, Lange L, Rueff F, et al. Provoking allergens and treatment of anaphylaxis in children and adolescents--data from the anaphylaxis registry of German-speaking countries. *Pediatric Allergy and Immunology.* 2011 Sep; 22(6):568-74.

[57] Rudders SA, Banerji A, Clark S, Camargo CA, Jr. Age-related differences in the clinical presentation of food-induced anaphylaxis. *The Journal of Pediatrics.* [Comparative Study Research Support, N.I.H., Extramural Research Support, Non-U.S. Gov't]. 2011 Feb; 158(2): 326-8.

[58] Sicherer SH, Munoz-Furlong A, Burks AW, Sampson HA. Prevalence of peanut and tree nut allergy in the US determined by a random digit dial telephone survey. *The Journal of Allergy and Clinical Immunology.* [Research Support, Non-U.S. Gov't]. 1999 Apr; 103(4):559-62.

[59] Tariq SM, Stevens M, Matthews S, Ridout S, Twiselton R, Hide DW. Cohort study of peanut and tree nut sensitisation by age of 4 years. *British Medical Journal.* [Research Support, Non-U.S. Gov't]. 1996 Aug 31; 313(7056):514-7.

[60] Pumphrey RS. Fatal anaphylaxis in the UK, 1992-2001. *Novartis Foundation symposium* 2004; 257:116-28; discussion 28-32, 57-60, 276-85.

[61] Nicolaou N, Murray C, Belgrave D, Poorafshar M, Simpson A, Custovic A. Quantification of specific IgE to whole peanut extract and peanut components in prediction of peanut allergy. *The Journal of Allergy and Clinical Immunology.* [Letter Research Support, Non-U.S. Gov't]. 2011 Mar; 127(3):684-5.

[62] Rabjohn P, Helm EM, Stanley JS, West CM, Sampson HA, Burks AW, et al. Molecular cloning and epitope analysis of the peanut allergen Ara h 3. *The Journal of Clinical Investigation.* [Research Support, Non-U.S. Gov't Research Support, U.S. Gov't, P.H.S.]. 1999 Feb; 103(4):535-42.

[63] Restani P, Ballabio C, Corsini E, Fiocchi A, Isoardi P, Magni C, et al. Identification of the basic subunit of Ara h 3 as the major allergen in a group of children allergic to peanuts. *Annals of Allergy Asthma and Immunology.* [Comparative Study Research Support, Non-U.S. Gov't]. 2005 Feb; 94(2):262-6.

[64] Sicherer SH, Sampson HA. Peanut allergy: emerging concepts and approaches for an apparent epidemic. *The Journal of Allergy and Clinical Immunology.* [Review]. 2007 Sep;120(3):491-503; quiz 4-5.

[65] Maleki SJ, Viquez O, Jacks T, Dodo H, Champagne ET, Chung SY, et al. The major peanut allergen, Ara h 2, functions as a trypsin inhibitor, and roasting enhances this

function. *The Journal of Allergy and Clinical Immunology.* [Research Support, U.S. Gov't, Non-P.H.S.]. 2003 Jul; 112(1): 190-5.

[66] Beyer K, Morrow E, Li XM, Bardina L, Bannon GA, Burks AW, et al. Effects of cooking methods on peanut allergenicity. *The Journal of Allergy and Clinical Immunology.* [Research Support, Non-U.S. Gov't]. 2001 Jun;107(6):1077-81.

[67] Shreffler WG, Castro RR, Kucuk ZY, Charlop-Powers Z, Grishina G, Yoo S, et al. The major glycoprotein allergen from Arachis hypogaea, Ara h 1, is a ligand of dendritic cell-specific ICAM-grabbing nonintegrin and acts as a Th2 adjuvant in vitro. *The Journal of Immunology.* [Research Support, N.I.H., Extramural Research Support, Non-U.S. Gov't]. 2006 Sep 15; 177(6): 3677-85.

[68] Asarnoj A, Ostblom E, Ahlstedt S, Hedlin G, Lilja G, van Hage M, et al. Reported symptoms to peanut between 4 and 8 years among children sensitized to peanut and birch pollen - results from the BAMSE birth cohort. *Allergy.* [Research Support, Non-U.S. Gov't]. 2010 Feb; 65(2): 213-9.

[69] Krause S, Reese G, Randow S, Zennaro D, Quaratino D, Palazzo P, et al. Lipid transfer protein (Ara h 9) as a new peanut allergen relevant for a Mediterranean allergic population. *The Journal of Allergy and Clinical Immunology.* 2009 Oct; 124(4): 771-8 e5.

[70] Nicolaou N, Poorafshar M, Murray C, Simpson A, Winell H, Kerry G, et al. Allergy or tolerance in children sensitized to peanut: prevalence and differentiation using component-resolved diagnostics. *The Journal of Allergy and Clinical Immunology.* [Research Support, Non-U.S. Gov't]. 2010 Jan; 125(1):191-7 e1-13.

[71] Nowak-Wegrzyn A, Bloom KA, Sicherer SH, Shreffler WG, Noone S, Wanich N, et al. Tolerance to extensively heated milk in children with cow's milk allergy. *The Journal of Allergy and Clinical Immunology.* [Research Support, N.I.H., Extramural]. 2008 Aug; 122(2):342-7, 7 e1-2.

[72] Asarnoj A, Nilsson C, Lidholm J, Glaumann S, Ostblom E, Hedlin G, et al. Peanut component Ara h 8 sensitization and tolerance to peanut. *The Journal of Allergy and Clinical Immunology.* 2012 Jun 26.

[73] Shreffler WG, Beyer K, Chu TH, Burks AW, Sampson HA. Microarray immunoassay: association of clinical history, in vitro IgE function, and heterogeneity of allergenic peanut epitopes. *The Journal of Allergy and Clinical Immunology.* [In Vitro Research Support, U.S. Gov't, P.H.S.]. 2004 Apr; 113(4):776-82.

[74] Flinterman AE, Knol EF, Lencer DA, Bardina L, den Hartog Jager CF, Lin J, et al. Peanut epitopes for IgE and IgG4 in peanut-sensitized children in relation to severity of peanut allergy. *The Journal of Allergy and Clinical Immunology.* [Research Support, N.I.H., Extramural Research Support, Non-U.S. Gov't]. 2008 Mar; 121(3):737-43 e10.

[75] Hourihane JO, Roberts SA, Warner JO. Resolution of peanut allergy: case-control study. *British Medical Journal* 1998 Apr 25; 316(7140):1271-5.

[76] Fleischer DM, Conover-Walker MK, Christie L, Burks AW, Wood RA. The natural progression of peanut allergy: Resolution and the possibility of recurrence. *The Journal of Allergy and Clinical Immunology.* [Research Support, Non-U.S. Gov't Research Support, U.S. Gov't, P.H.S.]. 2003 Jul; 112(1):183-9.

[77] Skolnick HS, Conover-Walker MK, Koerner CB, Sampson HA, Burks W, Wood RA. The natural history of peanut allergy. *The Journal of Allergy and Clinical Immunology.* 2001 Feb;107(2):367-74.

[78] Sicherer SH, Furlong TJ, DeSimone J, Sampson HA. The US Peanut and Tree Nut Allergy Registry: characteristics of reactions in schools and day care. *J. Pediatr.* 2001 Apr; 138(4):560-5.

[79] Sicherer SH. Clinical implications of cross-reactive food allergens. *The Journal of Allergy and Clinical Immunology.* [Research Support, Non-U.S. Gov't Research Support, U.S. Gov't, P.H.S.]. 2001 Dec; 108(6):881-90.

[80] Crespo JF, James JM, Fernandez-Rodriguez C, Rodriguez J. Food allergy: nuts and tree nuts. *Br J Nutr* 2006 Nov;96 Suppl 2:S95-102.

[81] Sicherer SH, Sampson HA. Food allergy. *The Journal of Allergy and Clinical Immunology.* [Review]. 2010 Feb; 125(2 Suppl 2):S116-25.

[82] Turner P, Ng I, Kemp A, Campbell D. Seafood allergy in children: a descriptive study. *Annals of Allergy Asthma and Immunology* [Research Support, Non-U.S. Gov't]. 2011 Jun; 106(6): 494-501.

[83] Sicherer SH, Munoz-Furlong A, Sampson HA. Prevalence of seafood allergy in the United States determined by a random telephone survey. *The Journal of Allergy and Clinical Immunology.* [Research Support, Non-U.S. Gov't Research Support, U.S. Gov't, P.H.S.]. 2004 Jul; 114(1):159-65.

[84] Sicherer SH. Risk of severe allergic reactions from the use of potassium iodide for radiation emergencies. *The Journal of Allergy and Clinical Immunology.* 2004 Dec; 114(6):1395-7.

[85] Hoffer V, Scheuerman O, Marcus N, Levy Y, Segal N, Lagovsky I, et al. Anaphylaxis in Israel: experience with 92 hospitalized children. *Pediatric Allergy and Immunology.* 2011 Mar; 22(2):172-7.

[86] Novembre E, Cianferoni A, Bernardini R, Mugnaini L, Caffarelli C, Cavagni G, et al. Anaphylaxis in children: clinical and allergologic features. *Pediatrics* 1998 Apr; 101(4):E8.

[87] Host A, Halken S. A prospective study of cow milk allergy in Danish infants during the first 3 years of life. Clinical course in relation to clinical and immunological type of hypersensitivity reaction. *Allergy* 1990 Nov; 45(8):587-96.

[88] Skripak JM, Matsui EC, Mudd K, Wood RA. The natural history of IgE-mediated cow's milk allergy. *The Journal of Allergy and Clinical Immunology..* [Research Support, N.I.H., Extramural Research Support, Non-U.S. Gov't]. 2007 Nov;120(5):1172-7.

[89] Wal JM. Bovine milk allergenicity. *Annals of Allergy Asthma and Immunology.* [Review]. 2004 Nov; 93(5 Suppl 3):S2-11.

[90] Macdougall CF, Cant AJ, Colver AF. How dangerous is food allergy in childhood? The incidence of severe and fatal allergic reactions across the UK and Ireland. *Archives of Disease in Childhood.* [Research Support, Non-U.S. Gov't]. 2002 Apr; 86(4):236-9.

[91] Boyano-Martinez T, Garcia-Ara C, Diaz-Pena JM, Martin-Esteban M. Prediction of tolerance on the basis of quantification of egg white-specific IgE antibodies in children with egg allergy. *The Journal of Allergy and Clinical Immunology.* 2002 Aug; 110(2):304-9.

[92] Savage JH, Matsui EC, Skripak JM, Wood RA. The natural history of egg allergy. *The Journal of Allergy and Clinical Immunology.* 2007 Dec; 120(6): 1413-7.

[93] Colver AF, Nevantaus H, Macdougall CF, Cant AJ. Severe food-allergic reactions in children across the UK and Ireland, 1998-2000. *Acta Paediatrica.* [Research Support, Non-U.S. Gov't].2005Jun;94(6):689-95.

[94] Mehl A, Wahn U, Niggemann B. Anaphylactic reactions in children--a questionnaire-based survey in Germany. *Allergy* 2005 Nov; 60(11): 1440-5.

[95] Eigenmann PA. Anaphylactic reactions to raw eggs after negative challenges with cooked eggs. *The Journal of Allergy and Clinical Immunology*. [Case Reports]. 2000 Mar; 105(3):587-8.

[96] Bernhisel-Broadbent J, Dintzis HM, Dintzis RZ, Sampson HA. Allergenicity and antigenicity of chicken egg ovomucoid (Gal d III) compared with ovalbumin (Gal d I) in children with egg allergy and in mice. *The Journal of Allergy and Clinical Immunology*. [Comparative Study Research Support, U.S. Gov't, P.H.S.]. 1994 Jun; 93(6):1047-59.

[97] Jarvinen KM, Beyer K, Vila L, Bardina L, Mishoe M, Sampson HA. Specificity of IgE antibodies to sequential epitopes of hen's egg ovomucoid as a marker for persistence of egg allergy. *Allergy*. [Research Support, N.I.H., Extramural Research Support, Non-U.S. Gov't]. 2007 Jul; 62(7):758-65.

[98] Leonard SA, Martos G, Wang W, Nowak-Wegrzyn A, Berin MC. Oral immunotherapy induces local protective mechanisms in the gastrointestinal mucosa. *The Journal of Allergy and Clinical Immunology*. [Research Support, N.I.H., Extramural Research Support, Non-U.S. Gov't]. 2012 Jun; 129(6):1579-87 e1.

[99] Foucard T, Malmheden Yman I. A study on severe food reactions in Sweden--is soy protein an underestimated cause of food anaphylaxis? *Allergy*. [Case Reports]. 1999 Mar; 54(3):261-5.

[100] Holzhauser T, Wackermann O, Ballmer-Weber BK, Bindslev-Jensen C, Scibilia J, Perono-Garoffo L, et al. Soybean (Glycine max) allergy in Europe: Gly m 5 (beta-conglycinin) and Gly m 6 (glycinin) are potential diagnostic markers for severe allergic reactions to soy. *The Journal of Allergy and Clinical Immunology*.. [Research Support, Non-U.S. Gov't]. 2009 Feb; 123(2):452-8.

[101] Savage JH, Kaeding AJ, Matsui EC, Wood RA. The natural history of soy allergy. *The Journal of Allergy and Clinical Immunology*.2010 Mar; 125(3):683-6.

[102] Matricardi PM, Bockelbrink A, Beyer K, Keil T, Niggemann B, Gruber C, et al. Primary versus secondary immunoglobulin E sensitization to soy and wheat in the Multi-Centre Allergy Study cohort. *Clinical and Experimental Allergy*. [Multicenter Study Research Support, Non-U.S. Gov't]. 2008 Mar; 38(3):493-500.

[103] Commins SP, Satinover SM, Hosen J, Mozena J, Borish L, Lewis BD, et al. Delayed anaphylaxis, angioedema, or urticaria after consumption of red meat in patients with IgE antibodies specific for galactose-alpha-1,3-galactose. *The Journal of Allergy and Clinical Immunology*. [Research Support, N.I.H., Extramural Research Support, Non-U.S. Gov't]. 2009 Feb; 123(2):426-33.

[104] Nunez R, Carballada F, Gonzalez-Quintela A, Gomez-Rial J, Boquete M, Vidal C. Delayed mammalian meat-induced anaphylaxis due to galactose-alpha-1,3-galactose in 5 European patients. *The Journal of Allergy and Clinical Immunology*. [Letter Research Support, Non-U.S. Gov't]. 2011 Nov;128(5):1122-4 e1.

[105] Mullins RJ, James H, Platts-Mills TA, Commins S. Relationship between red meat allergy and sensitization to gelatin and galactose-alpha-1,3-galactose. *The Journal of Allergy and Clinical Immunology*. [Research Support, N.I.H., Extramural]. 2012 May; 129(5): 1334-42 e1.

[106] Nish WA, Whisman BA, Goetz DW, Ramirez DA. Anaphylaxis to annatto dye: a case report. *Ann. Allergy* 1991 Feb; 66(2):129-31.

[107] Ebo DG, Ingelbrecht S, Bridts CH, Stevens WJ. Allergy for cheese: evidence for an IgE-mediated reaction from the natural dye annatto. *Allergy* 2009 Oct; 64(10):1558-60.

[108] Beaudouin E, Kanny G, Lambert H, Fremont S, Moneret-Vautrin DA. Food anaphylaxis following ingestion of carmine. *Annals of Allergy Asthma and Immunology.* 1995 May; 74(5):427-30.

[109] Yunginger JW, Jones RT, Kita H, Saito K, Hefle SL, Taylor SL. Allergic reactions after ingestion of erythritol-containing foods and beverages. *The Journal of Allergy and Clinical Immunology.* 2001 Oct; 108(4):650.

[110] Papanikolaou I, Stenger R, Bessot JC, de Blay F, Pauli G. Anaphylactic shock to guar gum (food additive E412) contained in a meal substitute. *Allergy* 2007 Jul; 62(7):822.

[111] James JM, Cooke SK, Barnett A, Sampson HA. Anaphylactic reactions to a psyllium-containing cereal. *The Journal of Allergy and Clinical Immunology.* 1991 Sep; 88 (3 Pt 1): 402-8.

[112] Cianferoni A, Novembre E, Mugnaini L, Lombardi E, Bernardini R, Pucci N, et al. Clinical features of acute anaphylaxis in patients admitted to a university hospital: an 11-year retrospective review (1985-1996). *Annals of Allergy Asthma and Immunology* [Research Support, Non-U.S. Gov't]. 2001 Jul; 87(1):27-32.

[113] Fisher MM. Clinical observations on the pathophysiology and treatment of anaphylactic cardiovascular collapse. *Anaesthesia and Intensive Care* 1986 Feb; 14(1):17-21.

[114] Pumphrey RS. Fatal posture in anaphylactic shock. *The Journal of Allergy and Clinical Immunology.* [Letter]. 2003 Aug;112 (2):451-2.

[115] Golden DB. Patterns of anaphylaxis: acute and late phase features of allergic reactions. *Novartis Foundation Symposium.* [Review]. 2004; 257:101-10; discussion 10-5, 57-60, 276-85.

[116] Jarvinen KM, Amalanayagam S, Shreffler WG, Noone S, Sicherer SH, Sampson HA, et al. Epinephrine treatment is infrequent and biphasic reactions are rare in food-induced reactions during oral food challenges in children. *The Journal of Allergy and Clinical Immunology.* 2009 Dec; 124(6):1267-72.

[117] Lieberman P. Biphasic anaphylactic reactions. *Annals of Allergy Asthma and Immunology.* [Review]. 2005 Sep; 95(3): 217-26; quiz 26, 58.

[118] Gupta P, Oegema TR, Jr., Brazil JJ, Dudek AZ, Slungaard A, Verfaillie CM. Structurally specific heparan sulfates support primitive human hematopoiesis by formation of a multimolecular stem cell niche. *Blood* 1998 Dec 15;92(12):4641-51.

[119] Grimshaw KE, King RM, Nordlee JA, Hefle SL, Warner JO, Hourihane JO. Presentation of allergen in different food preparations affects the nature of the allergic reaction--a case series. *Clinical and Experimental Allergy* [Clinical Trial Randomized Controlled Trial Research Support, Non-U.S. Gov't]. 2003 Nov; 33(11):1581-5.

[120] Palosuo K, Varjonen E, Kekki OM, Klemola T, Kalkkinen N, Alenius H, et al. Wheat omega-5 gliadin is a major allergen in children with immediate allergy to ingested wheat. *The Journal of Allergy and Clinical Immunology.* [Research Support, Non-U.S. Gov't]. 2001 Oct; 108(4): 634-8.

[121] Palosuo K, Varjonen E, Nurkkala J, Kalkkinen N, Harvima R, Reunala T, et al. Transglutaminase-mediated cross-linking of a peptic fraction of omega-5 gliadin enhances IgE reactivity in wheat-dependent, exercise-induced anaphylaxis. *The Journal*

of Allergy and Clinical Immunology. [Research Support, Non-U.S. Gov't]. 2003 Jun; 111(6):1386-92.

[122] Romano A, Di Fonso M, Giuffreda F, Papa G, Artesani MC, Viola M, et al. Food-dependent exercise-induced anaphylaxis: clinical and laboratory findings in 54 subjects. *International Archives of Allergy and Immunology* 2001 Jul; 125(3):264-72.

[123] Hanakawa Y, Tohyama M, Shirakata Y, Murakami S, Hashimoto K. Food-dependent exercise-induced anaphylaxis: a case related to the amount of food allergen ingested. The *British Journal of Dermatology.* 1998 May; 138(5): 898-900.

[124] Aihara M, Miyazawa M, Osuna H, Tsubaki K, Ikebe T, Aihara Y, et al. Food-dependent exercise-induced anaphylaxis: influence of concurrent aspirin administration on skin testing and provocation. *The British Journal of Dermatology.* 2002 Mar; 146(3):466-72.

[125] Aihara Y, Takahashi Y, Kotoyori T, Mitsuda T, Ito R, Aihara M, et al. Frequency of food-dependent, exercise-induced anaphylaxis in Japanese junior-high-school students. *The Journal of Allergy and Clinical Immunology.* [Research Support, Non-U.S. Gov't]. 2001 Dec; 108(6): 1035-9.

[126] Harada S, Horikawa T, Ashida M, Kamo T, Nishioka E, Ichihashi M. Aspirin enhances the induction of type I allergic symptoms when combined with food and exercise in patients with food-dependent exercise-induced anaphylaxis. *The British Journal of Dermatology.* [Case Reports Review]. 2001 Aug; 145(2):336-9.

[127] American College of Allergy A, Immunology. Food allergy: a practice parameter. *Annals of Allergy Asthma and Immunology* [Practice Guideline]. 2006 Mar; 96(3 Suppl 2):S1-68.

[128] Knight AK, Shreffler WG, Sampson HA, Sicherer SH, Noone S, Mofidi S, et al. Skin prick test to egg white provides additional diagnostic utility to serum egg white-specific IgE antibody concentration in children. *The Journal of Allergy and Clinical Immunology.* [Research Support, N.I.H., Extramural Research Support, Non-U.S. Gov't]. 2006 Apr; 117(4):842-7.

[129] Nowak-Wegrzyn A, Assa'ad AH, Bahna SL, Bock SA, Sicherer SH, Teuber SS. Work Group report: oral food challenge testing. *The Journal of Allergy and Clinical Immunology.* 2009 Jun; 123(6 Suppl):S365-83.

[130] Lin RY, Schwartz LB, Curry A, Pesola GR, Knight RJ, Lee HS, et al. Histamine and tryptase levels in patients with acute allergic reactions: An emergency department-based study. *The Journal of Allergy and Clinical Immunology.* [Research Support, U.S. Gov't, P.H.S.]. 2000 Jul; 106(1 Pt 1): 65-71.

[131] Keet C. Recognition and management of food-induced anaphylaxis. *Pediatric Clinics of North America.* [Research Support, N.I.H., Extramural Review]. 2011 Apr; 58(2):377-88, x.

[132] Sampson HA, Jolie PL. Increased plasma histamine concentrations after food challenges in children with atopic dermatitis. *The New England Journal of Medicine.* [Clinical Trial Controlled Clinical Trial Research Support, U.S. Gov't, P.H.S.]. 1984 Aug 9; 311(6): 372-6.

[133] Vadas P, Gold M, Perelman B, Liss GM, Lack G, Blyth T, et al. Platelet-activating factor, PAF acetylhydrolase, and severe anaphylaxis. *The New England Journal of Medicine.* 2008 Jan 3; 358(1):28-35.

[134] Simons FE. First-aid treatment of anaphylaxis to food: focus on epinephrine. *The Journal of Allergy and Clinical Immunology*. [Review]. 2004 May; 113(5):837-44.

[135] Brown SG. Cardiovascular aspects of anaphylaxis: implications for treatment and diagnosis. *Current Opinion in Allergy and Clinical Immunology*. [Comparative Study Review]. 2005 Aug; 5(4): 359-64.

[136] Clark S, Bock SA, Gaeta TJ, Brenner BE, Cydulka RK, Camargo CA, et al. Multicenter study of emergency department visits for food allergies. *The Journal of Allergy and Clinical Immunology*. [Multicenter Study Research Support, Non-U.S. Gov't Research Support, U.S. Gov't, P.H.S.]. 2004 Feb; 113(2):347-52.

[137] Braganza SC, Acworth JP, McKinnon DR, Peake JE, Brown AF. Paediatric emergency department anaphylaxis: different patterns from adults. *Archives of Disease in Childhood* 2006 Feb; 91(2):159-63.

[138] Stewart AG, Ewan PW. The incidence, aetiology and management of anaphylaxis presenting to an accident and emergency department. *QJM.*. [Research Support, Non-U.S. Gov't]. 1996 Nov; 89(11):859-64.

[139] Klein JS, Yocum MW. Underreporting of anaphylaxis in a community emergency room. *The Journal of Allergy and Clinical Immunology.*1995 Feb; 95(2):637-8.

[140] Gold MS, Sainsbury R. First aid anaphylaxis management in children who were prescribed an epinephrine autoinjector device (EpiPen). *The Journal of Allergy and Clinical Immunology* 2000 Jul; 106(1 Pt 1):171-6.

[141] Sicherer SH, Forman JA, Noone SA. Use assessment of self-administered epinephrine among food-allergic children and pediatricians. *Pediatrics* 2000 Feb; 105(2):359-62.

[142] Fleischer DM, Perry TT, Atkins D, Wood RA, Burks AW, Jones SM, et al. Allergic Reactions to Foods in Preschool-Aged Children in a Prospective Observational Food Allergy Study. *Pediatrics* 2012 Jun 25.

[143] Kambam JR, Merrill WH, Smith BE. Histamine 2 receptor blocker in the treatment of protamine related anaphylactoid reactions: two case reports. *CanadianJjournal of Anaesthesia = Journal canadien d'anesthesie*. [Case Reports]. 1989 Jul; 36(4):463-5.

[144] Douglas DM, Sukenick E, Andrade WP, Brown JS. Biphasic systemic anaphylaxis: an inpatient and outpatient study. *The Journal of Allergy and Clinical Immunology.* 1994 Jun; 93(6):977-85.

[145] Stark BJ, Sullivan TJ. Biphasic and protracted anaphylaxis. *The Journal of Allergy and Clinical Immunology*. [Comparative Study]. 1986 Jul; 78 (1 Pt 1): 76-83.

[146] Lieberman P. Anaphylaxis. *The Medical Clinics of North America*. [Review]. 2006 Jan; 90(1):77-95, viii.

[147] Simons E, Weiss CC, Furlong TJ, Sicherer SH. Impact of ingredient labeling practices on food allergic consumers. *Annals of Allergy Asthma and Immunology*. 2005 Nov; 95(5):426-8.

[148] Taylor SL, Hefle SL. Food allergen labeling in the USA and Europe. *Current Opinion in Allergy and Clinical Immunology*. [Research Support, Non-U.S. Gov't Review]. 2006 Jun; 6(3):186-90.

[149] Warner JO. European Food Labelling Legislation--a nightmare for food manufacturers and allergy sufferers alike. *Pediatr Allergy Immunol.* 2005 Feb; 16(1):1-2.

[150] Hefle SL, Furlong TJ, Niemann L, Lemon-Mule H, Sicherer S, Taylor SL. Consumer attitudes and risks associated with packaged foods having advisory labeling regarding the presence of peanuts. *The Journal of Allergy and Clinical Immunology*. [Research

Support, Non-U.S. Gov't Research Support, U.S. Gov't, Non-P.H.S.]. 2007 Jul; 120(1):171-6.

[151] Crotty MP, Taylor SL. Risks associated with foods having advisory milk labeling. *The Journal of Allergy and Clinical Immunology.* [Letter]. 2010 Apr; 125(4):935-7.

[152] Jones RT, Squillace DL, Yunginger JW. Anaphylaxis in a milk-allergic child after ingestion of milk-contaminated kosher-pareve-labeled "dairy-free" dessert. *Annals of Allergy.* [Case Reports Research Support, Non-U.S. Gov't]. 1992 Mar; 68(3):223-7.

[153] Fleischer DM, Perry TT, Atkins D, Wood RA, Burks AW, Jones SM, et al. Allergic reactions to foods in preschool-aged children in a prospective observational food allergy study. *Pediatrics* 2012 Jul; 130(1):e25-32.

[154] Furlong TJ, DeSimone J, Sicherer SH. Peanut and tree nut allergic reactions in restaurants and other food establishments. *The Journal of Allergy and Clinical Immunology.* 2001 Nov; 108(5):867-70.

[155] Ahuja R, Sicherer SH. Food-allergy management from the perspective of restaurant and food establishment personnel. *Annals of Allergy Asthma and Immunology.* 2007 Apr;98(4):344-8.

[156] Nowak-Wegrzyn A, Conover-Walker MK, Wood RA. Food-allergic reactions in schools and preschools. *Archives of Pediatrics and Adolescent Medicine.* [Research Support, Non-U.S. Gov't Research Support, U.S. Gov't, P.H.S.]. 2001 Jul; 155(7): 790-5.

[157] Rhim GS, McMorris MS. School readiness for children with food allergies. *Annals of Allergy Asthma and Immunology.* [Research Support, Non-U.S. Gov't]. 2001 Feb; 86(2): 172-6.

[158] Pulcini JM, Sease KK, Marshall GD. Disparity between the presence and absence of food allergy action plans in one school district. *Allergy and Asthma Proceedings.* 2010 Mar-Apr;31(2):141-6.

[159] Sicherer SH, Mahr T, American Academy of Pediatrics Section on A, Immunology. Management of food allergy in the school setting. *Pediatrics.* [Review]. 2010 Dec; 126(6):1232-9.

[160] Simons E, Sicherer SH, Simons FE. Timing the transfer of responsibilities for anaphylaxis recognition and use of an epinephrine auto-injector from adults to children and teenagers: pediatric allergists' perspective. *Annals of Allergy Asthma and Immunology.* 2012 May; 108(5):321-5.

[161] Young MC, Munoz-Furlong A, Sicherer SH. Management of food allergies in schools: a perspective for allergists. *The Journal of Allergy and Clinical Immunology.* [Review]. 2009 Aug; 124(2):175-82, 82 e1-4; quiz 83-4.

[162] Muraro A, Clark A, Beyer K, Borrego LM, Borres M, Lodrup Carlsen KC, et al. The management of the allergic child at school: EAACI/GA2LEN Task Force on the allergic child at school. *Allergy* 2010 Jun 1;65(6):681-9.

[163] Wainstein BK, Kashef S, Ziegler M, Jelley D, Ziegler JB. Frequency and significance of immediate contact reactions to peanut in peanut-sensitive children. *Clinical and Experimental Allergy.* 2007 Jun; 37(6):839-45.

[164] Simonte SJ, Ma S, Mofidi S, Sicherer SH. Relevance of casual contact with peanut butter in children with peanut allergy. *The Journal of Allergy and Clinical Immunology.* [Clinical Trial Randomized Controlled Trial Research Support, U.S. Gov't, P.H.S.]. 2003 Jul; 112(1):180-2.

[165] Roberts G, Golder N, Lack G. Bronchial challenges with aerosolized food in asthmatic, food-allergic children. *Allergy* 2002 Aug;57(8):713-7.
[166] Tonnel AB, Tillie-Leblond I, Botelho AD, De Blay F, Pauli G. Severe acute asthma associated with raw meat cutting. *Annals of Allergy Asthma and Immunology* [Case Reports Letter]. 2009 Apr; 102(4):348.
[167] Hallett R, Haapanen LA, Teuber SS. Food allergies and kissing. *The New England Journal of Medicine.* [Letter]. 2002 Jun 6;346(23):1833-4.
[168] Eriksson NE, Moller C, Werner S, Magnusson J, Bengtsson U. The hazards of kissing when you are food allergic. A survey on the occurrence of kiss-induced allergic reactions among 1139 patients with self-reported food hypersensitivity. *Journal of Investigational Allergology and Clinical Immunology..* [Research Support, Non-U.S. Gov't]. 2003; 13(3): 149-54.
[169] Maloney JM, Chapman MD, Sicherer SH. Peanut allergen exposure through saliva: assessment and interventions to reduce exposure. *The Journal of Allergy and Clinical Immunology.* 2006 Sep; 118(3):719-24.
[170] Sicherer SH, Furlong TJ, DeSimone J, Sampson HA. Self-reported allergic reactions to peanut on commercial airliners. *The Journal of Allergy and Clinical Immunology.* 1999 Jul; 104(1):186-9.
[171] Lieberman JA, Sicherer SH. Quality of life in food allergy. *Current Opinion in Allergy and Clinical Immunology.* [Review]. 2011 Jun; 11(3):236-42.
[172] Elliott SJ. Allergen immunotherapy: A practice parameter third update (vol 127, pg1, 2011). *The Journal of Allergy and Clinical Immunology.* 2011 Mar; 127(3):840-.
[173] Oppenheimer JJ, Nelson HS, Bock SA, Christensen F, Leung DY. Treatment of peanut allergy with rush immunotherapy. *The Journal of Allergy and Clinical Immunology.* 1992 Aug; 90(2):256-62.
[174] Sicherer SH, Sampson HA. Food allergy: recent advances in pathophysiology and treatment. *Annual Review of Medicine.* [Review]. 2009; 60:261-77.
[175] Nelson HS, Lahr J, Rule R, Bock A, Leung D. Treatment of anaphylactic sensitivity to peanuts by immunotherapy with injections of aqueous peanut extract. *The Journal of Allergy and Clinical Immunology.* 1997 Jun; 99(6 Pt 1): 744-51.
[176] Schofield. Egg Oral Immunotherapy. *Lancet* 1908; 1:716-17.
[177] Keet CA, Frischmeyer-Guerrerio PA, Thyagarajan A, Schroeder JT, Hamilton RG, Boden S, et al. The safety and efficacy of sublingual and oral immunotherapy for milk allergy. *The Journal of Allergy and Clinical Immunology.* 2012 Feb; 129(2):448-55, 55 e1-5.
[178] Burks AW, Jones SM, Wood RA, Fleischer DM, Sicherer SH, Lindblad RW, et al. Oral immunotherapy for treatment of egg allergy in children. *The New England Journal of Medicine.* 2012 Jul 19;367(3):233-43.
[179] Patriarca G, Nucera E, Roncallo C, Pollastrini E, Bartolozzi F, De Pasquale T, et al. Oral desensitizing treatment in food allergy: clinical and immunological results. *Aliment Pharmacol. Ther.* 2003 Feb; 17(3): 459-65.
[180] Meglio P, Bartone E, Plantamura M, Arabito E, Giampietro PG. A protocol for oral desensitization in children with IgE-mediated cow's milk allergy. *Allergy* 2004 Sep; 59(9):980-7.
[181] Morisset M, Moneret-Vautrin DA, Guenard L, Cuny JM, Frentz P, Hatahet R, et al. Oral desensitization in children with milk and egg allergies obtains recovery in a

significant proportion of cases. A randomized study in 60 children with cow's milk allergy and 90 children with egg allergy. *Eur. Ann. Allergy Clin. Immunol.* 2007 Jan; 39(1): 12-9.

[182] Staden U, Rolinck-Werninghaus C, Brewe F, Wahn U, Niggemann B, Beyer K. Specific oral tolerance induction in food allergy in children: efficacy and clinical patterns of reaction. *Allergy* 2007 Nov; 62(11): 1261-9.

[183] Longo G, Barbi E, Berti I, Meneghetti R, Pittalis A, Ronfani L, et al. Specific oral tolerance induction in children with very severe cow's milk-induced reactions. *The Journal of Allergy and Clinical Immunology.* 2008 Feb; 121(2): 343-7.

[184] Skripak JM, Nash SD, Rowley H, Brereton NH, Oh S, Hamilton RG, et al. A randomized, double-blind, placebo-controlled study of milk oral immunotherapy for cow's milk allergy. *The Journal of Allergy and Clinical Immunology.* 2008 Dec; 122(6):1154-60.

[185] Mempel M, Rakoski J, Ring J, Ollert M. Severe anaphylaxis to kiwi fruit: Immunologic changes related to successful sublingual allergen immunotherapy. *The Journal of Allergy and Clinical Immunology.* [Case Reports Letter Research Support, Non-U.S. Gov't]. 2003 Jun; 111(6): 1406-9.

[186] Enrique E, Pineda F, Malek T, Bartra J, Basagana M, Tella R, et al. Sublingual immunotherapy for hazelnut food allergy: a randomized, double-blind, placebo-controlled study with a standardized hazelnut extract. *The Journal of Allergy and Clinical Immunology.* [Randomized Controlled Trial]. 2005 Nov; 116(5):1073-9.

[187] Enrique E, Malek T, Pineda F, Palacios R, Bartra J, Tella R, et al. Sublingual immunotherapy for hazelnut food allergy: a follow-up study. *Annals of Allergy, Asthma and Immunology.* [Letter Randomized Controlled Trial]. 2008 Mar; 100(3):283-4.

[188] Kim EH, Bird JA, Kulis M, Laubach S, Pons L, Shreffler W, et al. Sublingual immunotherapy for peanut allergy: clinical and immunologic evidence of desensitization. *The Journal of Allergy and Clinical Immunology.* [Clinical Trial Randomized Controlled Trial Research Support, N.I.H., Extramural Research Support, Non-U.S. Gov't]. 2011 Mar; 127(3):640-6 e1.

[189] Thyagarajan A, Varshney P, Jones SM, Sicherer S, Wood R, Vickery BP, et al. Peanut oral immunotherapy is not ready for clinical use. *The Journal of Allergy and Clinical Immunology.* 2010 Jul; 126(1):31-2.

[190] Fisher HR, du Toit G, Lack G. Specific oral tolerance induction in food allergic children: is oral desensitisation more effective than allergen avoidance? a meta-analysis of published RCTs. *Archives of Disease in Childhood* 2011 Mar; 96(3):259-64.

[191] Kim JS, Nowak-Wegrzyn A, Sicherer SH, Noone S, Moshier EL, Sampson HA. Dietary baked milk accelerates the resolution of cow's milk allergy in children. *The Journal of Allergy and Clinical Immunology.* [Research Support, N.I.H., Extramural]. 2011 Jul; 128(1):125-31 e2.

[192] Huang F, Nowak-Wegrzyn A. Extensively heated milk and egg as oral immunotherapy. *Current Opinion in Allergy and Clinical Immunology* 2012 Jun; 12(3):283-92.

[193] Li XM, Srivastava K, Huleatt JW, Bottomly K, Burks AW, Sampson HA. Engineered recombinant peanut protein and heat-killed Listeria monocytogenes coadministration protects against peanut-induced anaphylaxis in a murine model. *The Journal of Immunology.* [Research Support, Non-U.S. Gov't Research Support, U.S. Gov't, P.H.S.]. 2003 Mar 15; 170(6): 3289-95.

[194] Li XM, Srivastava K, Grishin A, Huang CK, Schofield B, Burks W, et al. Persistent protective effect of heat-killed Escherichia coli producing "engineered," recombinant peanut proteins in a murine model of peanut allergy. *The Journal of Allergy and Clinical Immunology.* 2003 Jul; 112(1):159-67.

[195] MacGlashan DW, Jr., Bochner BS, Adelman DC, Jardieu PM, Togias A, McKenzie-White J, et al. Down-regulation of Fc(epsilon)RI expression on human basophils during in vivo treatment of atopic patients with anti-IgE antibody. *The Journal of Immunology.* [Clinical Trial Clinical Trial, Phase I Research Support, Non-U.S. Gov't Research Support, U.S. Gov't, P.H.S.]. 1997 Feb 1;158(3):1438-45.

[196] Leung DY, Sampson HA, Yunginger JW, Burks AW, Jr., Schneider LC, Wortel CH, et al. Effect of anti-IgE therapy in patients with peanut allergy. *The New England Journal of Medicine.* 2003 Mar 13; 348(11):986-93.

[197] Sampson HA, Leung DY, Burks AW, Lack G, Bahna SL, Jones SM, et al. A phase II, randomized, doubleblind, parallelgroup, placebocontrolled oral food challenge trial of Xolair (omalizumab) in peanut allergy. *The Journal of Allergy and Clinical Immunology.* [Clinical Trial, Phase II Letter Randomized Controlled Trial Research Support, N.I.H., Extramural Research Support, Non-U.S. Gov't]. 2011 May; 127(5):1309-10 e1.

[198] Li XM, Zhang TF, Huang CK, Srivastava K, Teper AA, Zhang L, et al. Food Allergy Herbal Formula-1 (FAHF-1) blocks peanut-induced anaphylaxis in a murine model. *The Journal of Allergy and Clinical Immunology.* 2001 Oct; 108(4): 639-46.

[199] Srivastava KD, Kattan JD, Zou ZM, Li JH, Zhang L, Wallenstein S, et al. The Chinese herbal medicine formula FAHF-2 completely blocks anaphylactic reactions in a murine model of peanut allergy. *The Journal of Allergy and Clinical Immunology* 2005 Jan; 115(1):171-8.

[200] Wang J, Patil SP, Yang N, Ko J, Lee J, Noone S, et al. Safety, tolerability, and immunologic effects of a food allergy herbal formula in food allergic individuals: a randomized, double-blinded, placebo-controlled, dose escalation, phase 1 study. *Annals of Allergy Asthma and Immunology.* [Clinical Trial, Phase I Randomized Controlled Trial Research Support, N.I.H., Extramural Research Support, Non-U.S. Gov't]. 2010 Jul; 105(1):75-84.

[201] Hol J, van Leer EH, Elink Schuurman BE, de Ruiter LF, Samsom JN, Hop W, et al. The acquisition of tolerance toward cow's milk through probiotic supplementation: a randomized, controlled trial. *The Journal of Allergy and Clinical Immunology.* 2008 Jun; 121(6):1448-54.

[202] Zhu FG, Kandimalla ER, Yu D, Agrawal S. Oral administration of a synthetic agonist of Toll-like receptor 9 potently modulates peanut-induced allergy in mice. *The Journal of Allergy and Clinical Immunology.* 2007 Sep; 120(3):631-7.

[203] Medeiros M, Jr., Figueiredo JP, Almeida MC, Matos MA, Araujo MI, Cruz AA, et al. Schistosoma mansoni infection is associated with a reduced course of asthma. *The Journal of Allergy and Clinical Immunology.* 2003 May; 111(5): 947-51.

[204] Bashir ME, Andersen P, Fuss IJ, Shi HN, Nagler-Anderson C. An enteric helminth infection protects against an allergic response to dietary antigen. *The Journal of Immunology.* 2002 Sep 15; 169(6):3284-92.

[205] Mangan NE, Fallon RE, Smith P, van Rooijen N, McKenzie AN, Fallon PG. Helminth infection protects mice from anaphylaxis via IL-10-producing B cells. *The Journal of Immunology*. 2004 Nov 15; 173(10):6346-56.

[206] Bager P, Arnved J, Ronborg S, Wohlfahrt J, Poulsen LK, Westergaard T, et al. Trichuris suis ova therapy for allergic rhinitis: a randomized, double-blind, placebo-controlled clinical trial. *The Journal of Allergy and Clinical Immunology*. [Randomized Controlled Trial Research Support, Non-U.S. Gov't]. 2010 Jan; 125(1):123-30 e1-3.

In: Anaphylaxis: Principles and Practice
Editor: M. Thirumala Krishna

ISBN: 978-1-62618-688-0

Chapter VI

Food-Dependent Exercise-Induced Anaphylaxis

Erick Prado de Oliveira[1,2*] and Roberto Carlos Burini[1]

[1]Centre for Physical Exercise and Nutrition Metabolism,
UNESP School of Medicine, Public Health Department,
São Paulo State, Brazil

[2]Department of Pathology, UNESP School of Medicine, Brazil

Abstract

The increase in sympathoadrenal activity is of major importance for the cardiovascular adaptation, thermoregulation and energy-yielding substrate in exercise. During exertion the blood flow to splanchnic organs is drastically reduced inducing changes in nutrient absorption, motility and mucosal integrity of the gastrointestinal (GI) tract. This reduced GI blood flow makes the gut mucosa susceptible to ischaemic injury, increases permeability and enhances occult blood loss as well as translocation of protective microbials and generation of endotoxins. Vigorous exercise and gut injury also facilitates allergen absorption from GI tract. Systemic reaction to exercise or 'physical allergy' occur in two distinct forms: cholinergic urticaria and exercise induced anaphylaxis (EIA). Symptoms of the former are usually limited to the skin whereas patients with EIA may present with a more severe systemic reaction. Food-dependent exercise-induced anaphylaxis (FDEIA) is a subtype of EIA and is related to prior consumption of food followed by exercise or other physical activity. Aspirin, nonsteroidal anti-inflammatory drugs, alcohol and menstruation are recognized cofactors. It has been suggested that exercise could increase basophil activation and histamine release by the increased osmolality, as well as trigger mast cell degranulation by decreased plasma pH. FDEIA can be of two subtypes - 'Specific FDEIA' relates to development of systemic reaction/anaphylaxis when consumption of a specific food allergen is followed by exercise as opposed to 'non-specific FDEIA', where symptoms

* Corrsponding author: Erick Prado de Oliveira. Faculdade Medicina - UNESP - 18.618-970 - Botucatu - SP - Brasil. Fax: +55 14 3811 6128. E-mail: erick_po@yahoo.com.br.

can appear after any meal followed by exercise, i.e., regardless the food eaten. 'Specific FDEIA' has been associated with cereals, seafood, peanut, eggs, milk and vegetables. Careful clinical history is 'key' to diagnosis of EIA and FDEIA. Management involves counseling patients regarding the condition, relevant avoidance measures and provision of written emergency treatment plan for anaphylaxis.

1. Introduction

High intensity short-duration exercise has been associated with 'physical allergy' due to exercise *per se* (exercise-induced anaphylaxis - EIA) or when preceded (~4-6 hours) by the ingestion of food/s and followed by exercise/physical activity (food-dependent exercise-induced anaphylaxis [FDEIA]). Aspirin/nonsteroidal anti-inflammatory drugs (NSAIDs), alcohol and menstruation are recognized cofactors for FDEIA [1]. Anaphylaxis associated with exercise can be fatal, with a mortality rate between 1 and 2%. About 5-15% of anaphylactic episodes are caused by or associated with exercise [2]. The prevalence of FDEIA is not well-documented, but it is estimated that a third to one half of EIA can be caused by FDEIA [3].

It has been hypothesised that high osmolality and lower plasma pH of high-intensity exercise are activators of basophil and mast cell degranulation. Exercise induces increased gastrointestinal permeability and enhanced absorption of food allergens (large peptides) leading to IgE mediated anaphylaxis in a sensitized individual. Although rare and unpredictable, this can be a fatal.

2. Pathophysiology

There is general consensus that histamine release is a key feature documented during EIA and FDEIA [3] and mast cells are the predominant cells involved in IgE-mediated anaphylaxis [4].

Mast cells have leading role in the initiation of a further cascade of pathological symptoms [3]. These cells tend not to circulate but reside in different anatomical sites with substantial differences in mediator content and sensitivity to agents that induce activation and mediator release [5]. Mast cells invade the connective and mucosal tissues as mast cell progenitors where they differentiate into phenotypically identifiable mast cells [6] which differ in their quantitative release of histamine and their metabolism of arachidonic acid to leukotriene C4 and B4 [7].

Usually the absorbed-food allergenic peptides are well tolerated in the gut by gut-specific mast cells but not by the phenotypically different mast cells of skin and/or skeletal muscle compartments [8]. Larger molecules such as allergenic peptides have greater access to the gut associated with an increased gastrointestinal permeability.

Increased permeability might also result in absorption of only partially digested allergenic proteins enhancing contact with the gut-associated immune system [3].

Tissue transglutaminase (TTG) is an enzyme that is localized beneath the gut epithelium and once activated it modifies specific glutamine residues (eg. wheat's omega-5 gliadin) which results in the formation of large peptide aggregates that leads to increased IgE cross-linking [9]. TTG expression is increased by inflammatory mediators, especially interleukin-6 [10].

The intestinal epithelium, the largest interface between the host and environment forms a selective barrier, which favors fluxes of ions and water movements and limits host contact with the massive intraluminal load of dietary antigens and microbes [11]. This barrier is not fully impermeable to macromolecules, in the steady state, the transpithelial passage of small amounts of food-derived antigens participates in the induction of a homeostatic immune response dominated by immune tolerance to dietary antigens [12]. Conversely, primary or secondary defects of the intestinal barrier can lead to excessive entrance of dietary-derived macromolecules which are putative contributors to the pathogenesis of a spectrum of human diseases, including food allergy [13].

The tight junctions in the gastrointestinal epithelium can become relaxed due thermal injury, alcohol intake and aspirin/NSAIDs [14].

The human low-affinity receptor for IgE (CD23) can mediate the transport of IgE immune complex (IgE IC) in food allergy. Immune sensitization, enhanced CD23 expression and allowed allergens complex with IgE to bypass epithelial lysosomal degradation, resulting in the entry of a large amount of intact allergens into the mucosa [15] and it is likely that IgE IC delivered to the lamina propria after epithelial transport can degranulate mast cells, underlining the ability of the IC to activate local immune cells. This mechanism could participate in the rapid onset of intestinal symptoms in IgE-dependent food allergy [11].

The pathophysiology of EIA and FDEIA is not fully understood. As both the food and the exercise are independently tolerated, this suggests a pliable state of immunological tolerance [16]. Different hypothesis concerning the possible influence of exercise on development of FDEIA symptoms include increased gastrointestinal permeability, blood flow redistribution, and most likely increased osmolality [3].

It is a suggestion that exercise could increase basophil activation and histamine releaseabilty by the increased osmolality as well as trigger mast cell degranulation by decreased pH. However, the increased histamine release in the FDEIA patients occurred at 340mOsM, a pathological (normal 280-290 mOsm) value that would not be achieved even through vigorous physical exercise. Similarly it has been reported that optimal mast cell degranulation occurs at a pH of 7.0 and that changes in pH is achieved only during very heavy exercises [16].

3. Diagnosis

A diagnosis of EIA is made based on clinical history and physical examination. Diagnosis is made if symptoms are associated with exercise - urticaria and/or angioedema or cardiovascular collapse, with or without other features affecting gastrointestinal and upper or lower airways [3].

If an association of anaphylactic symptoms with exercise is proven, it must be clearly stated whether it is food-dependent (FDEIA) or food-independent EIA [3]. Presence of specific IgE to relevant food should be demonstrated in patients with FDEIA. The role of co-factors such as aspirin/NSAIDs, alcohol and menstruation should be explored in the history.

Differential diagnosis should include disorders, such as idiopathic anaphylaxis, cholinergic and cold urticaria, mastocytosis, hereditary angiodoema, exercise-induced asthma and neoplasms [3]. The comparison between EIA and FDEIA are described on Table 1.

4. Exercise Induced Anaphylaxis

Systemic reactions to exercise occur in two distinct forms, cholinergic urticaria and exercise- induced anaphylaxis (EIA) [17]. Symptoms of cholinergic urticaria are usually limited to the skin and present with punctuate wheals with prominent erythematous flare triggered by exercise and increased body temperature. In contrast, the patient with EIA may present with symptoms of an acute systemic allergic reaction, including pruritus, flushing, urticaria, angiodoema, and in some cases, cardiovascular collapse [18].

EIA is a clinical syndrome in which anaphylaxis occurs in conjunction with exercise or other significant physical activity [19]. EIA is rare, unpredictable but potentially fatal syndrome. EIA is generally reported following submaximal exercise of a relatively short duration and has been described in either high-performance athletes and occasional exercisers [16]. Warm environment (64%), high humidity (32%), and cold environment (23%) have been reported to be associated with EIA [20]. It is important to emphasize that exercises in lower intensities decrease the likelihood of EIA and the episodes are not predictable [3].

5. Food-Dependent Exercise-Induced Anaphylaxis

In FDEIA, both the food allergen and exercise are independently tolerated. The clinical syndrome of FDEIA is typified by the onset of anaphylaxis during (or soon after) exercise that was preceded by the ingestion of the causal foods (Table 2) [16]. There is also related non-specific FDEIA in which the patient presents with anaphylactic symptoms after any meal followed by exercise, regardless of the food eaten [21] Furthemore, it is difficult to estimate the threshold for the food allergen and level of exercise that is required to trigger symptoms.

In a population of more than 76,000 Japanese high school students Aihara et al [22] found only 13 (0.017%) cases of FDEIA. The number of boys (n=11) was significantly higher than that of girls (n=2). In the subpopulation of patients with FDEIA, ingestion of causative food and physical effort are necessary to induce anaphylaxis. Wheat is the most frequent causative foodstuff in Japan [21], whereas lentil and chick pea (leguminosa family) are among the most frequent foods in the Mediterranean area [23]. Although wheat is the most commonly reported food allergen associated with FDEIA [22], other food allergens have also been implicated [19].

In Europeans tomatoes, cereals, and peanuts are the most frequent allergenic foods, whereas in the Japanese population, wheat is most common allergen. Other causative foods include seafood (specially shellfish), seeds, cow's milk, some vegetables and fruits (eg. oranges, onions, or grapes) [18, 24]. Some members of the Anacardiaceae family such as pistachio, cashew nut and mango, have been reported as causative allergens. The pistachio tree is native to western Asia and Asia minor [25]. Anaphylactic shock induced by exercise was also reported following ingestion of celery [18].

Table 1. Comparison of diagnosis of EIA and FDEIA

EIA	FDEIA
Diagnosis of EIA is made based on clinical history and physical examination	Diagnosis of FDEIA is made based on clinical history, physical examination and demonstration of relevant food specific IgE
The diagnosis of EIA is made if anaphylaxis is associated with exercise	Onset of anaphylaxis during (or soon after) exercise that was preceded by the ingestion of food up to 4-6 hours
A diagnosis of EIA should be made after FDEIA has been excluded.	

Table 2. Main allergens involved in FDEIA

Allergens
Cereals
Peanuts
Seafood
Nuts
Cow´s milk
Eggs
Vegetables
Fruits (oranges, onions, or grapes)

Prevalence of FDEIA is not well-documented, but it is estimated to make up one third to one half of all EIA patients [3] and EIA represents about 5% to 15% of all anaphylactic cases [21].

Wheat proteins are classified into three fractions according to their solubility: a) salt-soluble albumins and globulins; b) salt-insoluble gliadins and c) glutenins [26]. Eighty percent of the patients with wheat dependent EIA are sensitized to omega 5-gliadin and the remaining to glutenin [1]. Serum gliadin levels increase in accordance with allergic symptoms in patients with wheat dependent EIA strongly indicating that the blood antigen level is a key factor in induction of symptoms [27].

EIA does not differ significantly from that of anaphylaxis triggered by other factors. Four stages of an EIA [19], are described: prodromal, early, fully developed, and late. The prodromal symptoms manifest with fatigue and prostration and generalized pruritus with erythema. The early stage is characterized by generalized urticaria. If the event progresses, fully developed EIA includes gastrointestinal symptoms with abdominal cramps, nausea, and vomiting, as well as symptoms of upper airway obstruction with dyspnoea, stridor, and a feeling of choking. Symptoms of the late phase-frontal headache and fatigue may be present up to 72 hours after the onset of EIA. In a fully developed EIA attack, the spectrum of symptoms is wider and may be much more severe. Cardiovascular symptoms, including collapse or altered consciousness, are reported in one third of EIA patients, and fatalities or near fatalities are very rare [17].

In FDEIA, ingestion of causative food usually precedes exercise by minutes or 4-6 hours. However, some observations indicate that FDEIA may also occur if the food is ingested soon after the completion of exercise. Thus, it seems very likely that in FDEIA, it is not the sequence but rather the coincidence of triggering factors that is crucial [3].

6. Management of EIA and FDEIA

EIA occurs mainly in high intensity exercise and one intervention to prevent this event would be to perform exercise in lower intensities [21]. The FDEIA can be avoided with some important recommendations. Aspirin or NSAIDs and alcohol should not be taken in association with exercise. Furthermore, avoidance of exercise for 4 to 6 hours after possible allergen food intake is an important recommendation. There is some evidence that the sequence of FDEIA can be reversed, in other words, it means that anaphylaxis can occur with an intake of some foods after prolonged exercise. Thus, relevant allergen should be avoided up to 1 hour after the exercise, when the recovery of blood flow to viscera are almost complete and there is no increase in intestinal permeability [3, 16].

Pharmacologic interventions have been described to prevent anaphylaxis after exercise. After an intake of peaches before the exercise, the co-administration of cetirizine and montelukast showed a protective effect in the development of anaphylaxis [28]. Furthermore, the administration of sodium cromoglycate before the intake of wheat also prevented FDEIA [29]. Further large scale placebo controlled studies are required for confirmation. At the present time avoidance measures are 'key' to prevention of future episodes.

The acute treatment of EIA is not different of that other types of anaphylaxis [30].

Clinical Cases

Case 1. Food-dependent exercise-induced anaphylaxis to lentil and anaphylaxis to chickpea in a 17-year-old boy

Orhan et al. [23] reported a case of a 17-year-old boy who reported suffering from pruritus, diffuse warmth, and facial erythema followed by generalized urticaria, oedema of the eyelids, lips and tongue, wheezing, dyspnoea, and unconsciousness 30 to 60 minutes after beginning any kind of physical exertion immediately after ingestion of lentil soup. The boy experienced 4 episodes of exercise-induced anaphylaxis after ingestion of lentil and 2 episodes following ingestion of chickpea. Skin prick test to fresh lentil and chick pea were positive. Treadmill exercise challenge tests in the fasting state and 1 hour after a meal not containing lentil were negative. However, an exercise challenge test 1 hour after intake of lentil soup resulted in pruritus of the hands, forearms, shoulders, and back, urticarial lesions on the face and shoulders, mild angioedema of the lips, and mild hoarseness and cough that indicate that the patient had IgE-mediated FDEIA to lentil. This case reflects a case of food-dependent exercise-induced anaphylaxis due to lentil.

Comments: This case showed that when lentil was ingested 1 hour before the exercise, FDEIA occurred. The recommendation is to avoidance of lentil and chick pea 4-6 hours before and 1 hour after the exercise.

Case 2. Food-dependent exercise-induced anaphylaxis induced by low dose aspirin therapy

Fuji et al. [27] reported a case of a 63-year-old man who started on low dose aspirin therapy. After 4 months he had repeated episodes of generalized urticaria and lost consciousness while he was exercising after eating wheat. He was strongly positive for specific IgE to omega-5-gliadin on a CAPfluorescent enzyme immunoassay (FEIA). Therefore, a diagnosis of wheat-dependent exercise-induced anaphylaxis was made.

Comments: In this case the patient ingested low aspirin dose for cardiovascular disease prevention, however, even at this dose, aspirin probably increased the intestinal permeability which led to an enhanced the omega-5 gliadin absorption (wheat intake before physical activity). So, even at low doses, aspirin is a risk factor for FDEIA.

Clinical Pearls

- Vigorous exercise facilities allergen absorption from the GI tract. Specific FDEIA has been associated with cereals, seafood, peanut, tree nuts, eggs, milk and vegetables.
- Aspirin, NSAIDs, alcohol and menstruation are recognized cofactors in FDEIA.
- If a diagnosis of FDEIA has been made, then the allergen should be avoided both 4-6 hours prior to and an hour after exercise.

References

[1] Morita, E; Matsuo, H; Chinuki, Y; Takahashi, H; Dahlstrom, J; Tanaka, A. Food-dependent exercise-induced anaphylaxis -importance of omega-5 gliadin and HMW-glutenin as causative antigens for wheat-dependent exercise-induced anaphylaxis. *Allergol Int*, 2009, 58, 493-498.

[2] Du Toit, G. Food-dependent exercise-induced anaphylaxis in childhood. *Pediatr Allergy Immunol*, 2007, 18, 455-463.

[3] Barg, W; Medrala, W; Wolanczyk-Medrala, A. Exercise-induced anaphylaxis: an update on diagnosis and treatment. *Curr Allergy Asthma Rep*, 2011, 11, 45-51.

[4] Sheffer, AL; Tong, AK; Murphy, GF; Lewis, RA; McFadden, ER; Jr., Austen, KF. Exercise-induced anaphylaxis: a serious form of physical allergy associated with mast cell degranulation. *J Allergy Clin Immunol*, 1985, 75, 479-484.

[5] Galli, SJ. New concepts about the mast cell. *N Engl J Med*, 1993, 328, 257-265.

[6] Kitamura, Y; Fujita, J. Regulation of mast cell differentiation. *Bioessays*, 1989, 10, 193-196.

[7] Galli, SJ; Kalesnikoff, J; Grimbaldeston, MA; Piliponsky, AM; Williams, CM; Tsai, M. Mast cells as "tunable" effector and immunoregulatory cells: recent advances. *Annu Rev Immunol*, 2005, 23, 749-786.

[8] Cheng, CX; Li, YN; Ohno, H; Sawanobori, K; Li, YC; Shimada, O; Atsumi, S. Mast cells appearing in long-term skeletal muscle cell cultures of rat. *Anat Rec (Hoboken)*, 2007, 290, 1424-1430.

[9] Palosuo, K; Varjonen, E; Nurkkala, J; Kalkkinen, N; Harvima, R; Reunala, T; Alenius, H. Transglutaminase-mediated cross-linking of a peptic fraction of omega-5 gliadin enhances IgE reactivity in wheat-dependent, exercise-induced anaphylaxis. *J Allergy Clin Immunol*, 2003, 111, 1386-1392.

[10] Suto, N; Ikura, K; Sasaki, R. Expression induced by interleukin-6 of tissue-type transglutaminase in human hepatoblastoma HepG2 cells. *J Biol Chem*, 1993, 268, 7469-7473.

[11] Menard, S; Cerf-Bensussan, N; Heyman, M. Multiple facets of intestinal permeability and epithelial handling of dietary antigens. *Mucosal Immunol*, 2010, 3, 247-259.

[12] Strobel, S; Mowat, AM. Immune responses to dietary antigens: oral tolerance. *Immunol Today*, 1998, 19, 173-181.

[13] Cani, PD; Bibiloni, R; Knauf, C; Waget, A; Neyrinck, AM; Delzenne, NM; Burcelin, R. Changes in gut microbiota control metabolic endotoxemia-induced inflammation in high-fat diet-induced obesity and diabetes in mice. *Diabetes*, 2008, 57, 1470-1481.

[14] Oshima, T; Miwa, H; Joh, T. Aspirin induces gastric epithelial barrier dysfunction by activating p38 MAPK via claudin-7. *Am J Physiol Cell Physiol*, 2008, 295, C800-806.

[15] Bevilacqua, C; Montagnac, G; Benmerah, A; Candalh, C; Brousse, N; Cerf-Bensussan, N; Perdue, MH; Heyman, M. Food allergens are protected from degradation during CD23-mediated transepithelial transport. *Int Arch Allergy Immunol*, 2004, 135, 108-116.

[16] Robson-Ansley, P; Toit, GD. Pathophysiology, diagnosis and management of exercise-induced anaphylaxis. *Curr Opin Allergy Clin Immunol*, 2010, 10, 312-317.

[17] Castells, MC; Horan, RF; Sheffer, AL. Exercise-induced anaphylaxis (EIA). *Clin Rev Allergy Immunol*, 1999, 17, 413-424.

[18] Barg, W; Wolanczyk-Medrala, A; Obojski, A; Wytrychowski, K; Panaszek, B; Medrala, W. Food-dependent exercise-induced anaphylaxis: possible impact of increased basophil histamine releasability in hyperosmolar conditions. *J Investig Allergol Clin Immunol*, 2008, 18, 312-315.

[19] Castells, MC; Horan, RF; Sheffer, AL. Exercise-induced Anaphylaxis. *Curr Allergy Asthma Rep*, 2003, 3, 15-21.

[20] Kato, Y; Nagai, A; Saito, M; Ito, T; Koga, M; Tsuboi, R. Food-dependent exercise-induced anaphylaxis with a high level of plasma noradrenaline. *J Dermatol*, 2007, 34, 110-113.

[21] Choi, JH; Lee, HB; Ahn, IS; Park, CW; Lee, CH. Wheat-dependent, Exercise-induced Anaphylaxis: A Successful Case of Prevention with Ketotifen. *Ann Dermatol*, 2009, 21, 203-205.

[22] Aihara, Y; Takahashi, Y; Kotoyori, T; Mitsuda, T; Ito, R; Aihara, M; Ikezawa, Z; Yokota, S. Frequency of food-dependent, exercise-induced anaphylaxis in Japanese junior-high-school students. *J Allergy Clin Immunol*, 2001, 108, 1035-1039.

[23] Orhan, F; Karakas, T. Food-dependent exercise-induced anaphylaxis to lentil and anaphylaxis to chickpea in a 17-year-old boy. *J Investig Allergol Clin Immunol*, 2008, 18, 465-468.

[24] de Oliveira, EP; Burini, RC. Food-dependent, exercise-induced gastrointestinal distress. *J Int Soc Sports Nutr*, 2011, 8, 12.

[25] Porcel, S; Sanchez, AB; Rodriguez, E; Fletes, C; Alvarado, M; Jimenez, S; Hernandez, J. Food-dependent exercise-induced anaphylaxis to pistachio. *J Investig Allergol Clin Immunol*, 2006, 16, 71-73.

[26] Mittag, D; Niggemann, B; Sander, I; Reese, I; Fiedler, EM; Worm, M; Vieths, S; Reese, G. Immunoglobulin E-reactivity of wheat-allergic subjects (baker's asthma, food allergy, wheat-dependent, exercise-induced anaphylaxis) to wheat protein fractions with different solubility and digestibility. *Mol Nutr Food Res*, 2004, 48, 380-389.

[27] Fujii, H; Kambe, N; Fujisawa, A; Kohno, K; Morita, E; Miyachi, Y. Food-dependent exercise-induced anaphylaxis induced by low dose aspirin therapy. *Allergol Int*, 2008, 57, 97-98.

[28] Peroni, DG; Piacentini, GL; Piazza, M; Cametti, E; Boner, AL. Combined cetirizine-montelukast preventive treatment for food-dependent exercise-induced anaphylaxis. *Ann Allergy Asthma Immunol*, 2010, 104, 272-273.

[29] Sugimura, T; Tananari, Y; Ozaki, Y; Maeno, Y; Ito, S; Yoshimoto, Y; Kawano, K; Tanaka, S. Effect of oral sodium cromoglycate in 2 children with food-dependent exercise-induced anaphylaxis (FDEIA). *Clin Pediatr (Phila)*, 2009, 48, 945-950.

[30] Lieberman, P; Decker, W; Camargo, CA; Jr., Oconnor, R; Oppenheimer, J; Simons, FE. SAFE: a multidisciplinary approach to anaphylaxis education in the emergency department. *Ann Allergy Asthma Immunol*, 2007, 98, 519-523.

In: Anaphylaxis: Principles and Practice
Editor: M. Thirumala Krishna
ISBN: 978-1-62618-688-0

Chapter VII

Anaphylaxis during General Anaesthesia

Silvia Caimmi[1*], Naire Sansotta[2*], Diego G. Peroni[2] and Roberto Bernardini[3]
[1]Department of Pediatrics, University of Pavia, Italy
[2]Department of Pediatrics, University of Verona, Italy
[3]Pediatric Unit "San Giuseppe" Hospital, Empoli, Italy

1. Summary

Perioperative anaphylactic reactions are potential life-threatening immediate hypersensitivity reactions which are unrelated to the drug's pharmacological characteristics and correspond to immune-mediated allergic and non-immune-mediated so-called "pseudo-allergic or anaphylactoid" reactions. Their incidence and associated morbidity and mortality remain poorly defined. Perioperative anaphylaxis is becoming more common, probably due to more frequent use of general anaesthesia and the increasing complexity of the drugs employed. Moreover, current epidemiological data should be carefully evaluated since published studies relate to non-homogeneous populations and used differing definitions of drug hypersensitivity. Recognition and immediate treatment are particularly important because anaesthetized patients are at greater risk for adverse outcomes caused by physiological effects of anaesthesia. Several reports indicate that the relative risk of allergic reactions may vary with time, depending on changes in clinical practice as well as several environmental factors. Vigilance for signs of anaphylaxis and consideration of the risk factors, with possible modification of the agents used, are likely to reduce the morbidity and mortality associated with these reactions and socio-economic costs.

---

[*] These authors equally contributed to the chapter. The authors have no conflict of interest to declare.

2. Epidemiology

Drug hypersensitivity reactions are responsible for significant morbidity and mortality as well as socio-economic costs that have yet to be fully evaluated. Current epidemiological data have to be carefully interpreted since the various studies conducted so far have been on different populations (either adult or pediatric populations or both, in-patients or out-patients), gave different definitions of adverse drug reactions/drug allergy, and used different methods of data analysis. It should also be kept in mind that causality assessment (or drug imputability) mostly relies on personal clinical histories that are not accurate to definitively make a diagnosis of drug hypersensitivity reaction and cannot replace allergy testing [1-4].

Incidence of Reactions to Different Drugs

The majority of reports on the incidence of anaphylaxis are from France, Australia, the United Kingdom and New Zealand. Anaphylactic reactions have also been reported for smaller series in the United States. Nevertheless, the true incidence of anaphylactic reactions and their associated morbidity and mortality remain poorly defined. Moreover, although they are rare events, when an anaphylactic reaction occurs in the operating room, it may lead to death even when appropriately treated, with a mortality rate ranging from 3% to 9%; but the overall morbidity rate is unknown. Reports on the incidence of anaphylaxis are based on studies carried out in France, Australia, New Zealand, United Kingdom, Thailand, Spain and Norway. They reflect an active policy of systematic clinical and/or laboratory investigation of hypersensitivity reactions, or are the result of an analysis of databases on drug-related adverse events. According to these reports, the estimated incidence of all immune- and non-immune-mediated immediate hypersensitivity reactions was 1 in 5,000 to 1 in 13,000 anaesthetics in Australia, 1 in 5000 in Thailand, 1 in 4600 in France, 1 in 1250 to 1 in 5000 in New Zealand, and 1 in 3500 in England [5-9]. The estimated incidence of immune-mediated reactions seems to vary from 1 in 10,000 to 1 in 20,000 in Australia [10] and 1 in 13,000 in France [11], 1 in 10,263 in Spain [12], 1 in 5500 in Thailand [9] and 1 in 1700 to 1 in 20,000 in Norway [13]. A combined analysis of three different French data-bases, using a capture-recapture method, has allowed a nationally based estimate of incidence of IgE-mediated (immediate) reactions occurring during anaesthesia, stratified according to sex, age, and causal substance. This study has confirmed the general view that immediate-type hypersensitivity reactions are largely under-reported, with an incidence being estimated at 100.6 (76.2–125.3) per million procedures.

Almost all drugs and substances to which patients are exposed perioperatively have been known to cause allergic reactions. In all series, neuromuscular blocking agents (NMBAs) represent the most frequently incriminated substance ranging from 50 to 70%. The incidence of allergic reactions to latex largely depends on local Health and Safety policies applied in respective institutions. Reactions involving antibiotics are mainly due to penicillins and cephalosporins. These reactions have rapidly increased in the past decade, reflecting the increasing prevalence of allergy to these drugs in the general population as well as their increased use in perioperative antibiotic prophylaxis. Hypnotic agents, opioids, colloids, aprotinin, and protamine are less frequently attributed, whereas cases involving dyes, chlorhexidine, or nonsteroidal anti-inflammatory drugs (NSAIDs) have been reported with increasing frequency. Allergy to local anaesthetics appears truly uncommon [14].

In children, the various incriminated substances differ significantly from those for adult patients. The largest published study of allergic reactions in the perioperative period originates from France and latex was the most frequently incriminated substance (41.8%), followed by neuromuscular blocking agents [NMBAs] (32%) and antibiotics (9%). Interestingly, this study also provides an attractive hypothesis to explain the female predominance reported in all series. Indeed, in contrast with the results observed in adults, no significant differences were observed in regard to the sex distribution in children for both IgE- or non-IgE-mediated reactions.

This similar incidence of allergic and nonallergic reactions according to gender before adolescence strongly suggests a role for sex hormones in the increase of immediate hypersensitivity reactions to low-molecular- weight compounds [14]. In a Norwegian single-center study, NMBAs were the agents most commonly involved in anaphylactic reactions, with latex implicated in very few cases and with no causal agent identified in as much as one-third of the cases [13].

On the other hand, in a study conducted in two different Spanish centers, antibiotics were the main agents involved, followed by NMBAs [15]. From the different studies, it is evident that the incidence of anaphylaxis to vital dyes and chlorhexidine is currently increasing. Anaphylaxis may also occur with intravenous hypnotics, aprotinin, protamine and other drugs. Anaphylactic reactions to colloids remain relatively stable (around 4%), and gelatin is the volume expanding fluid most frequently involved.

Allergic reactions to local anaesthetics remain rather uncommon despite their frequent use. In fact, most of the adverse reactions to local anesthetics are related to inadvertent intravascular injection leading to excessive blood concentrations of the local anaesthetic; some reports related a reaction to the systemic absorption of epinephrine combined with the local anaesthetic. Allergic reactions to opioids are uncommon as well, and anaphylaxis to halogenated volatile anaesthetics has never been reported [16].

The observed incidence of reactions to corticosteroids varies from 0.5% to 5% [17].

Morbidity in anaphylaxis is mainly related to cerebral hypoxia occurring after an ineffective resuscitation. Perioperative anaphylactic reactions can be life-threatening particularly, if adequate treatment is not promptly started [18]. The mortality rate related to these reactions ranges from 3% to 6%, and an additional 2% of patients experience significant residual brain damage, as previously stated.

3. Risk Factors for Perioperative Anaphylaxis

Some conditions or characteristics affect the risk of developing reactions during anaesthesia [19].

There is not enough evidence that allergic reactions to anaesthetic drugs are associated with previous reactions to a drug that is unrelated with those used during the course of anaesthesia, with rare exceptions [19].

Demographic Features: Sex, Age, Family History

Anaphylaxis to sodium thiopental is 3 times more likely to occur in females and it is more common and severe in older patients mainly if associated chronic pulmonary or cardiovascular diseases [20]. However, age cannot be considered as a true risk factor since reactions to NMBAs have been reported in all ages, including in children as young as one year [21].

A family history of anaphylaxis has been suggested as important in one report of cousins who reacted to NMBAs, but no similar cases have been reported in the literature.

Atopic Diseases

In many large series of patients sensitised to a NMBAs, a disproportionate number of patients have histories of atopy, allergy or asthma. However, different studies have failed to demonstrate an increased risk of allergy to NMBAs in atopic patients [21]. Patients with food allergies may have decreased levels of enzyme [platelet activation factor acetyl hydrolase] that degrades platelet-activating factor, increasing the risk of anaphylaxis [20].

Propofol (2-6 diisopropylphenol) is an alkyl phenol in a lipid vehicle (soybean oil, egg lecithin, and glycerol). The main allergen of egg is ovalbumin (found in egg white) and the lecithin in propofol is derived from egg yolk protein [22]. However, there is insufficient evidence that propofol is more likely to provoke allergic reactions in subjects with egg and/or peanut allergy [23]. Patients with allergies to fruits (such as banana, pear, kiwi, fig, mango, passion fruit), nuts (peanuts, walnuts) have been associated with latex cross sensitivity [20].

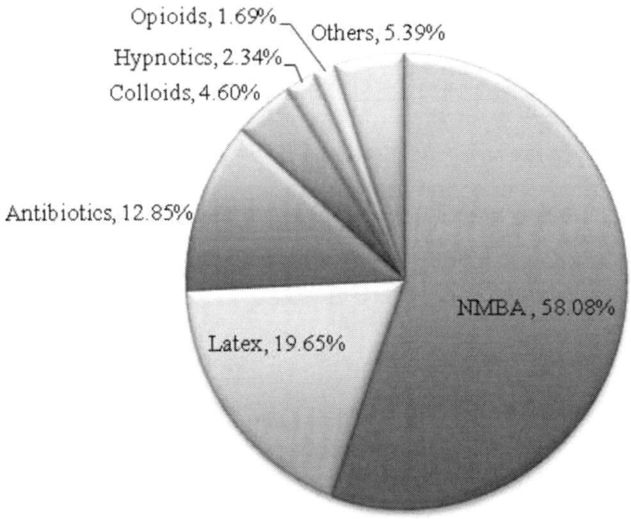

Figure 1. Perioperative anaphylaxis: causal agents [25].

Patients who are allergic to latex should be scheduled as first case of the day with all latex products removed from the room [24].

Previous Anaphylaxis

A history of perioperative anaphylaxis is the greatest risk factor for anaesthetic-induced anaphylaxis. Patients who have reported urticaria or angioedema during anaesthesia are at higher risk for another reaction. A family history of anaesthetic allergy or multiple drug allergy syndromes may also indicate the potential for hypersensitivity and should be considered in accordance with symptoms before testing [20].

Mast Cell Diseases

Patients with mastocytosis or clonal mast cell diseases can have exaggerated release of histamine, leukotrienes and prostaglandins during anaesthesia [20].

Drugs Mainly Involved: NMBAs and Antibiotics

In patients with a severe reaction to one or more muscle relaxants, subsequent administration of NMBAs was associated with clinical hypersensitivity reactions, ranging from anaphylaxis to minor adverse events, in about 58% of cases (Figure 1-2) [25].

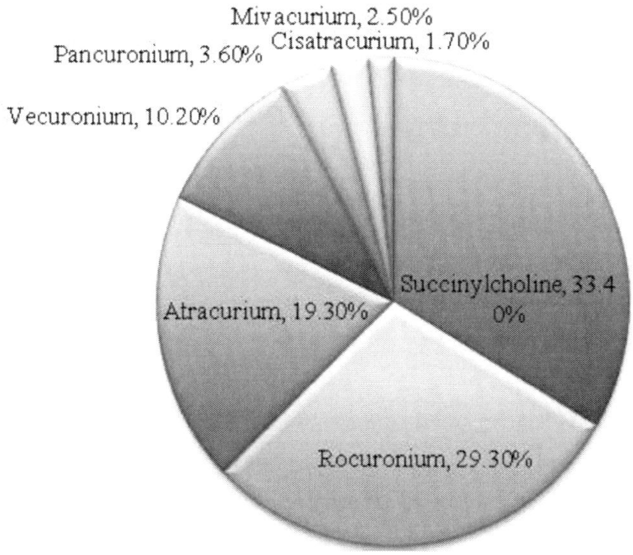

Figure 2. Neuromuscular blocking agents: involved drugs [25].

Therefore, an anaphylactic reaction to a NMBA is a positive risk factor for an allergic reaction to different NMBAs in future anaesthesia. Reactions to NMBA may develop at the first exposure. This may happen when a subject has been previously sensitized to cross reacting substances containing quaternary or tertiary ammonium ions such as other classes of drugs including acetylcholine, choline, morphine, neostigmine, pentolinium and pholcodine, cosmetics or detergents. There is no clear evidence that NMBAs crossreact with propofol [19].

Among antibiotics, penicillin and cephalosporin elicit approximately 70% of perioperative anaphylactic reactions [26].

In patients with allergy to penicillin there is a 3-10% risk of reaction with cephalosporin/s because they have a similar beta-lactam ring. Further cross reacting antibiotics with a β-lactam ring are piperacillin, ticarcillin, ertapenem, imipenem, and meropenem. Aztreonam is considered as a valid alternative in subjects allergic to penicillins and cephalosporins, with the sole exception of those patients with a proven allergy to ceftazidime [27]. Risk factors for an allergic reaction to penicillin or cephalosporin include a previous history of reaction and a positive skin test. Penicillin skin testing identifies patients with clinical hypersensitivity reactions in about 70% of cases [28]. Allergic reactions to other antibiotics, including vancomycin, bacitracin, clindamicin, gentamicin, and metronidazole are uncommon. It is unclear whether skin test results predict reactions to such antibiotics.

Recommendations

- A patient who has had a previous reaction to a drug should not receive the drug again except during a desensitization process.
- Alternatives should be used if a patient has an allergy to latex or a drug such as antibiotic or a non steroidal anti-inflammatory drug [20].

4. Pathophysiology of Drug Allergy

Anaphylaxis due to Drugs Administered in the Operating Room

The nomenclature task force set up by the European Academy of Allergy and Immunology (EAACI) has proposed that anaphylactic-type reactions be reclassified into allergic anaphylaxis and non-allergic anaphylaxis, allergic anaphylaxis being further subdivided into IgE-mediated and non-IgE-mediated reactions [29]. Immediate hypersensitivity reactions to anaesthetics and associated agents used during the perioperative period have been reported with increasing frequency in most developed countries. Most reactions either have an immunologic origin (IgE-mediated anaphylaxis) or are related to a directly stimulated release of histamine (anaphylactoid reactions) from mast cells. Cardiovascular collapse and bronchospasm appear more frequently in IgE-dependent reactions. The degree of severity of these reactions varies and does not allow clinical differentiation between IgE-mediated and non-IgE-mediated reactions, resulting from nonspecific mediator release, which actually accounts for 30%-40% of all perioperative hypersensitivity reactions [30].

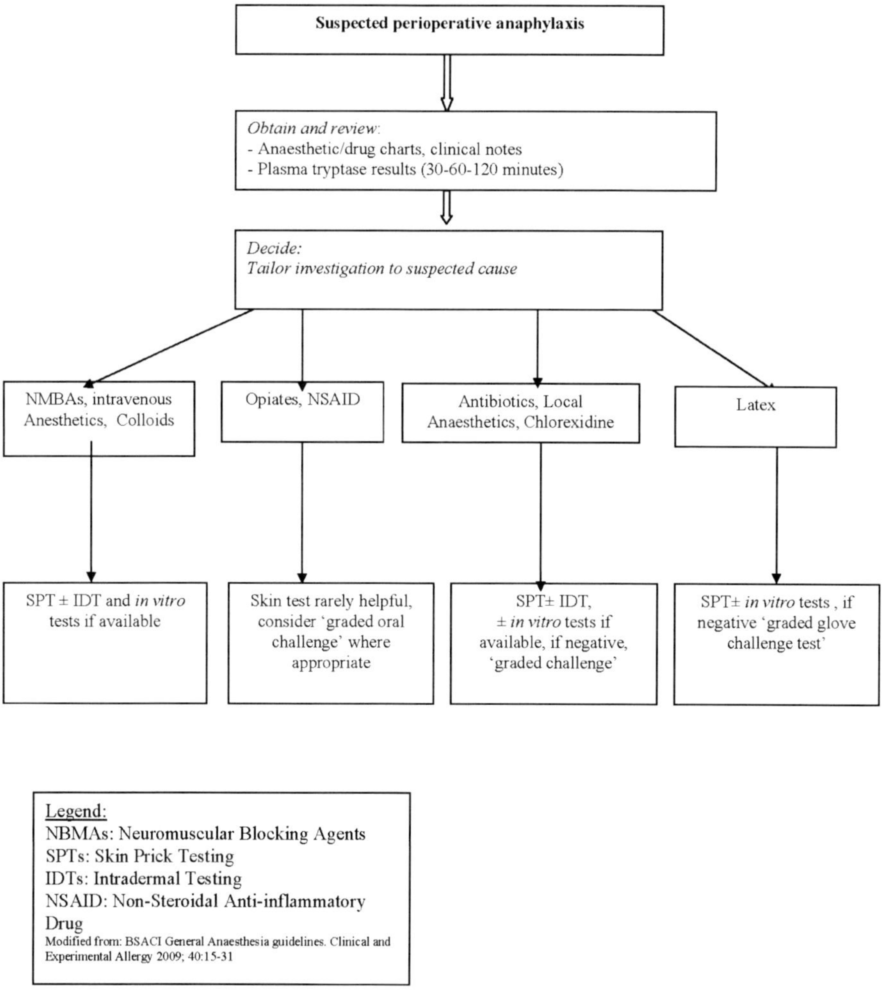

Figure 3. Investigation for suspected anaphylaxis during general anaesthesia.

Any suspected hypersensitivity reaction during anaesthesia must be thoroughly investigated to confirm the nature of the reaction, identify the culprit drug/agent, study cross-reactivity in cases of anaphylaxis to NMBAs and provide recommendations for future anaesthetic procedures. However, since, as previously stated, anaphylactic reactions cannot be clinically distinguished from non-immune-mediated reactions, any suspected episode must be extensively investigated using combined peri- and postoperative testing. In this way it should be possible to confirm the nature of the reaction, identify the causal agent and provide precise recommendation/s for future anaesthetic procedures. Cutaneous manifestations of anaphylaxis are less likely to be apparent when it occurs in a perioperative environment. The evaluation of IgE-mediated reactions to medications used during anaesthesia includes skin tests for a variety of anaesthetic agents (Figure 3 and Table 1). For example, thiopental allergy can be demonstrated by skin tests. Neuromuscular blocking agents such as succinylcholine may cause non-immunologic histamine release. Nevertheless, there have been few papers reporting cases of IgE-mediated reactions to these agents. Reactions to opioid analgesics are usually caused by the direct release of mast cell mediators rather than by IgE-dependent mechanism. Antibiotics that are administered perioperatively may cause immunologic or non-immunologic reactions; protamine can also cause severe systemic reactions through both IgE-mediated and non-immunologic mechanisms.

Table 1. 'Non-irritant' concentrations of anaesthetic agents for skin tests

DRUG	PRICK TEST		INTRADERMAL TEST	
	Dilution	Maximal concentration (mg/ml)	Dilution	Maximal Concentration (mcg/ml)
Hypnotics				
Etomidate	Undiluted	2	1/10	200
Midazolam	Undiluted	5	1/10	500
Propofol	Undiluted	10	1/10	1000
Thiopental	Undiluted	25	1/10	2500
Opioids				
Alfentanil	Undiluted	0.5	1/10	50
Fentanyl	Undiluted	0.05	1/10	5
Morphine	1/10	1	1/1000	10
Remifentanil	Undiluted	0.05	1/10	5
Sufentanil	Undiluted	0.005	1/10	0.5
Local anaesthetics				
Buvicaine	Undiluted	2.5	1/10	250
Lidocaine	Undiluted	10	1/10	1000
Mepivacaine	Undiluted	10	1/10	1000
Ropivacaine	Undiluted	2	1/10	200
Colloids				
Gelatin	Undiluted		undiluided	
Hydroxyethyl starch	Undiluted			
Dextran40/70	Undiluted	6-10	1/100	600-1000
Aprotinin	Undiluted	10000 IU/ml	1/100	100 IU/ml
Dyes				
Isosulfan	Undiluted	10	1/10	1000
Patent blue	Undiluted	25	1/10	2500
Methylene blue	Undiluted	10	1/100	100
Iodinate Contrast Media	Undiluted	300	1/10	30000
Chlohexidine	Undiluted	2%	1/100000	0.0002%
Muscle relaxants				
Atracurium	1/10	1	1/1000	10
Cisatracurium	Undiluted	2	1/100	20
Mivacurium	1/10	0.2	1/1000	2
Pancuronium	Undiluted	2	1/10	200
Rocuronium	Undiluted	10	1/100	100
Suxamethonium	1/5	10	1/500	100
Vecuronium	Undiluted	4	1/10	400

Modified from: Mertes PM et al. Hypersensitivity reactions to Neuromuscular blocking agents. Current Pharmaceutical Design 2008; 14:2809-25 [21]

Blood transfusions can elicit a variety of systemic reactions, some of which are IgE-mediated, while others are consequences of other immunologic mechanisms. Methylmethacrylate (bone cement) has been associated with different systemic reactions, including hypotension, although no IgE mechanism has been clearly documented. Nevertheless, when anaphylaxis occurs in a perioperative environment or during general anaesthesia, it has to be clear that its management is similar to the management of anaphylaxis in other situations [30].

Reactions Occurring in Radiology

Iodinated contrast media (ICM) were introduced since 1950s and are among the most common prescribed drugs. Severe and fatal reactions represent a serious problem, since more than 70 million applications of ICM are registered per year, worldwide. ICM are among the most commonly used injectable drugs administered in radiology and they may be injected during surgical procedures as well. Modern ICM can be introduced in the body through different routes, such as intravenously, intra-arterially, intrathecally and orally. ICM hypersensitivity reactions can be either immediate or non-immediate (occurring up to the seventh day after the injection) in susceptible individuals [31].

In a study by Katayama in Japan [32], allergic reactions were evaluated in 337,647 patients who received injections of ICM. The incidence of adverse reactions was 12.7% (0.22% of severe reactions for ionic products and 0.04% for non-ionic products); two reactions were fatal (incidence of 0.0006%). The least number of reactions have been reported with non ionic agents, and with dimers rather than monomers. The greater number of reactions, on the other hand, have been reported with hyperosmolar ionic monomers. (Table-2). The European Network of Drug Allergy (ENDA) reported that mild immediate reactions occur in 3.8%-12.7% of patients receiving intravenous injections of high-osmolar ionic ICM and in 0.7%-3.1% of patients receiving low-osmolar non-ionic ICM. Severe immediate reactions have been reported to occur with a frequency of 0.1%-0.4% for ionic ICM and with a frequency of 0.02%-0.04% for non-ionic ICM. The frequency of non-immediate adverse reactions ranges from 0.5% to 23%. This large variation may be due to the difficulty in verifying whether symptoms occurring hours or days after ICM exposure were actually caused by the ICM itself [33].

Table 2. Classification of Iodinated Contrast Media

Non ionic		**Ionic**	
Dimers	**Monomers**	**Dimers**	**Monomers**
Iodixanol	Iopamidol	Ioxaglate	Amidotrizoate
	Iohexol		Ioxitalamate
	Ioversol		
	Iopromide		
	Iomeprol		
	Iobitridol		

Although adverse reactions observed with non-ionic ICM are usually less severe than those with ionic ICM, their respective death rate does not significantly differ, being in the range of 1 every 100,000 examinations.

Non-immediate hypersensitive reactions occur at various rates and appear to be T cell mediated. Thus, they depend on the injected product and not on the osmolality, iodine content, or ionization of the drug.

Literature on secondary prevention by premedication is not clear enough to draw conclusions. The prophylactic use of corticosteroids and antihistamines remain controversial, and premedication practice varies from country to country. Moreover, several anaphylactic reactions have been reported despite optimal pre-treatment.

Reactions Occurring in Intraoperative Lymphatic Mapping

A literature review may reveal an impressive number of case reports of hypersensitivity reactions using everyday products containing blue dyes [34]. Considering the increasing use of blue dyes for lymphatic mapping for sentinel lymph node biopsy, the incidence of anaphylaxis to these drugs can be expected to increase. The mechanisms underlying the allergic reaction to patent blue remain unclear. Sensitization may originate from the widespread use of these dyes in cosmetics and other everyday life objects. Both direct mast cell and/or basophil activation and cross-linking of specific IgE antibodies are possible causative factors. Evidence supporting an IgE-mediated mechanism at least in some patients comes from two clinical reports, the first one demonstrating an immune mediated mechanism by a passive transfer test, the second one demonstrating the presence of specific IgE detected by an enzyme immune assay (EIA).

Since anaphylactic reactions involving methylene blue seem less common, it has been proposed as a possible alternative. Probably this small molecule does not bind to plasma proteins, thus reducing the risk of sensitization to a hapten-protein complex. This dye differs structurally from isosulfan blue and patent blue V and therefore, cross- reactivity is not expected. However, several cases of sensitization to both patent blue and methylene blue have been reported, suggesting a possible immunologic cross-reactivity between these dyes. These reports support the systematic investigation of a possible cross- reactivity before the use of an alternate dye. A negative skin test with methylene blue in case of hypersensitivity reaction to patent blue V or isosulfan blue encourage the use of former (methylene blue) for future sentinel lymph node mapping [34-38]. Skin prick tests should be performed at a concentration of 2.5 mg/ml and intradermal tests at 0.25 mg/ml [39].

5. Etiology

NMBAs, Latex, Antibiotics

The overall distribution of the various causal agents incriminated in anaphylaxis during anaesthesia is very similar in most reported series. It is very important to know the exact epidemiology of the different agents in order to reduce risk factors as much as possible. In general, NMBAs represent the most frequently involved substances with 50% to 70% of reactions occurring during anaesthesia, followed by latex and antibiotics. Anaphylaxis usually occurs shortly after induction when causal agents are NMBAs or antibiotics, but it may occur any time with all potentially allergenic agents. The incidence of latex-induced anaphylaxis has dramatically increased over the past two decades, especially in high-risk patients such as healthcare workers or children and adults requiring multiple surgical procedures. On the other hand, the incidence of anaphylaxis to NMBAs during anaesthesia has decreased in Norway since an over-the-counter cough syrup containing pholcodine, a morphine analogue, was withdrawn from the market in 2007.

Any drug containing pholcodine was withdrawn from the market in Sweden in 1989 when new guidelines for the treatment of coughs were published, and different and more effective pharmacological preparations had become available. The cough syrup was withdrawn from the market in Norway when doctors realized that anaphylactic reactions to NMBAs were over six times more common in the Norwegian population than in the Sweden [40]. Allergic reactions to NMBAs are almost exclusively IgE-mediated. Therefore, if an individual develops anaphylaxis to an NMBA, this implies the presence of specific IgE antibodies on his mast cells and basophils at the time of exposure and reaction. Howeever, up to 75% of reactions have been reported upon first known contact with an NMBA. Indeed, recent studies have suggested that sensitization to NMBAs in the Norwegian population is likely be due to exposure to pholcodine, responsible for a significant increase in specific IgEs to NMBAs in patients having experienced an allergic reaction to one of these drugs.

Hypnotics

Recently, in a French study, thiopental has been reported as being involved in less than 1% of allergic reactions [41]. Since Cremophor EL, as a solvent for some non-barbiturate hypnotics, has been avoided, many previously reported hypersensitivity reactions have actually disappeared. In recent French surveys, reactions to propofol accounted for less than 2.5% of allergic reactions, and to midazolam, etomidate or ketamine appear to be rare. Finally, no immune mediated immediate hypersensitivity reaction involving isoflurane, desflurane or sevoflurane has been reported despite the wide use of these drugs [2,41].

Opioids

Reactions to morphine, codeine phosphate, meperidine, fentanyl and its derivatives are uncommon. Since morphine is known to induce non specific histamine release, skin testing is carried out cautiously at concentrations that are known as not being sufficient to cause histamine release (Table-1). Because of the direct histamine releasing properties typical of opioids, distinction between anaphylaxis and non immune-mediated histamine release is not always easy. Only twelve cases have been recorded during the past 2 years in an epidemiologic survey conducted in France, nine of which being related to morphine administration [41].

Local Anaesthetics

Local anaesthetics include amine (lidocaine, mepivacaine, prilocaine, bupivacaine, levobupivacaine, ropivacaine), and ester derivatives (chloroprocaine, procaine, tetracaine). Allergic reactions to local anaesthetics are very rare despite their frequent use and anaphylaxis has decreased in frequency because of the decreasing use of the ester group of local anaesthetics. It is estimated that less than 1% of all reactions to local anesthetics have an immune-mediated mechanism [1,42]. The most common causes of adverse reactions reported to these drugs are inadvertent intravascular injection leading to excessive blood concentrations of the local anaesthetic, or systemic absorption of epinephrine combined with the local anesthetic with consequent sympathomimetic effects. Allergy to local anesthetics may also be due to methylparaben, paraben or metabisulfite used as preservatives in commercial preparations.

NSAIDs

Nonsteroidal anti-inflammatory drugs (NSAIDs) may cause reactions, by inhibition of cyclo-oxygenase, resulting in generation of leukotrienes. NSAIDs are increasingly recognized as a cause of non IgE-mediated anaphylactic reactions [43]. They may be administered both during surgery or together with pre-medication, depending on the procedure. The onset of the reaction is usually up to 10 minutes after intravenous administration and 30- 60 minutes (or sometimes longer) after oral administration. If the reaction occurs at the end of surgery, induction agents may be immediately excluded, and the main differential diagnosis include reactions to NSAIDs, latex, chlorhexidine or colloids. Clinical patterns of NSAIDs allergy include generalized pruritus, erythema, urticaria, angioedema, rhinorrhea, asthma and anaphylactic shock. Pyrazolones may precipitate reactions ranging from urticaria and angioedema to anaphylactic shock, presumably by immunological IgE- mediated mechanism. There are no reliable diagnostic tests for NSAID intolerance, so that the diagnosis remains essentially clinical, after having excluded other potential causes. However, the diagnosis can be confirmed by provocation test, but such a procedure should be considered only when the history is unclear and it is mostly needed to confirm tolerability of alternative compounds.

Chlorhexidine

Several cases of allergic reactions to antiseptics have been reported in Literature. They mainly concern allergic reactions to chlorhexidine after insertion of central venous catheters impregnated with this antiseptic, or after intrauretheral use or topical application. Chlorhexidine is a synthetic cationic bis-biguanide, introduced in 1954, widely used as a disinfectant and antiseptic in medical and non-medical environments [44]. Chlorhexidine may be found in many commercially available products, such as mouthwashes, antiseptic creams, and disinfectant solutions. In a medical environment, chlorhexidine is used in alcoholic or aqueous solutions for skin disinfection before invasive procedures, and as a disinfectant hand wash. Chlorhexidine is also present in potentially hidden forms, such as bactericidal coating for central venous catheters or as a component of urethral lubricants.

Several factors may confound the clinical diagnosis of anaphylaxis to chlorhexidine, mainly a delayed presentation, or the fact that chlorhexidine is not a drug administrated by an anaesthetist and that it may be present in a covert form. Symptoms related to chlorhexidine allergy may appear up to 40 minutes after exposure [45].

Ethylene Oxyde

Ethylene oxyde (ETO), an alkylating compound of high chemical reactivity, is widely used as a sterilization gas for various medical devices that are heat-sensitive, such as catheters, infusions sets, gloves, suture sets, surgical drapes and certain implantable materials such as ventriculoperitoneal shunts. This type of sterilization may cause rare but severe IgE-mediated allergic reactions, in sensitive patients, in particular in patients presenting with myelomeningocele or in hemodialysis, with a reported prevalence of sensitization in these groups of 23% and 12.1% respectively.

A Danish study has showed that sIgE to ETO can vary over time [46]. The fact that ETO is highly toxic, a hapten, and a gas, it makes it difficult to produce standardized material for skin tests, challenge studies, and *in vitro* tests.

6. Diagnosis

The clinical diagnosis of an immediate hypersensitivity reaction occurring during anaesthesia is generally considered to be a difficult task for clinicians. When anaphylaxis occurs during anaesthesia, it may present as cardiovascular collapse or airway obstruction, with or without associated cutaneous manifestations. The signs of anaphylaxis occurring during anaesthesia differ to some extent from the signs and symptoms that occur during anaphylaxis not associated with anaesthesia (for example, all early symptoms such as malaise, pruritus and dizziness are absent in anaesthetized patient). Close vigilance is therefore essential since most reactions should be well known to the anaesthetist even before they appear.

Several excellent guidelines for the investigation of suspected anaphylaxis have been recently published by anaesthesiology and/or allergy societies [14]. Any suspected hypersensitivity reaction during anaesthesia must be extensively investigated using combined perioperative and post operative testing to confirm the nature of reactions, to identify the responsible drug, to detect possible cross reactivity and to provide recommendations for future anaesthetic procedures [46].

The diagnostic strategy is based on a detailed history including concurrent morbidity, previous anaesthetic history, any known allergies and a combination of investigations performed both immediately and days to weeks later (Figure-3). Early tests are essentially designed to determine whether an immunologic mechanism is involved while skin tests attempt to identify the responsible drug [48].

Laboratory tests are valuable in the diagnosis of anaphylaxis, although no test is a specific and sensitive marker for an allergic hypersensitivity reaction, plasma tryptase has a low sensitivity but high specificity [49]. Detection of the causative allergen is based on retrospective analysis of the clinical manifestations and timing of the onset of symptoms (such as hypotension) after exposure to culprit drug/agent, the measurement of tryptase levels and signs and symptoms of the reaction [50]. However, skin testing should not be used for preoperative screening without a previous clinical history of hypersensitivity [20]. If anaphylaxis is suspected intraoperatively, serum markers of mast cell activation should be analyzed: histamine and tryptase. Tryptase confirms an immune mediated reaction because it is released by mast cells and basophils [51]. Although a rise in serum tryptase simply indicates mast cell degranulation and does not discriminate between allergic and non allergic anaphylaxis, it has been proposed that increased tryptase concentrations exceeding 25 mcg/l suggests an IgE mediated mechanism. A normal acute plasma tryptase, however does not exclude anaphylaxis. The concentrations of tryptase are often normal in mild reactions and elevated mainly in systemic reactions.

Biological evidence of anaphylaxis includes an increase in level of total tryptase and beta-tryptase within 30 to 120 minutes after the onset of symptoms. A baseline total tryptase level should be tested at ≥24 hours. Histamine concentrations are maximal almost immediately and decrease thereafter with a half life of about 20 min because it is degraded very quickly and so a serum histamine level is not a reliable marker. A 24-hour urine collection for histamine and N-methyl histamine levels may be diagnostic [50,52]. After a reaction during general anaesthesia, a diagnostic evaluation by an allergist-immunologist is recommended [51]. This would include thorough evaluation of medical and allergic history, comorbidities, scrutinisation of anaesthetic/drug charts, plasma tryptase levels (acute and baseline), and allergy testing (skin tests, *in vitro* tests and drug provocative tests when indicated) as dictated by the clinical scenario [53]. To gain information for perioperative anaphylaxis cases, several websites may be helpful to clinicians, such as the site of the Association of Anaesthetists of Great Britain & Ireland (http://www.aagbi.org). Skin testing by prick and intradermal injection of a dilute concentration of the allergen is recommended postoperatively to confirm the trigger [50]. Detailed recommendations of the maximum concentration to be used for most of the drugs and substances used in the perioperative period have been published [54] (Table-1). Currently, skin tests are the most reliable method to determine the trigger [14]. Skin prick and/or intradermal tests are usually performed 4-6 weeks after the acute reaction. Recent recommendations however suggest that skin testing can be performed immediately after a reaction. [55].

Significant progress had been made with *in vitro* tests relating to specific IgE measurements and basophil activation tests (BATs). The availability of radioimmunoassays for the range of drugs and agents involved in perioperative anaphylaxis remains limited. NMBAs, latex, thiopental, chlorexidine and some antibiotics are the few classes of drugs/agents for which these tests are available. Basophil activation assays (histamine release assay, BAT, and leukotriene release test) have been proposed as possible methods to investigate hypersensitivity reactions. These tests may be used when skin test results are difficult to interpret or not feasible. Although not currently widely used, these tests seem to have a good specificity and have been successfully used in several situations.

Drug provocation tests (DPT) have limited indications in perianaesthetic anaphylaxis. When the clinical history is compatible with the report of an immediate hypersensitivity reaction, these tests can be performed with drugs for which skin tests cannot be conducted or when skin tests are negative (local anaesthetics, antibiotics, or, exceptionally, latex) or not validated (NSAIDs). For anaesthetics, this gold standard allergy test cannot be employed because of pharmacological effects of these drugs. Thus, it is only possible to demonstrate sensitization to a drug indirectly, eg, by a positive skin test result or demonstration of specific IgE with no final confirmation. When the allergen is not present in a suitably reactive form (drug metabolites), only provocation tests can confirm the diagnosis. This is applicable when skin tests for ß-lactams are negative, as well as for some other non–ß-lactam antibiotics and NSAIDs. Tests are conducted at least 1 month after the hypersensitivity reaction using the same drug and often the same route of administration (if the preferred route of oral provocation is not suitable) as when the reaction occurred. They should be conducted under strict supervision and only in specialized centers with monitoring and resuscitation facilities.

Drugs are administered in a graded fashion starting at a small dose, with a minimum interval of 30 minutes between each step and escalation is performed if good tolerance is established at the previous dose and until the full therapeutic dose is reached [56].

Skin prick test with latex extracts are sensitive, specific and rapid. Significant variability in the allergen content of extracts continues to limit the reproducibility of the test. Diagnostic sensitivity of different latex extracts for SPTs could differ; ammoniated latex extracts have higher sensitivity if compared to non-ammoniated products [57]. If clinical history, SPT to latex and determination of specific serum IgE to latex are not sufficient to arrive at a correct diagnosis of latex allergy, an *in vivo* provocation tests may be used, which may include natural environmental exposure, glove use and rubbing tests and nasal, mucosal, conjunctival and bronchial provocation tests (Figure-3) [58]. The presence of specific IgE to latex is a marker of sensitization only without correlation with clinical reactivity [59]. In addition, serum-specific IgEs to recombinant allergens are a useful diagnostic tool to confirm the diagnosis of latex allergy (*Hevea brasilienses allergens*). Component-resolved diagnosis for latex allergens is indeed needed to assess the patient sensitization profile: in fact, the quantification of specific IgE responses to the spectrum of documented natural rubber latex allergens and the evaluation of a possible sensitization to cross-reactive carbohydrate determinants (CCDs) are necessary to reach a definitive diagnosis.

Hev b 1, 2, 5, 6.01 and 13 have been identified as major latex allergens and they should be present both in standardized latex extracts and *in vitro* allergosorbents. In particular, rHev b 6.01 and rHev b 5 specific IgE are considered as the major allergens to cause latex allergy. sIgE against rHev b1 and rHev b 3 are usually found in multi-operated patients; rHev b 8 is a helpful marker to highlight latex/pollen cross-reactivity, improving the specificity of the serological tests; CCDs have a minor role in patients presenting with clinical symptoms of latex allergy.

When a patient is thought to have presented a hypersensitivity reaction to an antibiotic, skin testing is the basic diagnostic tool. In both the ENDA document and the American practice parameters, skin testing were standardized for beta lactams but not for other antibiotics. For the procedure, it is recommended to perform prick testing first, and if results are negative, the intradermal test should be performed [56]. For the risk of a systemic reaction, certain precautions should be taken during skin testing, e.g. strict supervision in the hospital during and after (at least 1 hour) skin testing [60].

In vitro tests can be used: detection of specific IgE antibodies to betalactam antibiotics through immunoassays and detection on the basis of basophil activation on contact with the hapten, either by quantification of mediator release (histamine or leukotrienes) or basophil activation marker expression [56].

To confirm the diagnosis, drug provocation tests (DPT) could be used. A lower starting dose should be used in patients with severe reactions and the cumulative dose should be adapted for children or persons with kidney or liver disease. DPTs are also useful to assess cross-reactivity between different BLs.

In suspected case of muscle relaxant anaphylaxis, skin tests are ‘gold standard’ for diagnosis of NMBA allergy with high sensitivity. Standardized procedures and dilutions must be used for each tested agent in order to avoid false positive results due to any direct histamine releasing properties as it is the case for known histamine releasing compounds such as mivacurium, atracurium and tubocurarine (Table-1). Detailed recommendations for skin test dilutions of anaesthetic drugs including NMBAs have recently also been proposed by the SFAR (Société Française d’Anesthésie et de Réanimation) and SFAIC (Société Française d’Allergologie et d’Immunologie Clinique) [61]. IDTs should be undertaken if SPTs are negative for a drug suspected to be the cause. In patients who presented with an allergic reaction to NMBA, all neuromuscular blocking agents should be tested, because cross reactivity occurs commonly[62,63]. It was recently demonstrated that skin tests show an excellent negative predictive value (NPV) in patients with an allergic hypersensitivity reaction to NMBAs. Nevertheless, the number of patients included in the study was small, and larger studies are therefore needed to establish NPV of these tests [64].

Immediate hypersensitivity reactions to ICM are relatively rare in the perioperative period. They are mainly observed prior to surgery during radiologic investigations in emergency situations or during anaesthesia outside the operating room [65]. Several studies have shown that skin tests are useful tools for the diagnosis of ICM allergy, when the test is conducted within 2-6 months after the reaction, and the negative predictive value of ICM skin tests is 96.6%. However, further studies involving a larger sample size are required [66].

Skin tests should include skin prick tests, with the drug at the concentration commonly used for injections, followed by intradermal tests with the drug diluted at 10% of the commercially available concentration. If the patient's history is severe, both skin prick tests and intradermal tests should start at lower concentrations (0.1-1%).

Uncommon Agents

Hypnotics may be skin tested according to the concentration limits provided in Table 1.

Skin prick tests, possibly followed, when negative, by intradermal tests, are performed with phenylpiperidines (alfentanil, fentanyl, remifentanil, sufentanil). Cross-reactivity remains uncommon among phenylpiperidines [50].

Local anaesthetics may be skin tested without preservatives or epinephrine, according to the concentration limits provided in Table 1.

The clinical diagnosis of reactions elicited by dyes is difficult. Reactions are usually long lasting and relatively delayed (i.e. thirty minutes after injection), and justify a prolonged follow-up in an intensive care unit, if prolonged epinephrine administration is necessary [67]. Dyes may be skin tested by prick tests followed by intradermal tests (with maximum dilution of 1/100 for the histamine-releaser methylene blue, and of 1/10 for isosulfan/ patent blue) [50].

7. Prevention

The prevention of anaphylaxis after administration of general anaesthetics would require the identification of patients 'at risk', but this approach is not easy to implement considering the large number of drugs, diagnostic reagents, devices containing latex, antiseptics and blood products that are all routinely used in anaesthesia [68].

Any patient with a history of previous anaphylaxis or severe reaction during anaesthesia should be referred to an allergist for diagnostic evaluation. However, the identification of the triggering agent is not always feasible because of the low accuracy of tests [19].

Prevention of anaphylaxis has two major objectives: 1) preventing sensitization of a patient to a particular allergen, and 2) preventing, in a sensitized patient, the occurrence of an anaphylactic reaction to an introduced allergen that has already been presented to the immune system. In this regard, in the wake of the relatively high rate of sensitization in the absence of any prior exposure, optimal prevention of sensitization to NMBAs, even if their administration were to be radically curtailed, will be probably difficult to achieve [69].

In patients with an allergy to a particular antibiotic, the most important prevention represents avoidance of antibiotics with the same chemical structure. Allergic reactions to β-lactam drugs are the most frequent and more studied; and so the safest therapeutic approach to patients who are allergic to penicillin is to administer antibiotics that do not contain a β-lactam ring [19].

In case of latex allergy, primary prevention is achieved by reducing contact with latex products, while secondary prevention strategy must include a 'latex free environment', that should be established not only in the room or surgical suite but also in the ward and in all clinical settings [19].

Considering the relatively high rate of sensitisation without prior exposure, optimal prevention of sensitisation to NMBAs will be probably be difficult to achieve. Pre-treatment with corticosteroids or histamine receptor antagonists, by either H1 or H1 and H2 receptor antagonists remains controversial. Pre-treatment with H1 and H2 receptor antagonists has been found to reduce histamine mediated but not immune reactions [70]. Moreover, several anaphylactic reactions have been reported despite optimal pre-treatment [71]. Literature on secondary prevention by premedication is not clear enough to draw conclusions.

A careful clinical history has a critical role in identifying patients at increased risk of developing reactions during anaesthesia. Prevention of perioperative allergic reactions relies on the identification of the offending agent by an allergist. However, a guaranteed 'primary' or 'secondary' prevention is not possible to achieve, due to the relatively high rate of sensitization to anaesthetics in the absence of prior exposure or 'risk factors' and to the low diagnostic accuracy of IgE tests respectively [19].

8. Treatment

When a perioperative allergic reaction occurs, there is a wide spectrum of clinical features that may be recorded. Although the management of such reactions should be tailored to an individual patient, in order to achieve the best clinical outcome, the two therapeutic cornerstones are early and prompt administration of epinephrine and fluids. Epinephrine is a powerful and effective treatment in most cases of severe systemic reactions or anaphylaxis and the dose should be titrated carefully and may have to be repeated until the patients show a therapeutic response. Its α–agonist action reverses the vasodilatation and oedema typical of anaphylaxis, while its β-agonistic property act on the airways, increases the cardiac output and suppresses the release of inflammatory mediators such as leukotrienes and histamine. If administered early, intravenous doses of 10-25 μg of epinephrine in children and 10-50 μg in adults are sufficient to reverse anaphylaxis. The relatively rare fatalities in anaphylaxis are usually caused by a delay or a lack of administration of the drug [14].

Steroids and antihistamines are useful to treat symptoms included in the early symptoms of anaphylaxis, such as generalized cutaneous signs, erythema, urticaria and angioedema. However, both drugs are valid as a second line treatment for systemic reactions and severe forms of anaphylaxis, as they help preventing the appearance of edema and other cutaneous symptoms and a relapse of systemic (biphasic) reactions that may occur up to 24 hours after the initial reaction is recorded.

An early recognition of clinical features of perioperative allergy is essential in order to commence prompt and adequate treatment, to reduce symptoms, and to avoid both severe forms of anaphylaxis and myocardial ischemia and therefore to achieve a faster and better resolution of severe symptoms. Several recent case reports suggest that the administration of sugammadex, a chemically modified gamma-cyclodextrin used to quickly reverse the effects of the rocuronium–induced neuromuscular blockade, might be useful in mitigating recuronium-induced anaphylaxis. If the efficacy of sugammadex will be confirmed, the possibility of new therapies should be considered in cases of difficult-to-treat anaphylaxis [14].

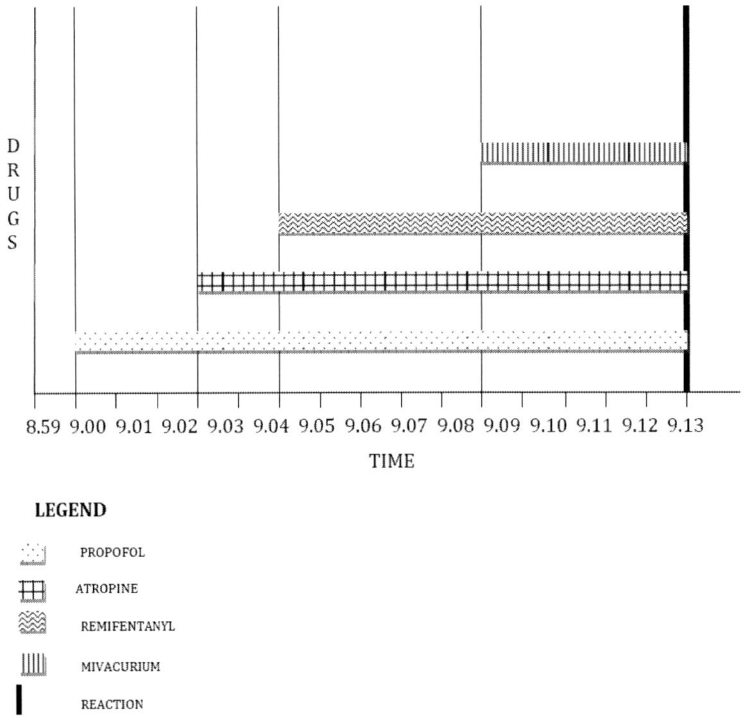

Figure 4. Case-1: Sequence of injection of the drugs before the allergic reaction. Fifteen minutes after induction, the patient presented a generalized erythema and urticaria.

Clinical Cases

Case 1

An 8-year old female patient was investigated for a history of an immediate hypersensitivity reaction occurred during general anaesthesia (Figure 4). She was anaesthetized for an adeno-tonsillectomy. After induction of the anaesthesia, she immediately developed generalized erythema and urticaria but showed no cardiorespiratory involvement. Symptoms settled after an i.v. injection of 10 mg of chlorphenamine.

She was not atopic and did not suffer from allergic conditions such as rhinitis, asthma, eczema, food or known drug allergy.

Investigations

1. Plasma tryptase taken during the reaction, 2 and 24 hours later were 14.9, 7.3, and 3 mcg/l, respectively.
2. Skin prick tests were negative for latex and drugs used during induction: propofol 10 mg/ml, atropine 0.25mg/ml, remifentanil 1 mg/ml and mivacurium 0.2 mg/ml. Intradermal test were positive to mivacurium at a concentration of 0.02 mg/ml, with an increase in wheal diameterof 6 mm. Intradermal tests were also positive to cis-atracurium and vecuronium, while they were negative to rocuronium (Table 3).

Table 3. Drugs concentrations and results of skin tests in the 1st case report

DRUG	Prick test	IDR 1/100	IDR 1/10
Propofol 10 mg/ml	neg	neg	neg
Atropine 0.25 mg/ml	neg	neg	neg
Remifentanil 1 mg/ml	neg	neg	neg
Mivacurium 0.2 mg/ml	neg	neg	pos
Cisatracurium 2 mg/ml	neg	pos	
Vecuronium 4 mg/ml	neg	neg	pos
Rocuronium 10 mg/ml	neg	neg	neg

The patient and her parents were properly informed of the results of the investigations and of the potential risk for a new episode of anaphylaxis during a future surgical intervention, unless a safe alternative neuro-muscular blocking agent was detected. We therefore continued our investigations, and were able to find a safe alternative and the patient received an ‘allergic patient identity card’, explaining the previous episode, the drugs to which she is allergic and the possible safe alternatives we found.

Case 2

A 15-years old female patient suffering from metrorrhagia needed to start therapy with iron supplements and progesterone. Nevertheless, since she reported two episodes of hypersensitivity reactions during previous surgeries, she was referred to our centre for an allergy work-up.

She was not atopic and did not suffer from allergic conditions including atopic eczema, allergic rhinoconjucntivitis or asthma. Both her reactions occurred during two surgical interventions for bilateral flat feet. The first one occurred 45 minutes after the beginning of the intervention on the first foot, and she presented with generalized urticaria associated with hypotension and tachycardia; the second one, occurring a year later, when she was being operated on the contralateral foot, and was characterized by urticaria, tachycardia, mild hypotension (90/50 mmHg) and bronchospasm, occurring 35 minutes after the beginning of the surgical procedure. Administered drugs included: propofol, fentanyl, sevoflurane, ceftriaxone and acetaminophen (Figure 5a and 5b).

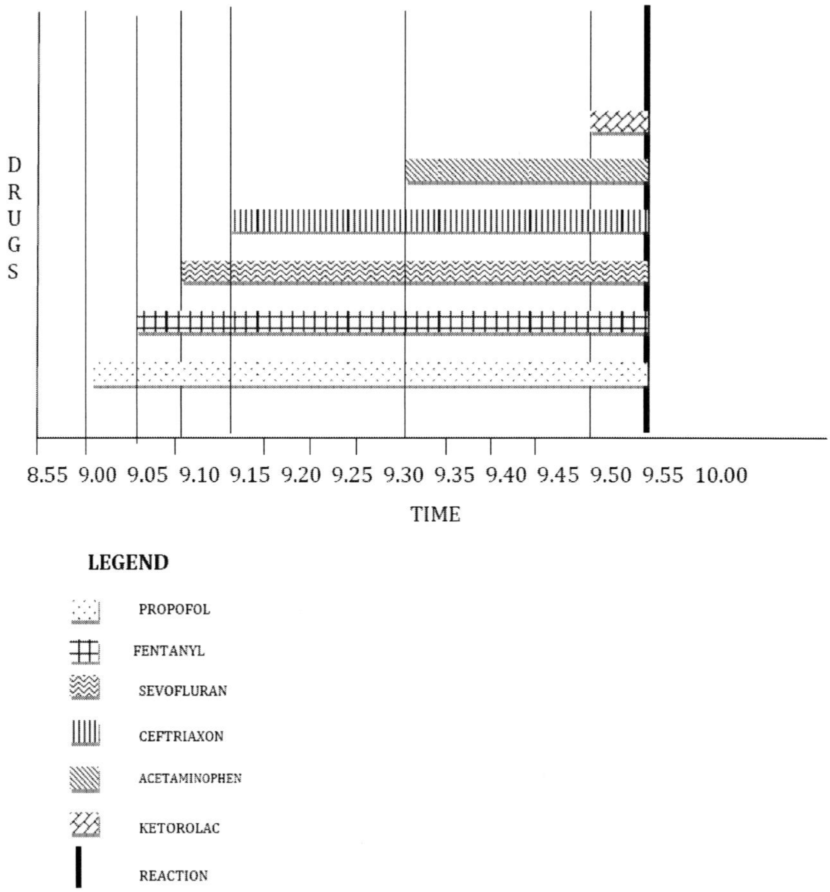

Figure 5a. Case 2: Sequence of injection of the drugs before the allergic reaction, during the first surgery for flat foot. Fourty-five minutes after the beginning of the intervention, the patient presented generalized urticaria associated with hypotension.

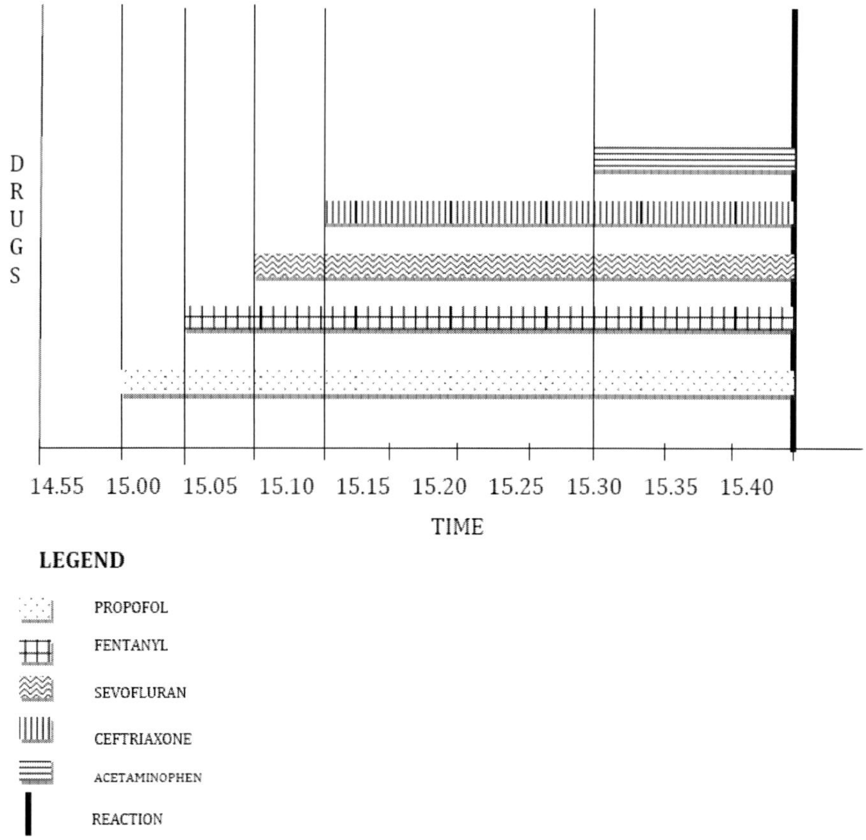

Figure 5b. Case 2: Sequence of injection of the drugs before the allergic reaction, during the second surgery for flat foot. Thirty-five minutes after the beginning of the intervention, the patient presented urticaria, tachycardia, mild hypotension (90/50 mmHg), and bronchospasm.

The first reaction was treated with methylprednisolone and ethylephrine chlorhydrate and the surgery was completed; nevertheless, during the second reaction, an injection of ketorolac at the end of the procedure worsened the angioedema of the hands and of the face. The symptoms disappeared after injection of methylprednisolone, adrenaline and nebulised salbutamol.

Investigations

1. Plasma tryptase taken during the reaction, and 2 and 24 hours later were 13.5, 6.8, and 2.3 mcg/l, respectively.
2. Skin prick tests were negative for latex, propofol 10 mg/ml, fentanyl (0.05 mg/ml) and ceftriaxone; intradermal test were positive for ceftriaxone (wheal increase of 5 mm of diameter) at a concentration of 2 mg/ml, but negative for all other administered drugs (Table 4). Basophil Activation Test was strongly positive for ceftriaxone as well.

Table 4. Drugs concentrations and results of skin tests, in the 2nd case report

DRUG	Prick test	IDR 1/100	IDR 1/10	IDR 1
Propofol 10 mg/ml	neg	Neg	neg	
Fentanyl 0.05mg/ml	neg	Neg	neg	
Ceftriaxone 2 mg/ml	neg	Neg	neg	pos

The patient was properly informed of the results of the investigations and of the potential risk for a new episode of anaphylaxis if re-exposed to ceftriaxone. We found an alternative beta-lactam (cefuroxime) that she might take, if needed, and we gave the patient an 'allergic patient identity card', explaining the previous episode, the drugs to which she is allergic and the possible safe alternatives.

Conclusion

Perioperative anaphylactic reactions are potentially life-threatening immediate hypersensitivity reactions, unrelated to the drug's pharmacological characteristics. They correspond to immune-mediated allergic and non immune-mediated "pseudo-allergic or anaphylactoid" reactions. Perioperative anaphylaxis has become more and more common, probably because of a more frequent use of general anaesthesia and of an increased complexity of the administered drugs. On the other side, it has to be stated that the real incidence of these reactions is still underestimated, since it is underreported. Neuromuscular blocking agents represent the most frequently involved allergens, followed by latex and antibiotics. Nevertheless, each drug or substance used during surgery may be involved in an anaphylactic reaction. Since the introduction in modern anaesthesic procedures of NMBAs, much progress has been made in the identification of adverse reactions to these agents, and in their potential mechanisms. However, despite the introduction of newer drugs in clinical practice, the incidence of serious immediate reactions has remained virtually unchanged.

Since no premedication may effectively prevent an allergic reaction, any suspected hypersensitivity reaction must be extensively investigated using combined peri and postoperative testing. Diagnosis relies on specific tryptase measurements, and evaluation of specific IgE levels (and basophil activation tests) right after the reaction, and skin tests 4-6 weeks after the anaphylaxis has occurred; serum tests should be repeated at this time as well.

Patients must be fully informed of the results of the allergy work-up, and advised to provide a detailed report prior to future anaesthesia. Vigilance for any signs of anaphylaxis and consideration of the risk factors, with possible modification of the administered agents, will likely reduce the morbidity and mortality associated with these reactions. The wearing of a warning bracelet as well as the possession of a warning card is strongly indicated in all patients reporting a previous allergic perioperative reaction.

Clinical Pearls

- An allergic evaluation is mandatory for all immediate hypersensitivity reactions and should be advised in case of delayed reactions as well.
- The incidence of IgE-mediated hypersensitivity reactions occurring during anaesthesia has been estimated being around 100.6 per million procedures.
- Clinical symptoms are the cornerstones of the evaluation of a drug hypersensitivity reaction.
- Neuromuscular blocking agents are most frequently involved during anaesthesia (50-70% of the reactions), followed by latex and antibiotics.
- Allergic reactions to local anaesthetics are very rare.
- Several excellent guidelines for the investigation of suspected allergic reactions have been recently published by anaesthesiology and/or allergy societies.
- Skin testing by prick or intradermal injection of a dilute concentration of the allergen is recommended 4-6 weeks after the surgery, to confirm the culpability of an allergen.
- Serial plasma tryptase levels should be measured after the reaction, since they actually document mast cell activation and may help to confirm an allergic reaction.
- The main risk factor for perioperative anaphylaxis is a previous immediate perioperative reaction.
- Literature on secondary prevention by premedication is not clear enough to draw conclusions.
- Epinephrine is a powerful and efficient treatment in most cases of severe systemic reactions or anaphylaxis.

References

[1] Laxemaire, MC; Mertes, PM. Anaphylaxis during anaesthesia. Results of a two-year survey in France. *Bt J Anaest*, 2001, 87, 549-58.

[2] Mertes, PM; Laxenaire, MC; Alla, F. Anaphylactic and anaphylactoid reactions occurring during anaesthesia in France in, 1999-2000. *Anesthesiology*, 2003, 99, 536-45.

[3] Florvaag, E; Jihansson, SG; Irgens, A; de Pater, GH. IgE – sensitization to cough suppressant pholcodine and the effects of its withdrawal from the Norwegian market. *Allergy*, 2011, 66, 955-60.

[4] Hayward, RA; Hofer, TP. Estimating hospital deaths due to medical errors: preventability is in the eye of the reviewer. *JAMA*, 2001, 286, 415-20.

[5] Laxenaire, MC. What is the real risk of drug hypersensitivity in anesthesia? Incidence. Clinical aspects. Morbidity-mortality. Substances responsible. *Ann Fr Anesth Reanim*, 2002, 21 Suppl 1, 38s-54s.

[6] Fisher, MM; More, DG. The epidemiology and clinical features of anaphylactic reactions in anaesthesia. *Anaesth Intensive Care*, 1981, 9(3), 226-34.

[7] Mertes, PM; Laxenaire, MC. Allergic reactions occurring during anaesthesia. *Eur J Anaesthesiol*, 2002, 19, 240-62.

[8] Watkins, J. Adverse anaesthetic reactions. An update from a proposed national reporting and advisory service. *Anaesthesia*, 1985, 40(8), 797-800.

[9] Thienthong, S; Hintong, T; Pulnitiporn, A. The Thai Anesthesia Incidents Study (THAI Study) of perioperative allergic reactions. *J Med Assoc Thai*, 2005, 88, Suppl 7, S128-33.

[10] Whittington, T; Fisher, MM. Anaphylactic and anaphylactoid reactions. Clinical Anaesthesiology. *Br Clin Anaesthesiol*, 1998, 12, 301-323.

[11] Laxenaire, MC. Epidémiologie des réactions anaphylactoïdes peranesthésiques. Quatrième enquête multicentrique (juillet 1994-décembre 1996). *Ann Fr Anesth Reanim*, 1999, 18, 796-809.

[12] Escolano, F; Valero, A; Huguet, J; Baxarias, P; de Molina, M; Castro, A; Granel, C; Sanosa, J; Bartolomé, B. Grupo de estudio de anafilaxia perioperatoria en Cataluña. Prospective epidemiologic study of perioperative anaphylactoid reactions occurring in Catalonia (1996-7). *Rev Esp Anestesiol Reanim*, 2002, 49(6):286-93.

[13] Harboe, T; Guttormsen, AB; Irgens, A; Dybendal, T; Florvaag, E. Anaphylaxis during anesthesia in Norway: A 6–year single-center follow-up study. *Anesthesiology*, 2005, 102, 897-903.

[14] Mertes, PM; Demoly, P; Malinovsky, JM. Hypersensitivity reactions in the anesthesia setting/allergic reactions to anesthetics. *Curr Opin Allergy Clin Immunol*, 2012, 12, 361-368.

[15] Lobera, T; Audicana, MT; Pozo, MD; Blasco, A; Fernandez, E; Canada, P; Gastaminza, G; Martinez-Albelda, I; Gonzalez-Mahave, I; Munoz, D. Study of hypersensitivity reactions and anaphylaxis during anesthesia in Spain. *J Investig Allergol Clin Immunol*, 2008, 18, 350-6.

[16] Mertes, PM; Laxenaire, MC. Allergy and anaphylaxis in anesthesia. *Minerva Anestesiol*, 2004, 70, 285-91.

[17] Venturini, M; Lobera, T; Del Pozzo, MD; Gonzalez, I; Blasco, A. Immediate hypersensitivity to corticosteroids. *J Investig Allergol Clin Immunol*, 2006, 16, 51-56.

[18] Fisher, MM; Baldo, BA. The incidence and clinical features of anaphylactic reactions during anesthesia in Australia. *Ann Fr Anesth Reanim*, 1993, 12, 97-104.

[19] Caffarelli, C; Stringari, G; Pajno, GB; Peroni, DG; Franceschini, F; Dello Iacono, I; Bernardini, R. Perioperative allergy: risk factors. *Int J Immunopathol Pharmacol*, 2011, 24 (3S):S27-34.

[20] Norred, CL. Anesthetic Induced Anaphylaxis. Update for nurse Anesthetists. *AANA Journal*, 2012, 80, 129-40.

[21] Mertes, PM; Gastin, A; Faivre, MC; Gueant, JL; et al. Hypersensitivity reactions to neuromuscular blocking agents. *Curr Pharm Des*, 2008, 14, 2809-25.

[22] Hofer, KN; McCarthy, MW; Buck, ML; Hendrick, AE. Possible anaphylaxis after propofol in a child with food allergy. *Annals of Pharmacotherapy*, 2003, 37, 398–401.

[23] Harper, NJN; Chairman, N; Dixon, T; Dugue´, P; Edgar, DM; Fay, A; Gooi, HC; Herriot, R; Hopkins, P; Hunter, JM; Mirakian, R; Pumphrey, RSH; Seneviratne, SL; Walls, AF; Williams, P; Wildsmith, JA; Wood, P. Ex Officio: Nasser AS; Powell RK; Mirakhur R; Soar J; Executive Officers, AAGBI. Suspected anaphylactic reactions associated with anaesthesia. Association of Anaesthetists of Great Britain and Ireland. *Anaesthesia*, 2009, 64, 199-211.

[24] Hepner, DL; Castells, MC. Latex allergy: an update. *Anesth Analg*, 2003, 96(4), 1219-29.

[25] Mertes, PM; Alla, F; Trèchet, P; Auroy, Y; Jougla, E; Groupe d'Etudes des Rèactions AnaphylactoidesParanesthésiques. Anaphylaxis during anesthesia in France: an 8-year national survey. *J Allergy Clin Immunol*, 2011, 128(2), 366-73.

[26] Ebo, DG; Fisher, MM; Hagendorens, MM; Bridts, CH; Stevens, WJ. Anaphylaxis during anaesthesia: diagnostic approach. *Allergy*, 2007, 62, 471–87.

[27] Romano, A; Gaeta, F; Valluzzi, RL; Caruso, C; Rumi, G; Bousquet, PJ. IgE-mediated hypersensitivity to cephalosporins: cross-reactivity and tolerability pf penicillins, monobactams, and carbapenems. *J Allergy Clin Immunol.*, 2010, 126(5):994-9.

[28] Torres, MJ; Romano, A; Mayorga, C. diagnostic evaluation of a large group of patients with immediate allergy to penicillins: the role of skin testing. *Allergy*, 2001, 56, 850-56.

[29] Johansson, SG; Bieber, T; Dahl, R; Friedmann, PS; Lanier, BQ; Lockey, RF; Motala, C; Ortega Martell, JA; Platts-Mills, TA; Ring, J; Thien, F; Van Cauwenberge, P; Williams, HC. Revised nomenclature for allergy for global use: Report of the Nomenclature Review Committee of the World Allergy Organization, October 2003. *J Allergy Clin Immunol*, 2004, 113, 832-36.

[30] Lieberman, P. Anaphylactic reactions during surgical and medical procedures. *J Allergy Clin Immunol*, 2002, 110, S64-69.

[31] Singh, J; Daftary, A. Iodinated contrast media and their adverse reactions. *J Nucl Med Technol*, 2008, 36, 69-74.

[32] Katayama, H; Yamaguchi, K; Kozuka, T; Takashima, T; Seez, P; Matsuura, K. Adverse reactions to ionic and nonionic contrast media. A report from the Japanese Committee on the Safety of Contrast Media. *Radiology*, 1990, 175, 621-28.

[33] Brockow, K; Christiansen, C; Kanny, G; Clément, O; Barbaud, A; Bircher, A; Dewachter, P; Guéant, JL; Rodriguez Guéant, RM; Mouton-Faivre, C; Ring, J; Romano, A; Sainte-Laudy, J; Demoly, P; Pichler, WJ. ENDA; EAACI interest group on drug hypersensitivity. Management of hypersensitivity reactions to iodinated contrast media. *Allergy*, 2005, 60, 150.

[34] Cimmino, VM; Brown, AC; Szocik, JF; Pass, HA; Moline, S; De, SK; Domino, EF. Allergic reactions to isosulfan blue during sentinel node biopsy--a common event. *Surgery*, 2001, 130, 439-42.

[35] Pevny, I; Bohndorf, W. Group allergy due to patent blue sensitization. *Med Klin*, 1972, 67, 698-702.

[36] Wohrl, S; Focke, M; Hinterhuber, G; Stingl, G; Binder, M. Near-fatal anaphylaxis to patent blue V. *Br J Dermatol*, 2004, 150, 1037-38.

[37] Mertes, PM; Malinovsky, JM; Mouton-Faivre, C; Bonnet- Boyer, MC; Benhaijoub, A; Lavaud, F; Valfrey, J; O'Brien, J; Pirat, P; Lalourcey, L; Demoly, P. Anaphylaxis to dyes during the perioperative period: reports of 14 clinical cases. *J Allergy Clin Immunol*, 2008, 122, 348-52.

[38] Keller, B; Yawalkar, N; Pichler, C; Braathen, LR; Hunger, RE. Hypersensitivity reaction against patent blue during sentinel lymph node removal in three melanoma patients. *Am J Surg*, 2007, 193, 122-24.

[39] Haque, RA; Wagner, A; Whisken, JA; Nasser, SM; Ewan, PW. Anaphylaxis to patent blue V: a casa series and proposed diagnostic protocol. *Allergy.*, 2010, 65, 396-400.

[40] Baldo, BA; Fisher, MM; Pham, NH. On the origin and specificity of antibodies to neuromuscular blocking (muscle relaxant) drugs: an immunochemical perspective. *Clin Exp Allergy*, 2009, 39, 325-44.

[41] Mertes, PM; Laxenaire, MC. Anaphylactic and anaphylactoid reactions occurring during anaesthesia in France. Seventh epidemiologic survey (January 2001-December 2002). *Ann Fr Anesth Reanim*, 2004, 23, 1133-43.

[42] Fisher, MM; Bowey, CJ. Alleged allergy to local anaesthetics. *Anaesth Intensive Care*, 1997, 25, 611-14.

[43] Nizankwska-Mogilnicka, E; Bochenek, G; Mastalerz, L; Swierczynska, M; Picado, C; Scadding, G; Kowalski, ML; Setkowicz, M; Ring, J; Brockow, K; Bachert, C; Wohrl, S; Dalén, B; Szczeklik, A. EAACI/GA2LEN guideline: aspirin provocation tests for diagnosis of aspirin hypersensitivity. *Allergy*, 2007, 62, 1111-18.

[44] Garvey, LH; Kroigaard, M; Poulsen, LK; Skov, PS; Mosbech, H; Venemalm, L; Degerbeck, F; Husum, B. IgE-mediated allergy to chlorhexidine. *J Allergy Clin Immunol*, 2007, 120, 409-15.

[45] Parkes, AW; Harper, N; Herwadkar, A; Pumphrey, R. Anaphylaxis to the chlorhexidine component of Instllagel: a case series. *Br J of Anesthesia*, 2009, 120, 65-68.

[46] Opstrup, MS; Mosbech, H; Garvey, LH. Allergic sensitization to ethylene oxide in patients with suspected allergic rractions during surgery and anesthesia. *J Investig Allergol Clin Immunol*, 2010, 20, 267-72.

[47] Kroigaard, M; Garvey, LH; Gillbert, L. Dcandinavian clinical practise guidelines on the diagnosis, management and follow-up of anaphylaxis during anesthesia. *Acta Anaesthesiol Scand*, 2007, 51, 655-70.

[48] Mertes, PM. Perioperative anaphylaxis. *Immunol Allergy Clin N Am*, 2009, 429-51

[49] Harper, NJN; Dixon, T; Dugué, P; et al; and the Working Party of the Association of Anaesthetists of Great Britain and Ireland. Guidelines: suspected anaphylactic reactions associated with anaesthesia. *Anaesthesia.*, 2009, 64, 199-211.

[50] Dewachter, P; Mouton-Faivre, D; Emala, CW. Anaphylaxis and anesthesia: controversies and new insights. *Anesthesiology.*, 2009, 111, 1141-50.

[51] Dewachter, P; Mouton-Faivre, C; Castells, MC; Hepner, DL. Anesthesia in the patient with multiple drug allergies: are all allergies the same? *Curr Opin Anaesthesiol.*, 2011, 24, 320-25.

[52] Dong, SW; Mertes, PM; Petitpain, N; Hasdenteufel, F; Malinovsky, JM. Hypersensitivity reactions during anaesthesia. Results from the ninth French Survey (2005-2007). *Minerva Anestesiologica*, 2012, 78, 868-78.

[53] Ewan, PW; Dugué, P; Mirakian, R; Dixon, TA; Harper, JN; Nasser, SM. BSACI guidelines for the investigation of suspected anaphylaxis during general anesthesia. *Clin Exp Allergy.*, 2010, 40, 15-31.

[54] Peroni, D; Sansotta, N; Bernardini, R; Cardinale, F; Paravati, F; Franceschini, F; Boner, AL. Perioperative allergy. *Int J Immunopsthol Pharmacol*, 2011, 24(3S), 69-74.

[55] Soetens, F; Rose, M; Fisher, M. Timing of skin testing after a suspected anaphylactic reaction during anaesthesia. *Acta Anaesthesiol Scan*, 2012, 56, 1042-46.

[56] Caimmi, S; Caimmi, D; Lombardi, E; Crisafulli, G; Franceschini, F; Ricci, G; Marseglia, GL. Antibiotic allergy. *Int J Immunopathol Pharmacol*, 2011, 24(3S), S47-53.

[57] Bernardini, R; Catania, P; Caffarelli, C; Cardinale, F; Franceschini, F; Pelosi, U. Peroni DG. Perioperative latex allergy. *Int J Immunopathol Pharmacol*, 2011, 24 (3S): S55-60.

[58] Nucera, E; Pollastrini, E; Sabato, V; Colagiovanni, A; Aruanno, A; Rizzi, A; Buonomo, A; Pecora, V; Lombardo, C; Astorri, AL; Rossi, G; Patriarca, G; Schiavino, D. Challenge tests in the diagnosis of latex allergy. *Int J Immunopathol Pharmacol*, 2010, 23, 543-52.

[59] Novembre, E; Bernardini, R; Brizzi, I; Bertini, G; Mugnaini, L; Azzari, C; Vierucci, A. The prevalence of latex allergy in children seen in a university hospital allergy clinic. *Allergy*, 1997, 52, 101-05.

[60] Torres, MJ; Blanca, M. The complex clinical picture of b-lactam hypersensitivity: penicillins, cephalosporins, monobactams, carbapenems, and clavams. *Med Clin N Am*, 2010, 94, 805-20.

[61] Mertes, PM; Laxenaire, MC; Lienhart, A; et al. Reducing the risk of anaphylaxis during anaesthesia: guidelines for clinical practice. *J Investig Allergol Clin Immunol*, 2005, 15, 91-101.

[62] Dewachter, P; Mouton-Faivre, C; Pertek, JP. Boudaa C; Mertes PM. Value of skin tests for the choice of a neuromuscular blocking agent after an anaphylactic reaction. *Ann Fr Anesth Reanim*, 2005, 24, 543-46.

[63] Peroni, DG; Sansotta, N; Bernardini, R; Crisafulli, G; Franceschini, F; Caffarelli, C; Boner, AL. Muscle relaxants allergy *Int J Immunopathol Pharmacol*, 2011, 24 (3S), S35-46.

[64] Ramirez, LF; Pereira, A; Chirac, AM; Bonnet-Boyer, MC; Demoly, P. Negative predictive value of skin tests to neuromucular blocking agents. *Allergy*, 2012, 67(3), 439-41.

[65] Brockow, K; Chistiansen, C; Kanny, G; Clément, O; Barbaud, A; Bircher, A; Dewachter, P; Guéant, JL; Rodriguez Guéant, RM; Mouton-Faivre, C; Ring, J; Romano, A; Sainte-Laudy, J; Demoly, P; Pichler, WJ; ENDA; EAACI interest group on drug hypersensitivity. Management of hypersensitivity reactions to iodinated contrast media. *Allergy*, 2005, 60, 150-58

[66] Caimmi, S; Benyahia, B; Suau, D; Bousquet-Rouanet, L; Caimmi, D; Bousquet, PJ; Demoly, P. Clinical value of negative skin tests to iodinated contrast media. *Clin Exp Allergy*, 2010, 40, 805-10.

[67] Mertes, PM; Malinovsky, JM; Mouton-Faivre, C; Bonnet-Boyer, MC; Benhaijoub, A; Lavaud, F; Valfrey, J; O'Brien, J; Pirat, P; Lalourcey, L; Demoly, P. Anaphylaxis to dyes during the perioperative period: reports of 14 clinical cases. *J Allergy Clin Immunol*, 2008, 122, 348-52.

[68] Liccardi, L; Lobefalo, G; Di Florio, E; Di Iorio, C; Occhiochiuso, L; Romano, L; Savoia, G; Massa, RM; D'Amato, G. on behalf of the Cardarelli Hospital Radiocontrast Media and Anesthetic-Induced Anaphylaxis Prevention (CHRAIAP) Working Group. *J Investig Allergol Clin Immunol*, 2008, Vol. 18(1), 1-11.

[69] Caimmi, S; Caimmi, D; Cardinale, F; Indinnimeo, L; Crisafulli, G; Peroni, DG; Marseglia, GL. Antibiotic allergy. *Int J Immunopathol Pharmacol*, 2011, 24 (3S), S47-53.

[70] Mertes, PM; Aimone-Gastin, I; Guéant-Rodriguez, RM; Mouton-Faivre, C; Audibert, G; O'Brien, J; Frendt, D; Brezeanu, M; Bouaziz, H; Guéant, JL. Hypersensitivity reactions to neuromuscular blocking agents. *Curr Pharm Des.*, 2008, 14(27), 2809-25.

[71] Caimmi, S; Caimmi, D; Cardinale, F; Indinnimeo, L; Crisafulli, G; Peroni, DG; Marseglia, GL. Perioperative allergy: un common agents. *Int J Immunopathol Prharmacol*, 2011, 24(3S), S 61-68.

In: Anaphylaxis: Principles and Practice
Editor: M. Thirumala Krishna
ISBN: 978-1-62618-688-0

Chapter VIII

Non Steroidal Anti-Inflammatory Drug-Induced Anaphylaxis

Mario Sánchez-Borges*[*], *Fernan Caballero Fonseca*, *and Arnaldo Capriles-Hulett
Allergy and Clinical Immunology Department,
Centro Médico-Docente La Trinidad, Caracas, Venezuela

Abstract

Aspirin (ASA) and nonsteroidal anti-inflammatory drugs (NSAIDs) constitute the second most frequent cause of adverse reactions to drugs. Various clinical pictures can be induced by NSAIDs, including systemic reactions. Severity of the clinical picture is variable, but often the clinical manifestations are so severe that life may be endangered. The mechanisms of anaphylaxis induced by ASA/NSAIDs are incompletely understood at present time, and include allergic, IgE-mediated reactions, observed in patients reacting to a single drug, as well as non allergic hypersensitivity reactions exemplified by those observed in patients cross-reactive to various NSAIDs of a different chemical structure. The diagnosis of NSAID-induced anaphylaxis relies heavily on the medical history, and in selected cases is confirmed by skin tests and oral provocation. Patient management is based on the pharmacologic pattern of the reaction, and consists of drug avoidance and, in cross-reactive patients, the use of alternative NSAIDs that do not inhibit cyclooxygenase-1.

Introduction

According to the Nomenclature Committee of the World Allergy Organization, anaphylaxis is a serious life-threatening generalized or systemic hypersensitivity reaction [1].

[*] Corresponding author: Mario Sánchez-Borges, MD, Sexta transversal urbanización Altamira, piso 8, consultorio 803, Caracas 1060, Venezuela; Telephone/FAX: +58-212-2615284; e-mail: sanchezbmario@gmail.com.

In many geographical locations foods are the most common triggers of anaphylaxis, although drugs are also involved with high frequency [2,3]. Adverse drug reactions affect 10-20% of hospitalized patients and more than 7% of the general population [3]. Drug-induced anaphylaxis can occur at any age, but is more common in middle-aged and the elderly.

It has been estimated that average consumption of nonsteroidal anti-inflammatory drugs (NSAIDs) all over the world is as high as 80 tablets per person per year [4] and each year human beings consume around 40,000 metric tons of aspirin (ASA), an amount which is equivalent to about 120 billion aspirin tablets [5]. These figures do not include other NSAIDs that are also potential inducers of severe adverse effects. The use of these medications is actively promoted through the press and the massive communication media, and they are sold without prescription in most countries.

In a previous study we calculated that 13.3 tablets of ibuprofen per adult per year and about 8.69 mL of the drug per child per year were consumed in Venezuela in 2004 [6]. The magnitude of the population exposed to aspirin and NSAIDs is so huge that it is not surprising that hypersensitivity reactions to this group of medications occur so frequently and constitute a major motive for consultation to general practitioners as well as allergists, dermatologists and other specialists.

Among drugs, antibiotics (mainly beta lactams and increasingly others) are the most common cause of hypersensitivity reactions, followed by non steroidal anti-inflammatory drugs (NSAIDs) [7]. The prevalence of aspirin hypersensitivity in the general population ranges between 0.5 % and 1.9 % [8], while reactions to the new and more selective NSAIDs are observed less frequently. However, in a series of 200 patients with suspected hypersensitivity to cyclooxygenase (COX) inhibitors, anaphylaxis accounted for 3.5 % of the reactions [9], whereas in children with suspected hypersensitivity to COX inhibitors, anaphylaxis accounted for 5.9 % of the cases [10]. Additionally, in a tertiary care hospital in Korea ASA/NSAIDs were the commonest etiologic agents of hypersensitivity [11].

While all NSAIDs are able to cause selective NSAID reactions, some studies suggested that the use of heteroaryl acetic group of NSAIDs such as naproxen, diclofenac, and ibuprofen confers a higher risk of anaphylactic reactions than other groups of NSAIDs [12].

Table 1. Classification of NSAIDs according to their chemical structure

Chemical group	Drugs
Alkanones	Nabumetone
Antranilic acids (phenamates)	Meclophenamic acid, mefenamic acid
Arylpropionic acids	Fenoprofen, flurbiprofen, ibuprofen, ketoprofen, naproxen, oxaprozin
Enolic acids	Piroxicam, tenoxicam, phenylbutazone, oxyphenbutazone
Heteroaryl acetic acids	Diclofenac, ketorolac, tolmetin
Indol/indene acetic acids	Etodolac, indomethacin, sulindac
Para-aminophenol derivatives	Acetaminophen
Pyrazol derivatives	Aminopyrin, antipyrin, dipyrone
Salicilic acid derivatives	Aspirin, choline/magnesium trysalycilate, diflunisal, olsalazine, salycilsalycilic acid, salsalate, sodium salycilate, sulfasalazine

Pyrazolones are most often implicated in IgE-mediated anaphylaxis to NSAIDs [13]. This chapter presents a review of NSAID-induced anaphylaxis, one of the most severe forms of immediate reactions to these drugs.

Other life-threatening reactions of the delayed type of hypersensitivity, mediated by T cells specifically recognizing NSAID antigens, which are clinically manifested as Stevens-Johnson Syndrome (SJS), Toxic Epidermal Necrolysis (TENs), and other severe bullous diseases are out the scope of this article and have been recently summarized [14]. It is noteworthy to mention that the first adverse reaction induced by ASA was reported by Hirchsberg in 1902, soon after acetylsalicylic acid was synthesized [15].

Pharmacologic Overview of NSAIDs

Arachidonic acid derived from cell membrane phospholipids through the action of phospholipases is metabolized to produce potent inflammatory mediators by two enzymatic pathways. Cyclooxygenases (COX) mediate the production of prostaglandins. On the other hand, 5-lipooxygenase (5-LO) and 5-LO activating protein (FLAP) catalyze the synthesis of cysteinyl leukotrienes LTC4, LTD4 and LTE4.

There exist two main isoforms of COX. Cyclooxygenase-1, the constitutive isoenzyme, is present in all cells and its action is inhibited by ASA and all "classic" NSAIDs. The inducible form, COX-2, is present exclusively in inflammatory and immune system cells and is inhibited by classic and also by the newer preferential (nimesulide, meloxicam) and selective (coxibs: rofecoxib, valdecoxib, etoricoxib, parecoxib and lumiracoxib) COX-2 inhibitors.

Classic NSAIDs have been classified according to their chemical structure in 7 groups (Table 1). On the other hand, the degree of inhibition for COX isoenzymes is used to classify NSAIDs according to their selectivity for COX-1 or COX-2 isoforms (Table-2). Recently, new COX isoenzymes which are preferentially inhibited by pyrazolones, acetaminophen and antipyrine have been described as COX-1 variants and designated as COX-2b or COX-3 [16,17].

Epidemiology of Anaphylaxis Induced by NSAIDs

Since in general most adverse reactions to drugs are not usually reported, the prevalence of systemic reactions to NSAIDs remains largely unknown. The observation has been made that NSAIDs are the leading cause of anaphylaxis in ambulatory patients seen in emergency services [18]. In a study published by Kemp et al more than half of drug-induced anaphylactic episodes were attributed to NSAIDs. It was a retrospective review of medical records from 266 patients with anaphylaxis in which drugs were involved in 52 cases (19.5 %) and NSAIDs in 27 (10.1%) [19]. Previously, Strom et al had observed that 35 out of 52000 patients exposed to NSAIDs between February 1982 and January 1983 experienced symptoms of anaphylaxis [20]. In a recent report from our institution which included 2421 outpatients consulting to an allergology clinic 179 subjects with anaphylaxis (7.39 %) were identified. Drugs were the commonest cause of anaphylaxis, accounting for 98 episodes

(54.7%) and in this group NSAIDs constituted the first etiologic agents (87 out of 98 cases, 87.7%) [21].

In a recently published Latin American survey drugs were the first cause of anaphylaxis (31.2 %), followed by foods (23.3 %), and insect stings (14.8 %). Among drugs, NSAIDs were involved in 72.7 % of cases, and antibiotics in 18.1 % [3]. In 191 children foods induced 36.1 % of reactions, drugs caused 53 reactions (27.7 %), and insects 26.2 %, and among drugs NSAIDs were responsible for 36 reactions (67.9 %) and antibiotics were involved in 13 (24.5 %) [22].

In a prospective study Quiralte et al submitted 223 NSAID-sensitive patients to single-blinded placebo-controlled oral challenges (SBPCOC) with NSAIDs. Fifty patients in that cohort (22.4 %) developed anaphylaxis during the provocation tests [12]. These investigators also indicated that some patients with a history of urticaria induced by a single NSAID developed selective systemic reactions during subsequent exposures to specific NSAIDs. In other patients multiple NSAID-induced systemic responses during SBPCOC were observed.

All NSAIDs can induce anaphylaxis and glafenine (presently discontinued) and diclofenac have been associated with an increased frequency of admission due to anaphylaxis [23]. As previously mentioned, the risk for anaphylactic reactions is higher with the use of heteroaryl acetic acids [24]. The risk is also increased in female subjects, in patients with acute pain [20], in atopic individuals [25], and in patients with mastocytosis and/or increased basal serum tryptase levels [26,27]. Finally, anaphylaxis to COX-2 inhibitors is rarely reported; in fact, in a review by our group which included reports on adverse reactions to coxibs published in the literature between 2001 and 2004, only six cases of anaphylaxis were present [28].

Table 2. Classification of NSAIDs according to their selectivity for COX isoenzymes

Weak COX inhibitors
Acetaminophen, salsalate
Inhibitors of COX-1 and COX-2
Piroxicam, indomethacin, sulindac, tolmetin, ibuprofen, naproxen, fenoprofen, meclofenamate, mefenamic acid, diflunisal, ketoprofen, diclofenac, ketorolac, etodolac, nabumetone, oxaprozin, flurbiprofen
Preferential COX-2 inhibitors
Nimesulide, meloxicam
Selective COX-2 inhibitors
Celecoxib, rofecoxib, valdecoxib, etoricoxib, parecoxib, lumiracoxib

Pathogenesis

In a recent paper, the European Network of Drug Allergy (ENDA), the Interest Group on Drug Hypersensitivity of the European Academy of Allergy and Clinical Immunology, and the European Network on Hypersensitivity to aspirin and nonsteroidal anti-inflammatory drugs (HANNA) proposed an updated classification of hypersensitivity reactions to NSAIDs. This classification is based on timing, clinical picture, and pharmacologic pattern of the reaction. Reactions are divided in immediate (occurring after minutes to several hours of exposure to the drug) and delayed (appearing more than 24 hours after exposure).

Immediate reactions include Aspirin exacerbated respiratory disease (AERD), Aspirin-exacerbated cutaneous disease (AECD) [29], urticaria and angioedema induced by multiple NSAIDs in patients with no underlying disease, and urticaria, angioedema and anaphylaxis induced by a single drug [30]. AERD is characterized by the classic "ASA triad" composed of chronic rhinosinusitis with nasal polyposis, chronic asthma, and acute respiratory reactions (bronchoconstriction) induced by ASA and other COX-1 inhibitors. AECD is present in patients with chronic spontaneous urticaria and angioedema who experience exacerbations of the chronic cutaneous disease when exposed to ASA and classic NSAIDs.

In a study by Quiralte et al as many as 30 % of patients with a history of NSAID hypersensitivity appeared to be single-drug reactors [12]. In such cases, specific IgE synthesis is induced by the NSAID which functions as hapten and binds to a carrier protein. An immediate hypersensitivity reaction can occur when this sensitized individual is again exposed to the same or a structurally similar NSAID. Patients with this type of reaction are tolerant to other NSAIDs of a different chemical structure, and show a clinical picture and reaction time that resembles an IgE-mediated allergic reaction. Positive immediate-type skin tests to the drug and drug-specific IgE in the serum have been demonstrated in patients with single drug-induced reactions to pyrazolones [13,31], and a strong genetic association with HLA-DQ and HLA-DR polymorphisms has been observed in patients with pyrazolone hypersensitivity [32].

Although not included in the above mentioned classification, it is theoretically possible that some patients exhibit systemic non allergic hypersensitivity reactions to various COX-1 inhibitors of different chemical composition, and these reactions (previously denominated as pseudoallergic or anaphylactoid) [18] are likely to be mediated through inhibition of cyclooxygenase-1, in the same fashion as urticaria/angioedema of AECD and AERD are produced [1,12].

COX-1 inhibition leads to a decreased synthesis of PGE2 (which under physiological conditions inhibits mast cell mediator release) and increased cysteinyl leukotriene production [33]. Under these circumstances leukotrienes mediate various inflammatory and tissue effects which result in the symptoms of anaphylaxis.

Clinical Picture

Frequent symptoms and signs of anaphylaxis are observed in the skin (the most commonly involved organ), the respiratory and gastrointestinal tracts, the central nervous and the cardiovascular systems. Those have been reviewed recently by the Anaphylaxis Committee of the World Allergy Organization [34]. Clinical criteria for diagnosing anaphylaxis have been established and include any *one* of the following three:

1. Acute onset of an illness (minutes to several hours) with involvement of the skin, mucosal tissue, or both (eg. generalized hives, pruritus or flushing, swollen lips-tongue-uvula)

   AND AT LEAST ONE OF THE FOLLOWING:

1) Respiratory compromise (eg. dyspnea, wheeze-bronchospasm, stridor, reduced peak expiratory flow, hypoxemia)
2) Reduced blood pressure or associated symptoms of end-organ dysfunction (eg. hypotonia [collapse], syncope, incontinence)

2. Two or more of the following that occur rapidly after the exposure to a *likely* allergen for that patient (minutes to several hours):
   - Involvement of the skin-mucosal tissue (eg. generalized hives, itch-flush, swollen lips-tongue-uvula)
   - Respiratory compromise (eg. dyspnea, wheeze-bronchospasm, stridor, reduced peak expiratory flow, hypoxemia)
   - Reduced blood pressure or associated symptoms (eg. hypotonia [collapse], syncope, incontinence)
   - Persistent gastrointestinal symptoms (eg. crampy abdominal pain, vomiting)
3. Reduced blood pressure after exposure to a *known* allergen for that patient (minutes to several hours):
   - Infants and children: low systolic blood pressure (age-specific) or greater than 30 % decrease in systolic blood pressure
   - Adults: systolic blood pressure of less than 90 mm Hg or greater than 30 % decrease from that person's baseline [34].

Clinical manifestations of anaphylaxis triggered by ASA and other NSAIDs are usually not different to those of anaphylaxis induced by other causes. Most commonly the skin and the respiratory tract are involved with sudden onset of symptoms such as urticaria, angioedema, pruritus, flushing, breathlessness, wheezing, dysphonia, stridor, cough, rhinorrhoea, and tearing temporally associated with ASA/NSAID administration. Other organs may be compromised, including the gastrointestinal tract, the central nervous and cardiovascular systems.

Facial (periorbital) and laryngeal angioedema associated to ASA/NSAID hypersensitivity are highly prevalent in various cohorts of patients as has been observed, for example, by Quiralte et al [35]. The reasons explaining this preferential clinical expression are presently not elucidated.

Additionally, aspirin has been shown to enhance allergic reactions and anaphylaxis to foods, especially wheat, in food allergic patients [36-48]. Trying to explain the reasons why aspirin can exacerbate IgE-mediated allergic reactions Suzuki and Ra proposed that aspirin potentiation of IgE-mediated allergic reactions is not related to inhibition of prostaglandin synthesis; these authors proposed that ASA-induced release of cysteinyl leukotrienes by mast cells is mediated by dihydropiridine-sensitive L-type calcium channels [49]. Other pathways of interaction linking aspirin and IgE-mediated allergic inflammation have been recently summarized by our group, and include genetic factors, inhibition of COX-1, and stimulation of other inflammatory pathways [50].

Next we present and discuss a case of anaphylaxis induced by diclofenac in a young male atopic patient.

Case 1

A 20-years-old male patient developed facial angioedema, breathlessness, cough, dysphonia, and generalized urticaria 20 minutes after taking orally 50 mg of potassium diclofenac for headache.

The patient was taken to the emergency room, and nebulized fenoterol/ipratropium bromide was administered without inducing any improvement of his respiratory symptoms. Further deterioration with respiratory failure rapidly ensued and prompted patient's transfer to the intensive care unit (ICU) where intubation was performed. General and respiratory support was given and the patient was discharged from the ICU after two days of hospitalization.

Further questioning revealed a previous history of asthma and dipyrone-induced angioedema. His mother has a history of allergic asthma and rhinitis. Allergologic evaluation was done 5 months after the acute episode. Physical examination was within normal limits with the exception of bilateral inflammation of the nasal mucosa with oedema, a pale-gray aspect of the mucosa, and with abundant crystalline secretion. Immediate-type skin prick tests were positive for cat (3 mm wheal), *Dermatophagoides pteronyssinus* (10 mm), *Dermatophagoides farinae* (10 mm), and *Blomia tropicalis* (13 mm), and negative for molds, pollens, dog, cockroach, and foods. Increased levels of serum specific IgE for *Dermatophagoides pteronyssinus* and *farinae*, quantified by means of immunoenzymatic assay, were present.

Controlled oral provocation tests with alternative drugs were carried out. Celecoxib (200 mg) and meloxicam (15 mg) were tolerated during these challenges. The recommendation was given to the patient to avoid all COX-1 inhibitors and to use only the above mentioned COX-2 inhibitors celecoxib and meloxicam for the relief of pain and inflammation.

It was concluded that this is an atopic patient cross-reactive to NSAIDs (dypirone and diclofenac) who experienced an anaphylactic reaction triggered by potassium diclofenac.

Comments: 1. This patient developed a very severe, life-threatening reaction. Due to ethical reasons related with the severity of the reaction it was not considered safe to perform a confirmatory test with diclofenac. The advice for avoidance of all "classic" NSAIDs was based on the cross-reactivity to two NSAIDs, dipyrone and diclofenac, shown by the patient. COX-2 inhibitors are tolerated by the majority of patients sensitive to COX-1 inhibitors, but it is advised to perform provocation tests to demonstrate tolerance before recommending the use of inhibitors of COX-2 to these patients [51,52]. This patient received a preferential (meloxicam) and a selective (celecoxib) COX-2 inhibitor without showing any adverse effect.

2. Another issue that we would like to emphasize regarding this patient is the presence of a history of asthma and rhinitis, with proven sensitization to inhalant allergens (cat and mites).

We have shown that NSAID hypersensitivity occurs more frequently in atopic patients [25]. The reasons for this association are not presently clear, but various possible mechanisms have been hypothesized [50].

Diagnosis

The medical history is paramount to suspect NSAID-induced anaphylaxis. Acute systemic allergic reaction with symptoms such as urticaria, angioedema, flushing, dyspnoea, dysphonia, dysphagia, hypotension, generalized itching, and wheezing temporarily associated with ASA/NSAID administration require a careful assessment and prompt treatment for a favourable outcome.

Other possible etiologic factors, including other drugs, and differential diagnosis from other conditions simulating anaphylaxis should be considered. Those include common conditions (spontaneous urticaria, acute asthma, syncope, aspiration of a foreign body, myocardial infarction, stroke, seizures), postprandial syndromes (oral allergy syndrome, sulfites, scombroid poisoning), excess of endogenous histamine (mastocytosis, clonal mast cell disorders, basophilic leukemia), non organic diseases (vocal cord dysfunction, hyperventilation, psychosomatic episodes), various forms of shock [hypovolemic, cardiogenic, distributive (spinal cord lesion), septic] ingestion of monosodium glutamate (Chinese restaurant syndrome), flushing syndromes (perimenopausal, carcinoid, autonomic epilepsy, medullar carcinoma of thyroid), and miscellaneous causes [non allergic angioedema (Hereditary angioedema)], Red man syndrome (induced by vancomycin), and phaeochromocytoma.

Due to the life-threatening nature of this condition, oral provocation tests are generally not employed for the confirmation of NSAID-induced anaphylaxis. In some selected patients who require the drug for the treatment of chronic diseases such as coronary artery disease or arthropathy, or in those in which the cause of systemic symptoms are not clear, oral challenges could be performed by allergy specialists in the hospital, with easy access to equipment and medications for the treatment of systemic reactions should they occur. Different protocols of aspirin challenge are used in North America and Europe, as described in a recent review [29], and those procedures can be adapted in order to perform the challenge with other NSAIDs.

Immediate-type skin tests have been used to assess reactions to a single drug, which are presumably mediated by drug-specific IgE antibodies, and especially for the evaluation of possible pyrazolone-triggered anaphylaxis [13,53]. Skin tests and *in vitro* tests for the investigation and quantification of NSAID-specific IgE have not been adequately standardized and show low sensitivity. They are used more often as research tools and rarely for routine diagnosis.

Since there are ethical limitations to submit patients with anaphylaxis to *in vivo* challenges with NSAIDs, investigators have developed new *in vitro* techniques which could be helpful to confirm ASA/NSAID hypersensitivity without exposing the patient to the unnecessary risks implied by *in vivo* testing. For example, the basophil activation test (BAT) that utilizes a Fluorescence-activated cell sorter (FACS) to measure CD63 (activation marker expression on basophils) expression has been used for the detection of hypersensitivity to pyrazolones and other NSAIDs. According to some studies this test might be useful, especially if performed early after the reaction [54,55]. Specificity of this test is good but sensitivity varies among different laboratories [56].

Case 2

A 13-year old male patient was referred in July 2011 for allergologic evaluation after complaining of breathlessness, dysphonia, cough and urticarial rash on upper extremities and trunk which began 15 minutes after the ingestion of dipyrone (500 mg). The mother reported that at 9 years he had developed generalized urticaria during treatment with penicillin and dipyrone for acute upper respiratory infection. Two years later he received orally a combination of hyoscine and dipyrone for abdominal cramps and again wheals on upper and lower limbs, face and chest occurred. Before present consultation the patient took acetaminophen and nimesulide without experiencing any adverse effects. Other than allergic rhinitis, chickenpox and one episode of urinary tract infection, patient's and parent's interrogation did not disclose a history of other important previous diseases. His mother also has allergic rhinitis.

Physical examination: Nasal mucosa bilaterally pallid, oedematous, with abundant clear secretion. Acne on facial (forehead) and back skin. No other abnormalities.

Skin testing: Prick and intradermal skin tests (IDT) with benzylpenicillin, penicillin major/minor determinants were negative as were serum specific IgE to penicillin. Dipyrone: prick and IDT tests were positive at 1:1000 and 1:100 dilutions. Prick tests also positive for *Dermatophagoides pteronyssinus* (7 mm wheal), *Dermatophagoides farinae* (10 mm) and *Blomia tropicalis* (12 mm), negative to other inhalant allergens (pollens from grasses, weeds and trees, cat and dog dander, molds, feathers and cockroach.

Oral provocation tests (according to protocol shown in reference 29): Negative for Aspirin (up to 650 mg) and Diclofenac (up to 50 mg).

Comments: 1. Diagnosis: **Single-drug-induced anaphylaxis** (from dipyrone) in an atopic patient with **Allergic rhinitis**. Suspected from clinical history and confirmed by skin testing. Although he had previously tolerated acetaminophen and nimesulide, oral provocation tests with aspirin and diclofenac confirmed that the patient was allergic to a single NSAID.

2. Skin testing with penicillin was done for the purpose of discarding other possible drug allergies.

Recommendations: Written instructions were given to avoid pyrazolones (aminopyrine, antipyrine, chlormezanone, dipyrone, feprazone, oxyphenbutazone, phenylbutazone, and sulfinpyrazone). No restrictions for NSAIDs from other chemical groups.

Management (Figure 1)

Once the diagnosis of anaphylaxis caused by ASA or NSAIDs is confirmed, patient management will depend on the severity of the clinical picture and the pharmacologic pattern of the reaction. For patients who experience a first reaction or more than one episode triggered by the same or various closely related drugs it is important to ascertain the possibility of cross reactions to other chemical groups. In such cases, a provocation test with a second non-related NSAID is recommended. If this test is positive, the patient should be managed as a cross-reactor (see below). If the test is negative, the patient could receive NSAIDs of a different chemical structure to the one implicated in the original reaction, with avoidance of the culprit and related/similar NSAIDs (Table 1).

Patients who have reacted to various NSAIDs of a diverse chemical composition (cross-reactors) should avoid all "classic" COX-1 inhibitors. A confirmatory challenge with a COX-1 inhibitor can be done if the etiology of the reaction is doubtful. Otherwise, a provocation test with alternative non COX-1 inhibitors (or weak COX-1 inhibitors) including preferential and selective COX-2 inhibitors is performed. Patients showing negative challenge results can be treated with non COX-1 inhibitors and monitored periodically for NSAID tolerance, whereas patients reacting to non COX-1 inhibitors would belong to a high risk phenotype for NSAID sensitivity and should be managed with other analgesic and anti-inflammatory therapies different to NSAIDs (Figure 1) [57]. Desensitization procedures, as utilized in patients with aspirin-exacerbated respiratory disease, are not presently recommended for patients with NSAID-induced anaphylaxis.

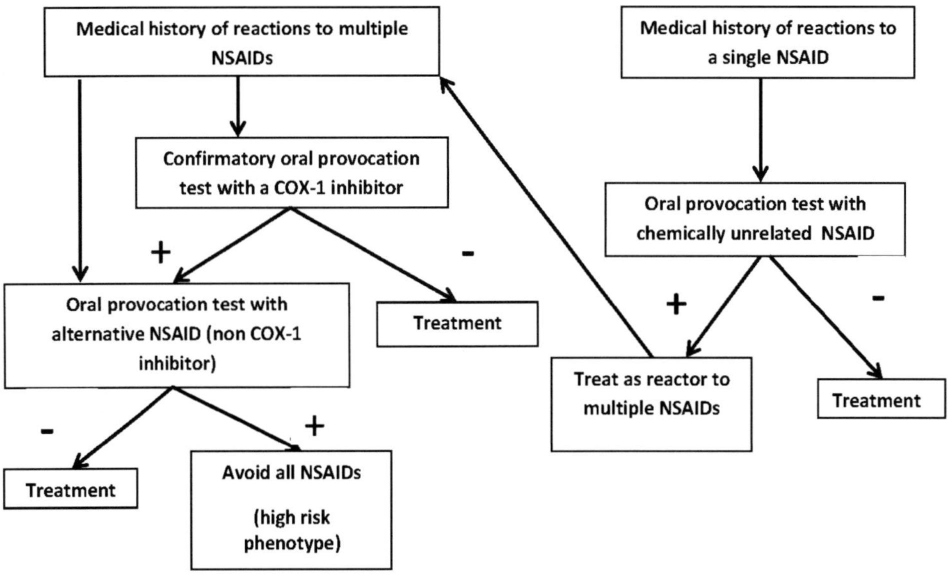

Figure 1. Algorithm for the management of patients with anaphylaxis induced by NSAIDs.

Conclusion

Aspirin and NSAIDs are drugs widely used in all continents. Not surprisingly, they constitute one of the most frequent etiologic agents inducing drug hypersensitivity, including severe systemic reactions and anaphylaxis. Allergic, IgE-mediated reactions to a single NSAID are observed more frequently in patients exposed to pyrazolones, and absolute avoidance to drugs from such chemical group are recommended in such cases. For patients who react to various COX-1 inhibitors of different chemical groups (cross-reactors), management includes avoidance of classic NSAIDs and substitution with weak COX-1 inhibitors such as acetaminophen or preferential and selective COX-2 inhibitors after tolerance is confirmed by means of oral challenge.

- **Clinical Pearls** After antibiotics, aspirin and NSAIDs are the second most common cause of drug-induced anaphylaxis.
- Anaphylaxis to NSAIDs can be allergic, mediated by drug-specific IgE (observed in single reactors), or non allergic, likely to be mediated by inhibition of COX-1 (observed in cross reactor patients).
- Severity of the reactions is variable and may be life-threatening.
- Aspirin intake can exacerbate allergic reactions to foods, especially wheat.
- ASA/NSAID anaphylaxis is a clinical diagnosis based on occurrence of symptoms with temporal association, and in selected patients confirmed by skin tests or provocation tests.
- Patient management is based on the recognition of the pharmacologic pattern of the reaction, and consists of drug avoidance and in cross reactive patients the use of alternative NSAIDs with low COX-1 inhibitory properties.

References

[1] Johansson, SGO; Bieber, T; Dahl, R; Friedmann, PS; Lanier, BQ; Lockey, RF; Motala, C; Ortega, Martell, JA; Platts-Mills, TA; Ring, J; Thien, F; Van Cauwenberge, P; Williams, HC. Revised nomenclature for allergy for global use: Report of the Nomenclature Review Committee of the World Allergy Organization, October 2003. *J Allergy Clin Immunol*, 2004, 113, 832-6.

[2] Simons, FER. Anaphylaxis: Recent advances in assessment and treatment. *J Allergy Clin Immunol*, 2009, 124, 625-36.

[3] Sole, D; Ivancevich, JC; Sánchez-Borges, M; Coelho, MA; Rosario, NA; Ardusso, LR; Bernd, LA. Latin American Anaphylaxis Working Group. Anaphylaxis in Latin America: A report of the Online Latin American Survey on Anaphylaxis (OLASA). *Clinics (Sao Paulo)*, 2011, 66, 943-7.

[4] Vane, JR. The fight against rheumatism: From willow bark to COX-1 sparing drugs. *J Physiol Pharmacol*, 2000, 51, 573-86.

[5] Warner, TD; Mitchell, JA. Cyclooxygenase-3 (COX-3): Filling in the gaps toward a COX continuum? *Proc Natl Acad Sci*, USA, 2002, 99, 13371-3.

[6] Sánchez-Borges, M; Capriles-Hulett, A; Caballero-Fonseca, F. Risk of skin reactions when using ibuprofen-based medicines. *Expert Opin Drug Saf*, 2005, 4, 837-48.

[7] Gomes, ER; Demoly, P. Epidemiology of hypersensitivity drug reactions. *Curr Opin Allergy Clin Immunol*, 2005, 5, 309-16.

[8] Settipane, RA; Constantine, HP; Settipane, GA. Aspirin intolerance and recurrent urticarial in normal adults and children. Epidemiology and review. *Allergy*, 1980, 35, 149-54.

[9] Schubert, B; Grosse Perdekamp, MT; Pfeuffer, P; Raith, P; Bröcker, EB; Trautmann, A. Nonsteroidal anti-inflammatory drug hypersensitivity: Fable or reality? *Eur J Dermatol*, 2005, 15, 164-7.

[10] Titchen, T; Cranswick, N; Beggs, S. Adverse reactions to nonsteroidal anti-inflammatory drugs, COX-2 inhibitors and paracetamol in a pediatric hospital. *Br J Clin Pharmacol*, 2005, 59, 718-23.

[11] Choi, JH; Shin, YS; Suh, CH; Nahm, DH; Park, HS. The frequency of adverse drug reactions in a tertiary care hospital in Korea. *Korean J Med*, 2004, 67, 290-6.

[12] Quiralte, J; Blanco, C; Delgado, J; Ortega, N; Alcantara, M; Castillo, R; Anguita, JL; Sáenz de San Pedro, B; Carrillo, T. Challenge-based clinical patterns of 223 Spanish patients with nonsteroidal anti-inflammatory drug-induced reactions. *J Investig Allergol Clin Immunol*, 2007, 17, 182-8.

[13] Himly, M; Jahn-Schmid, B; Pittertschatscher, K; Bohle, B; Grubmayr, K; Ferreira, F; Ebner, H; Ebner, C. IgE-mediated immediate type hypersensitivity to the pyrazolone drug propyphenazone. *J Allergy Clin Immunol*, 2003, 111, 882-8.

[14] Sánchez-Borges, M. Clinical management of nonsteroidal anti-inflammatory drug hypersensitivity. *WAO Journal*, 2008, 1, 29-33.

[15] Hirschberg: Mitteilung über einen Fall von Nebenwirkung des Aspirin. *Dtsch Med Wochenschr*, 1902, 28, 416.

[16] Chandrasekharan NV; Dai H; Roos KL; Evanson NK; Tomsik J; Elton TS; Simmons DL. COX-3, a cyclooxygenase-1 variant inhibited by acetaminophen and other analgesic/ antipyretic drugs: cloning, structure and expression. *Proc Natl Acad Sci*, USA 2002, 99, 13926-31.

[17] Simmons DL; Botting RM; Robertson PM; Madsen ML; Vane JR. Induction of an acetaminophen-sensitive cyclooxygenase with reduced sensitivity to nonsteroidal anti-inflammatory drugs. *Proc Natl Acad Sci*, USA 1999, 96, 3275-80.

[18] Berkes EA. Anaphylactic and anaphylactoid reactions to aspirin and other NSAIDs. *Clin Rev Allergy Immunol*, 2003, 24, 137-48.

[19] Kemp SF; Lockey RF; Wolf BL; Lieberman P. Anaphylaxis: A review of 266 cases. *Arch Intern Med*, 1995, 155, 1749-54.

[20] Strom BL; Carson JL; Morse ML; West SL; Soper KA. The effect of indication on hypersensitivity reactions associated with zomepirac sodium and other non steroidal anti-inflammatory drugs. *Arthritis Rheum*, 1987, 30, 1142-8.

[21] Sánchez-Borges, M. Etiology and clinical picture of anaphylaxis in ambulatory patients from Caracas, Venezuela. *J Investig Allergol Clin Immunol*, 2010, 20, 623-4.

[22] Sole, D; Ivancevich, JC; Sánchez-Borges, M; Coelho, MA; Rosario, NA; Ardusso, LR; Bernd, LA. Latin American Anaphylaxis Working Group. Anaphylaxis in Latin American children and adolescents: the Online Latin American Survey on Anaphylaxis (OLASA). *Allergol Immunopathol (Madr)*, 2011 Nov 21. [Epub ahead of print].

[23] Van der Klauw, MM; Stricker, BH; Herings, RM. A population based case-cohort study of drug-induced anaphylaxis. *Br J Clin Pharmacol*, 1993, 35, 400-8.

[24] Van Puijenbroek, EPEA; Meyboom, RH; Leufkens, HG. Different risks for NSAID-induced anaphylaxis. *Ann Pharmacother*, 2002, 36, 24-9.

[25] Sánchez-Borges, M; Capriles-Hulett, A. Atopy is a risk factor for non-steroidal anti-inflammatory drug sensitivity. *Ann Allergy Asthma Immunol*, 2000, 84, 101-6.

[26] Rueff, F; Przybilla, B; Bilo, MB; Muller, U; Scheipl, F; Aberer, W; Birnbaum, J; Bodzenta-Lukaszyk, A; Bonifazi, F; Bucher, C; Campi, P; Darsow, U; Egger, C; Haeberli, G; Hawranek, T; Körner, M; Kucharewicz, I; Küchenhoff, H; Lang, R; Quercia, O; Reider, N; Severino, M; Sticherling, M; Sturm, GJ; Wüthrich, B. Predictors of severe systemic anaphylactic reactions in patients with Hymenoptera venom allergy: importance of baseline serum tryptase- a study of the European Academy of Allergology and Clinical Immunology Interest Group on Insect Venom Hypersensitivity. *J Allergy Clin Immunol*, 2009, 124, 1047-54.

[27] Bonadonna, P; Perbellini, O; Passalacqua, G; Caruso, B; Colarossi, S; Dal Fior, D; Castellani, L; Bonetto, C; Frattini, F; Dama, A; Martinelli, G; Chilosi, M; Senna, G; Pizzolo, G; Zanotti, R. Clonal mast cell disorders in patients with systemic reactions to Hymenoptera stings and increased serum tryptase levels. *J Allergy Clin Immunol*, 2009, 123, 680-6.

[28] Sánchez-Borges, M; Capriles-Hulett, A; Caballero-Fonseca, F. Adverse reactions to selective cyclooxygenase-2 inhibitors (coxibs). *Am J Ther*, 2004, 11, 494-500.

[29] Sánchez-Borges, M. NSAID hypersensitivity (respiratory, cutaneous, and generalized anaphylactic symptoms). *Med Clin N Am*, 2010, 94, 853-64.

[30] Kowalski, ML; Makowska, JS; Blanca, M; Bavbek, S; Bochenek, G; Bousquet, J; Bousquet, P; Celik, G; Demoly, P; Gomes, ER; Nizankowska-Mogilnicka, E; Romano, A; Sánchez-Borges, M; Sanz, M; Torres, MJ; De Weck, A; Szczeklik, A; Brockow, K. Hypersensitivity to nonsteroidal anti-inflammatory drugs (NSAIDs)- Classification, diagnosis and management: Review of the EAACI/ENDA and GA2LEN/HANNA. *Allergy*, 2011, 66, 818-29.

[31] Czerniawska-Mysik, G; Szczeklik, A. Idiosyncrasy to pyrazolone drugs. *Allergy*, 1981, 36, 381-4.

[32] Kowalski, ML; Woszczek, G; Bienkiewicz, B; Mis, M. Association of pyrazolone drug hypersensitivity with HLA-DQ and –DR antigens. *Clin Exp Allergy*, 1998, 28, 1153-8.

[33] Picado, C. The role of cyclooxygenase in acetylsalicylic acid sensitivity. *Allergy Clin Immunol Int: J World Allergy Org*, 2006, 18, 154-7.

[34] Simons, FER; Ardusso, L; Bilo, MB; El-Gamal, YM; Ledford, DK; Ring, J; Sánchez-Borges, M; Senna, GE; Sheik, A; Thong, BY. World Allergy Organization Guidelines for the assessment and management of anaphylaxis. *J Allergy Clin Immunol*, 2011, 127, 587-93, e1-e20.

[35] Quiralte, J. Aspirin-induced isolated periorbital angioedema. *Ann Allergy Asthma Immunol*, 1998, 81 (5 Pt 1):459.

[36] Cant, AJ; Gibson, P; Dancy, M. Food hypersensitivity made life threatening by ingestion of aspirin. *Br Med J*, 1984, 288, 755-6.

[37] Paul, E; Gall, HM; Müller, I; et al. Dramatic augmentation of a food allergy by acetylsalicylic acid. *J Allergy Clin Immunol*, 2000, 105, 884.

[38] Aihara, M; Miyazawa, M; Osuna, H; et al. Food-dependent exercise-induced anaphylaxis: Influence of concurrent aspirin administration on skin testing and provocation. *Br J Dermatol*, 2002, 146, 466-72.

[39] Fujita, H; Osuna, H; Kanbara, T; et al. Wheat anaphylaxis enhanced by administration of acetyl salicylic acid or by exercise. *Arerugi*, 2005, 54, 1203-7.

[40] Inomata, N; Nakamura, K; Yamane, Y; et al. Enhancement of nonsteroidal anti-inflammatory drugs and preventive effect of antihistamines and disodium cromglycate on wheat allergy. *Arerugi*, 2006, 55, 1304-11.

[41] Nakamura, K; Inomata, N; Ikezawa, Z. Dramatic augmentation of wheat allergy by aspirin in a dose-dependent manner. *Ann Allergy Asthma Immunol*, 2006, 97, 712-3.

[42] Vidal, C; Bartolomé, B; González-Quintela, A; et al. Prawns, barnacles and nonsteroidal anti-inflammatory drugs: Effect modifiers or diagnostic confounders. *J Investig Allergol Clin Immunol*, 2007, 17, 113-8.

[43] Fujii, H; Kambe, N; Fujisawa, A; Kohno, K; Morita, E; Miyachi, Y. Food-dependent exercise-induced anaphylaxis induced by low dose aspirin therapy. *Allergol Int*, 2008, 57, 97-8.

[44] Inoue, Y; Adachi, A; Ueno, M; et al. The inhibition effect of a synthetic analogue of prostaglandin E1 to the provocation by aspirin in patients with wheat-dependent exercise-induced anaphylaxis. *Arerugi*, 2009, 58, 1418-25.

[45] Matsuo, H; Kaneko, S; Tsujino, Y; et al. Effects of non-steroidal anti-inflammatory drugs (NSAIDs) on serum allergen levels after wheat ingestion. *J Dermatol Sci*, 2009, 53, 241-3.

[46] Matsukura, S; Aihara, M; Sugawara, M; et al. Two cases of wheat-dependent anaphylaxis induced by aspirin administration but not by exercise. *Clin Exp Dermatol*, 2010, 35, 233-7.

[47] Izumi, K; Aihara, M; Ikezawa, Z. Effects of non steroidal anti-inflammatory drugs (NSAIDs) on immediate-type food allergy. Analysis of Japanese cases from 1998 to 2009. *Arerugi,* 2009, 58, 1629-39.

[48] Shirai, T; Matsui, T; Uta, T; Chida, K; Nakamura, H. Nonsteroidal anti-inflammatory drugs enhance allergic reactions in a patient with wheat-induced anaphylaxis. *Allergy*, 2003, 58, 1071-81.

[49] Suzuki, Y; Ra, C. Analysis of the mechanism for the development of allergic skin inflammation and the application for its treatment: Aspirin modulation of IgE-dependent mast cell activation. Role of aspirin-induced exacerbation of immediate allergy. *J Pharmacol Sci*, 2009, 110, 233-44.

[50] Sánchez-Borges, M; Fernández-Caldas, E; Capriles-Hulett, A; Caballero-Fonseca, F. Mite-induced inflammation: more than allergy. *Allergy Rhinol*, 2012, 3, 1-5.

[51] Sánchez-Borges, M; Capriles-Hulett, A; Caballero-Fonseca, F; Perez, R. Tolerability to new COX-2 inhibitors in NSAID-sensitive patients with cutaneous reactions. *Ann Allergy Asthma Immunol*, 2001, 87, 201-4.

[52] Sánchez-Borges, M; Capriles-Hulett, A; Caballero-Fonseca, F. Cutaneous hypersensitivity reactions to inhibitors of cyclooxygenase-2. Results from 307 oral provocation tests and review of the literature. *Allergy Clin Immunol Int: J World Allergy Org*, 2007, 19, 44-9.

[53] Kowalski, ML; Bienkiewicz, B; Woszczek, G. Diagnosis of pyrazolone drug sensitivity: clinical history versus skin testing and in vitro testing. *Allergy Asthma Proc*, 1999, 20, 347-52.

[54] Gamboa, PM; Sanz, ML; Caballero, MR; Antepara, I; Urrutia, I; Jauregui, I; González, G; Diéguez, I; De Weck, AL. Use of CD63 expression as a marker of in vitro basophil activation and leukotriene determination in metamizol allergic patients. *Allergy*, 2003, 58, 312-7.

[55] Gómez, E; Blanca-Lopez, N; Torres, MJ; Requena, G; Rondon, C; Canto, G; Blanca, M; Mayorga, C. Immunoglobulin E-mediated immediate allergic reactions to dipyrone: value of basophil activation test in the identification of patients. *Clin Exp Allergy*, 2009, 39, 1217-24.

[56] Gamboa, P; Sanz, ML; Caballero, MR; Urrutia, I; Antépara, I; Esparza, R; de Weck, AL. The flow-cytometric determination of basophil activation induced by aspirin and other non-steroidal anti-inflammatory drugs (NSAIDs) is useful for in vitro diagnosis of the NSAID hypersensitivity syndrome. *Clin Exp Allergy*, 2004, 34, 1448-57.

[57] Sánchez-Borges, M; Capriles-Hulett, A; Caballero-Fonseca, F. A novel phenotype of NSAID hypersensitivity: The high risk patient. *J World Allergy Org*, 2009, 2, 17-9.

In: Anaphylaxis: Principles and Practice
Editor: M. Thirumala Krishna
ISBN: 978-1-62618-688-0

Chapter IX

Hymenoptera Sting Anaphylaxis

M. Beatrice Bilo*[*]*, Leonardo Antonicelli and Floriano Bonifazi

Allergy Unit - Department of Immunology, Allergy and Respiratory Diseases, University Hospital Ospedali Riuniti di Ancona, Ancona, Italy

Abstract

Insect sting allergy remains an important cause of morbidity and mortality all over the world. For patients with sting systemic reactions, prevention of future systemic reactions goes through the correct use of epinephrine by the Emergency Department doctors, the referral to an allergist for diagnosis and prescription of specific immunotherapy, if needed, and the proper techniques for self administration of epinephrine. However, compliance with international guidelines for the treatment of anaphylaxis, also in the specific case of insect-sting anaphylaxis, appears to be very low. Even recent epidemiological studies continue to reveal the poor management of venom-allergic patients and the startling lack of awareness of efficacy of venom immunotherapy.

Nevertheless, hymenoptera sting hypersensitivity and venom immunotherapy represent an excellent model for the study of anaphylaxis and immune tolerance. In recent years, new insights have emerged into both the immunological mechanisms of venom immunotherapy and the natural history and risk factors of severe systemic reactions in untreated as well as treated patients.

The availability of high quality venom extracts for use in the diagnosis and treatment of insect venom allergy has dramatically improved the prognosis and the health-related quality of life of venom-allergic patients. Subcutaneous venom immunotherapy is probably the most effective form of specific allergen immunotherapy. However, neither the efficacy nor the safety of the treatment are optimal, especially as regards to bee venom immunotherapy, and so there is considerable room for further improvement in these all-important areas. A number of new strategies for venom immunotherapy, mostly

[*] Corresponding author: Allergy Unit - Department of Immunology, Allergy and Respiratory Diseases, University Hospital Ospedali Riuniti di Ancona, Ancona, Italy; Tel. +39 071 5963804 Fax +39 071 5963253; b.bilo@ospedaliriuniti.marche.it.

based on genetic engineering, have been described; unfortunately, so far only a few of them have been used in humans.

Introduction

Hymenoptera stings are responsible for significant morbidity and deterioration in health-related quality of life (HRQL) due to the allergic reactions they cause, the most severe of which can culminate in fatal anaphylaxis [1-3].

Though the study of Hymenoptera sting allergy has unraveled most of the dilemmas in the immunology, pathophysiology, diagnosis and treatment of anaphylaxis, some mysteries of the natural history of venom sensitization and risk factors for an unfavourable outcome in both treated and untreated patients remain to be elucidated. Moreover, the general population and especially healthcare workers need to be made more aware of the disease and the availability of venom immunotherapy (VIT) as epidemiological studies continue to reveal that a substantial number of patients admitted to the emergency department had a known history of a previous generalized allergic sting reaction/s [4], and that auto-injectable epinephrine was not made available and importantly they were not undergoing VIT [5].

Taxonomy

Figure 1 shows the taxonomy of Hymenoptera [1,6]. Worldwide the hymenoptera belong to the suborder *Aculeate*, which groups the superfamilies *Apidea* and *Vespidae*. The family ***Apidae*** is made up of honeybees *(Apis mellifera)* which are brown in colour and moderately hairy and bumble-bees *(*Genus *Bombus)* which are bigger than honeybees, much more hairy and characterized by the distinct yellow or white bands on their abdomen.

The family ***Vespidae*** is divided into the *Vespinae* and *Polistinae* subfamilies, with differences at the junction of the thorax and abdomen. Whilst *Vespinae* have a truncated junction, *Polistinae* are more oval in shape. *Vespidae* are almost hairless and have black and yellow striped abdomen.

Vespula, Dolichovespula and *Vespa* make up the three genera of the *Vespinae.* The *Vespula spp* (*V. germanica* and *V. vulgaris) are* the most important species in Europe and easily distinguished from insects of the genus *Vespa* (Hornets) by their smaller size, but much harder from those of the genus *Dolichovespula* by the shorter distance between their eyes and upper jaws (short-headed wasps).

Dolichovespula media, D. saxonica and *D. sylvestris* are the commoner species of the genus *Dolichovespula* in Europe. In the genus *Vespa*, *Vespa crabro* (European hornet) is most prevalent in Europe.

In Europe *P. nimpha, P. gallicus,* and above all *P. dominulus* are widespread especially in the Mediterranean areas.

In central and northern Europe vespid (mainly *Vespula spp*) and honeybee stings are the most prevalent, whereas in the Mediterranean area stings from *Polistes and Vespula* are more frequent than honeybee stings; bumble-bee stings are rare throughout Europe and constitute more of an occupational hazard [1].

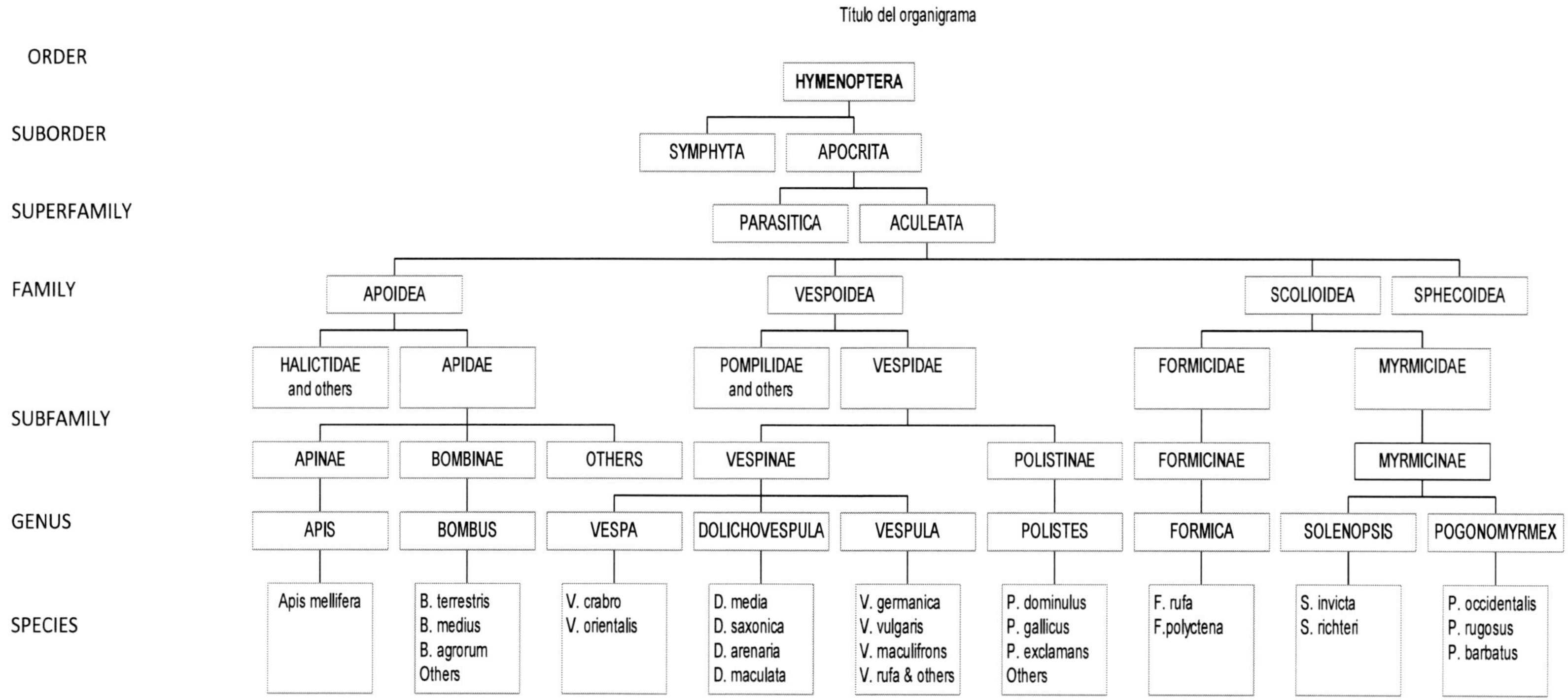

Figure 1. Taxonomy of Hymenoptera.

Table 1. Vespid species in the USA and Europe [7]

Genus	Species Europe	Popular Name Europe	Species USA	Popular Name USA
Polistes	Gallicus Dominulus	Wasp	Annularis Fuscatus Exclamans	Paper wasp
Vespula	Vulgaris Germanica Rufa	Wasp	Vulgaris Germanica Maculifronts	Yellow jacket
Dolichovespula	Media Saxonica	Wasp	Maculata Arenaria	Hornet
Vespa	Crabro Orientalis	Hornet	Crabro	European hornet

Several of the European species of the vespid family differ from those found in the USA (Table 1) [7]. Furthermore, common names for vespids in the USA and Europe are different and may lead to confusion (Table 1). Also, in the United States stinging hymenoptera include the fire ant (*Solenopsis invicta*), and while fire ants may be seen in Australia the jack jumper ant (*Myrmecia pilosula*) seems to pose more of a threat. In Europe allergic reactions from ant stings are an extremely rare occurrence and only a few cases have been reported, mostly to *Formica rufa*, which do not fall within the scope of this chapter.

Entomology, Behaviour of Insects and Risk of Stings

Social *Aculeatae* insects have developed a division of labour, in which sterile females form a class of workers, whose activities include nest-building, brood care, and defence of the nest or hive. The stinger of female workers is formed from the ovipositor and is not usable for the laying of eggs. The female *Aculeatae* stinging apparatus consists of a supporting stiletto and two lancets covering a poison canal. The venom is produced in the acid gland and stored in the venom sac, from which it is squeezed. Since the sting lancet has barbs, especially in bees, it easily embeds itself deep into the elastic skin of mammals, but not into the chitinous surface of other insects. Bees can therefore remove their stinger from other insects, though not from the soft skin of their human victims because of multiple small barbs.

Knowledge of insect behaviour and biology may help to identify the stinging insect, thereby making it easier to avoid further stings. Insects which forage on human foods pose the greatest threatas they not only attack in the vicinity of the nest site but further afield wherever man is going about his everyday routine business. Human food mainly attracts *Vespula spp.* However, sweets and fruits also attract honeybees and other insects.

Apidae: Honey bees and bumble-bees tend only to sting to defend themselves or when a critical distance from the nest is exceeded. Honeybees are bred by man all over the world for pollination, honey and wax production. Bumble-bees are increasingly used in green houses for their efficiency as pollinators of certain plants. The entire colony usually survives through winter and even on warm winter days honeybees may leave the hive and sting. Unlike vespids, large colonies of honey bees already exists early on as springtime making their stings common at this time of year.

Vespidae: Since only the queen survives the winter, larger populations are only observed in summer, which is when most vespid stings occur. By preference *Vespula* build their nests underground, in attics or shelters. *V. germanica* and *V. vulgaris* are more aggressive. Stings may often occur for no obvious reason. *Dolichovespula* nests are often built hanging freely from tree branches or under the eaves of house roofs. Stings are rare and occur almost exclusively in the vicinity of the nests. *Vespa crabro* (European hornet) build their nests in hollow tree-trunks or in birds' nesting-boxes. Hornet stings are rare and occur almost exclusively in the vicinity of the nests.

European species of *Polistes* are well adapted to the climate of the Mediterranean basin. However, small colonies of *Polistes* may be observed all over Europe except for the British Isles. Their paper nests hang from tree branches or roofs, only contain one womb and few individuals.

Venom Allergens

The amount of venom injected from a sting varies from one species to another and even within the same species. Honeybees (HBs) release from 50 to 140 μg of venom protein per sting, venom sacs may however contain up to more than 300 μg of venom. Bumble-bee stings release 10 to 31 μg of venom. In contrast *Vespinae* are capable of repeated stings and generally inject less venom per sting: *Vespula* stings release 1.7 to 3.1 μg of venom, *Dolichovespula* stings 2.4 to 5.0 μg and *Polistes* stings from 4.2 to 17 μg of protein.

The amount of venom injected by a single European hornet sting is still unknown though the dry weight of venom per sac was found to be 260 μg [1]. Hymenoptera venoms are a mixture of proteins, which can cause sensitization, and other molecules such as peptides and other low molecular weight components (e.g. biogenic amines, carbohydrates, lipids) many of which are pharmacologically active [8,9]. Accurate knowledge of the venom composition and structure of allergens is a prerequisite for correct diagnosis and treatment of insect venom allergy. The sequences and structures of the majority of major venom allergens have been cloned and sequenced (http://www.allergen.org); several major allergens have been expressed in recombinant form. The major allergens of Vespula venom (VV) are phospholipase A1 (Ves v1) and antigen 5 (Ves v5). Phospholipase A1 is a non-glycosylated, 34 kd enzyme which is not structurally related to HB venom phospholipase A2. Antigen 5 is a non-glycosylated, 23 kd allergen with unknown biological activity, and is also specific for VV as compared to HB venom [9] (Table 2).

Hyaluronidase (Ves v2) is a 38 kd, glycosylated enzyme which cross-reacts with HB venom hyaluronidase (HYA) because of 50% structural homology. Despite this, one recent report highlighted that much of this cross-reactivity arises from cross-reactive carbohydrate determinants (CCDs) [10] and not from homology of peptides. Cross-reactive carbohydrate determinants are not only found in insects but also in plant allergens and are generally considered to be of little clinical relevance. Moreover, only 10 to 15% of Vespula allergic patients are estimated to have specific IgE against the HYA protein, suggesting that it is a minor VV allergen [10].

Table 2. Allergens of *Vespula vulgaris* venom [Original]

Allergen	Biochemical Name	Molecular Weight (kDa)	Major/Minor
Ves v 1	Phospholipase A1B	35	Major
Ves v 2a Ves v 2b	Hyaluronidase Hyaluronidase*	42 42	Minor
Ves v 3	Dipeptidylpeptidase IV	100	Minor
Ves v 4	CUB-protease	42	?
Ves v 5	Antigen 5	25	Major
Ves v 6	Vitellogenin	200	?

* Putative isoform of Ves v 2a without enzymatic activity.

More recently, a glycosylated 100 kd VV allergen was identified as a dipeptidylpeptidase (Ves v3) [11], which is probably a minor allergen and may cross-react with the dipeptidylpeptidase (Api m5) of BV.

Vespula venom contains a number of low molecular weight components including histamine, serotonin, catecholamines, carbohydrates, amino acids, polyamines and volatile pheromones. Several VV kinins, oligopeptides, whose biological activities are similar to that of bradykinin, mastoparan, and a mast cell degranulating tetradecapeptide have been described. Much of mastoparan's biological activity is akin to that of the modulation of regulatory G-proteins, calmodulin, phospholipases and protein kinases [9]. Despite the obvious geographical differences, the overall composition of allergenic compounds is similar in all vespids venoms [12], the most common allergens of which are phospholipase A1, antigen 5 and HYA. In the case of Polistes, whilst HYA is the major allergen of P. *annulus* (seen in USA), serine-protease is the major determinant of P. *dominulus* (seen in Europe) (Table 3) [13]. To date a total of 12 HB venom allergens are known (Table 4). The most important HB allergen is phospholipase A2 (PLA2), also referred to as Api m 1, which is a glycoprotein with 134 amino acid residues. In addition to the IgE response it elicits, it may trigger an immediate immune response, by increasing leukotriene production [9]. Another well-known HB venom allergen, hyaluronidase (HYA) (also called Api m 2) [9], a 43 kd glycosylated enzyme, is able to enhance the penetration of venom components through the issue fluid. As mentioned above, much of the cross-reactivity between yellow jacket and honeybee HYAs occurs through CCDs [10] It would therefore seem reasonable to assume that antibody binding to HYA from other types of Hymenoptera such as honeybee in many cases may be due to CCDs. Future studies will have to critically reinvestigate the role of hyaluronidase in HB venom allergy, in which Api m 2 is considered the second-most important allergen after PLA2 (Table 4).

Table 3. Allergens of *Polistes dominulus* venom [Original]

Allergen	Biochemical Name	Molecular Weight (kDa)	Major/Minor
Pol d 1	Phospholipase A1	34	Major
Pol d 4	Serine protease	33	?
Pol d 5	Antigen 5	23	Major

Table 4. Allergens of honeybee venom [Original]

Allergen	Biochemical Name	Molecular Weight (kDa)	Major/Minor
Api m 1	Phospholipase A2	16	Major
Api m 2	Hyaluronidase	39	Major (?)
Api m 3	Acid phosphatase	43	Minor
Api m 4	Melittin	2.8	Minor
Api m 5	Low Dipeptidylpeptidase IV	102	?
Api m 6	Cysteine-rich trypsin inhibitor	8	Minor
Api m 7	CUB serine protease	39	?
Api m 8	Carboxylesterase	70	Minor
Api m 9	Serine carboxylesterase	60	?
Api m 10	Icarapin	50-55	?
Api m 11	Major royal jelly protein	50	?
Api m 12	Vitellogenin	200	?

Melittin (Api m 4) peptide, with a molecular weight of 2.84 kd, is the most important and abundant peptide in HB venom, even though only 28% of patients have specific immunoglobulin E (IgE) antibodies against this peptide [9]. Melittin can trigger lysis of a wide range of cells, including mast cells, which can lead to the release of histamine and other intracellular components into surrounding tissue. Other HB venom allergens have also been identified (Table 4). A recent study revealed that Api m 10 seems to be a genuine HB venom allergen with IgE sensitizing potential in a significant percentage of allergic patients, and that three therapeutical HB venom extracts lacked detectable amounts of this component [14].

Other low molecular weight components of HB venom are histamine, dopamine, noradrenalin, free amino acids, lipids, pheromones, and the peptides apamine, mast cell degranulating peptide/MCD-peptide, pertiapin, secapin [9]

Bumble-bee venom contains phospholipase A_2 (Bom p 1), protease (Bom p 4), hyaluronidase, acid phosphatase and several other proteins not found in honeybee venom [15]. Allergens encountered from mainly non-European Hymenoptera are extensively described elsewhere [16].

Cross-Reactivity between Venoms

Available data suggest that venoms and major allergens of different honeybees worldwide are similar and that the structure of the major allergen phospholipase A_2 is highly identical [6,16]. By contrast, variability of allergens within bumble-bee venoms is higher [11]. Immunological cross-reactivity exists between honeybee and bumble-bee venoms and many patients present with concurrent sensitization [15].

Because of the similar venom composition and structure homology of single allergens, cross-reactivity within vespids is high [1]. The antigen 5 and phospholipase allergens from different *Vespula* species show identities up to 95 %. Correspondingly, different *Vespula* venoms strongly cross-react. There is also substantial cross-reactivity between *Vespula*, *Vespa*, and *Dolichovespula* venoms.

Cross-reactivity of the *Vespinae* (*Vespula*, *Dolichovespula*, and *Vespa*) with paper wasps (*Polistes*) is generally lower than the cross-reactivity within the *Vespinae*. Indeed, antigen 5 and phospholipases from Vespula species and Polistes species only have a sequence identity of around 50%.

Cross-reactivity among European species of Polistes (*P. dominulus, P. gallicus*) is extremely high, whereas that between European and American species is weaker [1]. In particular, Antigen 5 and phospholipase from *P. dominulus* differ significantly in their aminoacid sequence from those of North American Polistes venoms [17], while serine proteases from North American and European paper wasps seem to be highly cross-reactive [13]. Cross-reactivity between HYAs of HB and yellow jacket has been extensively discussed in this chapter.

Clinical Presentation

Reactions to Hymenoptera stings are grouped by normal local reactions, large local reactions (LLRs), systemic toxic reactions, systemic anaphylactic reactions, and unusual reactions.

The most frequent clinical patterns of hymenoptera venom allergy (HVA) are LLRs and systemic reactions (SRs). The former is commonly defined as a swelling exceeding 10 cm in diameter lasting 24h. The underlying mechanisms of LLRs seem to be allergic IgE-mediated in some patients, cell-mediated in others or a combination of both [1].

In SRs, which are mostly IgE-mediated, the skin, gastrointestinal, respiratory and cardiovascular systems may be involved. Other mechanisms such as concomitant activation of complement, coagulation pathways and the kallikrein-kinin contact system have however been suggested [18]. In patients with mastocytosis with a negative allergological work-up, possible role of a toxic mediator release from mast cells has been discussed. Some authors [19] however question these 'pseudo-allergic' sting reactions, suggesting that the poor sensitivity of the diagnostic tests may distort findings.

Various classifications of the degree of severity of SRs have been proposed and those of H. Mueller and Ring are the most commonly referred to framework [1] (Table 5). Mueller's however fails to take into account the possible absence of cutaneous symptoms and that an isolated cardiovascular event might be the only allergic sting-induced manifestation, while the Ring's focuses almost entirely on the cardiovascular collapse, on the basis that it this event that is more severe than respiratory compromise. Using a universal definition of anaphylaxis like that recently proposed by the National Institute of Allergy and Infectious Disease (NIAID) and the Food Allergy and Anaphylaxis Network symposia (FAAN) [20] (Table 6) would enable uniform reporting of cases and establishing a more accurate picture of the severity of insect sting reactions. In a recent retrospective cohort study of emergency department (ED) admissions, the 2006 clinical criteria for the diagnosis of anaphylaxis also promulgated in the World Allergy Organisation (WAO) Anaphylaxis Guideline published in 2011 [18] were found to be highly sensitive [21].

Most often, the onset of symptoms occur within a few minutes to an hour following the sting, though in extremely rare cases symptoms have been known to appear hours or even days later.

Table 5. (a) Classification of systemic reactions to insect stings by H. L. Mueller, (b) classification of systemic reactions modified according to J. Ring (1)

Grade	Symptoms
(a)	
Grade I	Generalized urticaria, itching, malaise and anxiety
Grade II	Any of the above plus two of more of the following: angioedema, chest constriction, nausea, vomiting, diarrhea, abdominal pain, dizziness
Grade III	Any of the above plus two or more of the following: dyspnea, wheezing, stridor, dysarthria, hoarseness, weakness, confusion, feeling of impending disaster
Grade IV	Any of the above plus two or more of the following: fall in blood pressure, collapse, loss of consciousness, incontinence, cyanosis.
(b)	
Grade I	Generalised skin symptoms (e.g. flush, generalised urticaria, angioedema)
Grade II	Mild to moderate pulmonary, cardiovascular, and/or gastrointestinal symptoms
Grade III	Anaphylactic shock, loss of consciousness
Grade IV	Cardiac arrest, apnoea

Table 6. Clinical Criteria for Diagnosing Anaphylaxis [20]

Anaphylaxis is highly likely when any one of the following three criteria is fulfilled
1. Acute onset of an illness (minutes to several hours) with involvement of the skin, mucosal tissue, or both (eg, generalized urticaria, itching or flushing, swollen lips-tongue-uvula) AND AT LEAST ONE OF THE FOLLOWING: A) Respiratory compromise (eg, dyspnea, wheeze-bronchospasm, stridor, reduced PEF, hypoxemia) B) Reduced blood pressure or associated symptoms of end-organ dysfunction (eg. hypotonia [collapse], syncope, incontinence)
2. Two or more of the following that occur rapidly after exposure to a likely allergen for that patient (minutes to several hours) A) Involvement of the skin-mucosal tissue (eg, generalized urticaria, itch-flush, swollen lips-tongue-uvula) B) Respiratory compromise (eg, dyspnea, wheeze-bronchospasm, stridor, reduced peak expiratory flow [PEF], hypoxemia) C) Reduced blood pressure or associated symptoms (eg, hypotonia [collapse], syncope, incontinence) D) Persistent gastrointestinal symptoms (eg, crampy, abdominal pain, vomiting)
3. Reduced blood pressure after exposure to known allergen for that patient (minutes to several hours) A) Infants and children: low systolic blood pressure (age-specific) or greater than 30% decrease in systolic blood pressure* B) Adults: systolic blood pressure of less than 90 mm Hg or greater than 30% decrease from that person's baseline

PEF, peak expiratory flow.

* Low systolic blood pressure for children is defined as less than 70 mm Hg from 1 month to 1 year, less than (70 mm Hg + [2 x age]) from 1 to 10 years, and less than 90 mm Hg from 11 to 17 years.

Normally, recovery from anaphylaxis is within a few hours. 'Biphasic reactions' are another rare occurrence where there is an early onset followed by an apparent recovery and a subsequent relapse after 4-24 hours. Fatal reactions after insect stings occur but are rare. Autopsies after fatal sting reactions revealed significant cardiopulmonary co-morbidity in 50 % or even in majority of victims.

Epidemiology of Hymenoptera Venom Allergy

Depending on climate, 56.6-94.5% of interviewees remember being stung by a Hymenoptera insect at least once in their lives [22]. The prevalence of sensitization (indicated by a positive skin test and/or the detection of serum specific IgE in patients with no previous case history) is estimated at between 9.3 % and 28.7% in the adult population which is related to the degree of exposure to stings (in 30 % to 60% of beekeepers) and to the insect distribution and behaviour. The prevalence of LLRs in the general population ranges from 2.4% to 26.4 %, up to 38 % in beekeepers [23]. What accounts for such a wide variation remains to be unraveled, although the difference in definition of an LLR and quantifying the degree of exposure may be contributing factors.

Population-Based Studies of Insect Sting Induced-Systemic Reactions

In the USA the prevalence of SRs among adults ranges from 0.5% up to 3.3% [2].

European epidemiological studies report a prevalence of SRs between 1.5 % and 8.9 % [6,22].

Table 7 shows studies on the prevalence of SRs over the last decade, among which 0.6% to 25% cases of anaphylaxis were reported [24-30].

The prevalence of SRs in paediatric subjects seems to be lower. The degree of variability in the prevalence of SRs can essentially be accounted for by variables including the lack of an universal definition of anaphylaxis, a standard system of classification for allergic reactions, differences in data collection, the venoms used in diagnostic tests, differences between the populations studied, their professions and hobbies, and sting exposure [22].

The prevalence of SRs among beekeepers falls between 4.4 % and 38% [23].

Bumblebee anaphylaxis is rare due to their non-aggressiveness, although occupationally exposed people such as gardeners and horticultural workers in tomato farms are particularly at risk, epidemiological data are lacking [15].

Epidemiological Data Extrapolated from Anaphylaxis Studies due to Any Cause

Analysis of the latest population-based studies of anaphylaxis (irrespective of trigger) as well as the anaphylaxis registries of Latin American and German-speaking countries, conducted over a two to ten year span, revealed that insect sting was responsible for 0.3-37.5% of the total number of cases reported (Table 8) [31-37].

Table 7. Prevalence of Hymenoptera venom allergy: Epidemiological studies for the last decade [original]

References	Country	Study population	Number of subjects	Systemic reactions (%)	Severe Systemic reactions (%)	Skin test and/or Serum IgE positivities in systemic reactors (%)
Incorvaia [24]	Italy	Factory workers Foresters	462 112	2.8 4.5	Not specified	Not done
Navarro [25]	Spain	Working population (Ford Factory)	1,064	2.3	0.6 (IV grade Mueller's class.)	100 (IDT and serum IgE)
Nittner-Marszalska [26]	Poland	General population	169	8.9	0.6 (IV grade Mueller's class.)	53.3 (IDT /or serum IgE)
Fernandez [27]	Spain	Rural area population	145	2.8	25 (IV grade Mueller's class.)	50 (serum IgE)
Graif [28]	Israel	High school children	10,021	6.5 (moderate to severe)	2.5	Not done
Onbasi [29]	Turkey	General population	709	5.4	1.2	Not done
Marques [30]	Spain	General population	4,991	1	16	Not specified

PT: prick testing ; IDT: intradermal testing.

Table 8. Insect sting anaphylaxis: data extrapolated from studies of anaphylaxis due to any cause of anaphylaxis for the last years [original]

First author, year	Country	Type of study	Period of study	Study population	No. of cases of anaphylaxis	Insect sting (%)	No. of fatalities
Yang [31]	Korea	R (inpatients, outpatients, ED)	6 yrs 6 months	Children and adults	138	11.8	1*
De Swert [32]	Belgium	P	2 yrs	Children	64	7.3	0
Decker [33]	Rochester (Minnesota)	P	10 yrs	Children and adults	211	18.5	0
Tejedor Alonso [34]	Alcorcon (Spain)	P (inpatients, outpatients, ED, GPs)	2 yrs	Children and adults	336	0.3	0
Orhan [35]	Turkey	R	10 yrs	Children	224	37.5	1**
Solè [36]	Latin America§ (OLASA)	P	2 yrs	Children and adolescents	191	26.2	0
Hompes [37]	Germany° (Anaphylaxis registry)	P	4 yrs	Children and adolescents	197	24	0

R= retrospective P= Prospective; * Death not due to an insect sting; ** Death due to honeybee sting.

§OLASA: Online Latin American Survey of anaphylaxis (outpatients seen by the specialist).

° Voluntary anaphylaxis registry of German-speaking countries.

This figure is somewhat different from that reported by previous studies (7.3-59%) [6]. The Alcorcon [34] and Minnesota [33] findings are of particular note in that there was just one Hymenoptera-induced episode of sting-induced anaphylaxis in Spain (0.3%) compared with 18.5% in Minnesota. Possible explanations are the urban setting of Alcorcon and the colony collapse in Spain.

In contrast, in a recent multi-centre, retrospective, case study performed in Turkish children Hymenoptera stings were responsible for 37.5% of cases of anaphylaxis, and mainly due to HB stings, one of which registered as fatal [35].

Over the last decade, in ED studies of anaphylaxis 'due to any cause', the prevalence of insect sting- induced anaphylaxis has been estimated between 1.5% and 34% [22]. Many factors may underlie these disparate estimates and include the lack of standard diagnostic guidelines, the diverse population profiles, different International Classification of Disease, 9th Revision, Clinical Modification (ICD-9-CM) codes and other system codes, geography or allergen exposure. Moreover, in ED studies, the aetiology of anaphylaxis is based on the assessment of ED admissions rather than the confirmatory diagnostic test of an accurate allergy evaluation.

Emergency Department Admissions after Insect Stings

The largest multi-centre study of individuals presenting to the ED with insect sting allergic reactions was conducted in 15 North American EDs [4] under the ICD-9-CM code. Of the total number of admissions, 358 (58%) were local reactions, diagnosed as rashes, hives or swelling confined to or contiguous with the sting site. Two hundred and fifty nine (42%) were SRs, of which 70 (27%) were mild, 143 (55%) moderate and 46 (18%) severe [4].

Biphasic Anaphylactic Reactions

A biphasic anaphylactic reaction (BAR) occurs in 1–20% of cases of anaphylaxis but seems to be uncommon with insect stings as it is generally associated with the most severe reactions [38]. Indeed, among 46 cases of the BARs reported in six papers, hymenoptera stings were responsible for about 20% [22]. In a more recent study in Turkish children one BAR was observed in about 3% of anaphylaxis cases [35], suggesting that the phenomenon is less frequent in children than in adults. Fatalities can occur, but are extremely rare in insect sting BAR.

Mortality

The incidence of insect sting mortality from early anaphylaxis ranges from 0.03 to 0.48 fatalities per 1,000,000 inhabitants per year [7].

The USA Center for Disease Control estimates an average annual rate of 90-100 deaths due to venom anaphylaxis [39]. The German Federal Office of Statistics reported 335 deaths between 1990 and 2006 after hymenoptera stings [40].

In Italy, available Italian Institute of Statistics (ISTAT) data dating from 1994 up to 2003 reports 94 cases of insect sting deaths as defined by the ICD-9-CM code 989.5 (insect sting allergy) [22]. However, underestimates are common worldwide, with many sting fatalities being misdiagnosed [22,39]. The latest individual country studies on fatal anaphylaxis indicate that the percentage of fatal stings is around 20% of all fatal anaphylaxis causes [22].

In Pumphrey's study, out of 212 cases of fatal anaphylaxis 47 (22%) were due to insect stings (29 wasp, four bee and 14 unidentified) [41]. Death commonly resulted from shock 10–15 min after the sting and in a quarter of cases from angioedema of the upper airways. Although fatalities occurred mostly in the over 40-year-olds, children are also at risk. Fifteen percent of fatal stings occurred at work, 32% in the garden, 34% at home and 5% in bed [40].

Natural History and Risk Factors

In contrast to a high prevalence of sensitization to hymenoptera venom in adults, SRs only occur in a small proportion. Why only some sensitized patients develop SR or a LLR to a future sting has not been elucidated. A distinction needs to be drawn between factors that are associated with a higher risk of stings from those that influence the outcome and severity of a reaction. This subchapter will focus on the latter.

Factors Influencing the Severity of an Allergic Reaction (Table 9)

Age. In children, about 60% of SRs are mild and are generally cutaneous, whereas in about 70% of adults symptoms are respiratory and/or cardiovascular. Elderly patients more often develop severe SRs [42,43], where the fatality rate is higher than in children and young adults [22]. Children with cutaneous SRs have a lower rate of recurrence over time than adults, while those with moderate to severe SRs continue to have a high risk of reactions even 15–20 years later [44].

Severity of the preceding reaction. In general, after a LLR, between 5% and 15% of subjects develop an SR when re-stung. Whilst the estimated risk of a SR is linked to severity, age and the sting interval, adults with a recent history of severe anaphylaxis are estimated to have a 40–60% chance of reacting to a re-sting, as opposed to those with mild SRs who have a 20% chance of subsequent SRs [45]. Even though in general the risk of recurrence of SRs is linked to the severity of the previous reaction, it seems that a less severe preceding SR produces a booster effect which may predispose the patient to subsequent severe reactions [42]. However, the absence of urticaria/angioedema during anaphylaxis and a time interval < 5 minutes from the sting to the onset of symptoms appear to be further risk factors for a severe SR [43].

Atopy. Currently, there is no evidence of a higher risk of severe reactions in atopic patients. In contrast, atopy may increase the severity of SRs in beekeepers and their family members. It has been suggested that whilst they work at their hives, atopic beekeepers with allergic rhino-conjunctivitis or asthma are more prone to sensitization than non-atopic beekeepers [23], either due to exposure to airborne inhalants or multiple stings.

Gender. Even though the vast majority HVA studies demonstrate that men are more prone than women, there exists controversial data on the prevalence of HVA between genders. Despite this, the latest studies on fatal anaphylaxis from individual countries report that most fatalities occured in male patients [22].

Sting site. The belief that sting reactions located in the head, neck or throat are more severe than those in the extremities, whether fatal or not, needs further confirmation [22]

Insects. According to sting challenge studies non VIT treated bee venom-allergic patients are at a greater risk of a SR on re-sting (44 – 52%) than those who are vespid venom allergic (24 – 25%) [22]. However, the well-known association between bee allergy and more severe SRs could be untrue for field stings, as demonstrated by a European prospective multicentre study in which vespid venom allergy was significantly associated with severe reactions after a field sting [42].

Table 9. Factors influencing the severity of Hymenoptera stings [22]

History of prior severe sting reaction (with respiratory or cardiovascular symptoms), older age
Insect type (honeybee, European hornet)
Pre-existing disease: cardiovascular disease, asthma
Drugs: particularly beta blockers (also eye drops), angiotensin-converting enzyme inhibitors
Sting site (e.g., head)*
Mast cell diseases, elevated baseline serum tryptase concentration

* Not confirmed by all studies.

It may be that less HB venom is delivered at a field sting as most sting victims attempt to rapidly remove the stinger.

The relative risk for life-threatening sting reactions in the Mediterranean area is about three times higher for hornet (Vespa *crabro*) stings than for honeybee or wasp stings [7].

Besides patients suffering from mast cell diseases, anaphylaxis is usually confined to individuals with an allergy to a specific insect species.

Cardiovascular diseases and therapies. Pre-existing cardiovascular diseases are risk factors for particularly severe and fatal anaphylactic sting reactions. Beta-blockers do not seem to increase the overall risk of a SR, but may make it more severe or refractory. A recent study confirmed that treatment with angiotensin-converting enzyme inhibitors (ACEI) is a risk factor for SRs [42]. However, cardiovascular diseases are much more frequent than anaphylaxis and because of the effectiveness of beta-blockers, in cases of comorbidity a careful risk analysis is required [42].

Elevated baseline serum tryptase, mast cell diseases. Particularly severe cardiovascular, even fatal sting reactions may occur in patients with mast cell diseases [19] and monoclonal mast cell activation syndrome [47]. Certain genetic factors may be associated with indolent systemic mastocytosis that may pre-dispose to severe SRs [48]. Even in HVA patients who have not been diagnosed with mastocytosis, a baseline serum tryptase concentration (BSTC) > 5 mcg/l for adults [42] and > 7.5 mcg/l for children [49] seem to be the most useful predictors of severe SRs.

Other potential risk factors. Besides elevated basal serum tryptase levels, severe or fatal anaphylaxis might be associated with defects in mediator degradation pathways, resulting, for example, in elevated baseline levels of bradykinin (because of low serum ACE activity) and platelet-activating factor (PAF) (because of low serum PAF acetylhydrolase activity) [18,50].

Risk factors for biphasic anaphylactic and fatal sting reactions. Several risk factors for biphasic and protracted reactions emerge from the literature that probably apply to insect sting anaphylaxis and include a more rapid onset of anaphylaxis, delayed use of epinephrine, an inadequate amount of administered epinephrine given for the first response, the requirement of large doses of epinephrine, cardiovascular and respiratory diseases and concurrent therapy with beta-blockers [40].

Possible factors for fatal stings include a positive history of hymenoptera allergy (but not always), male gender, age over 40 years, probably because of comorbid cardiovascular diseases, perhaps the sting site (head or neck), bee and European hornet stings, mast cell diseases and the delayed administration or non-use of epinephrine [7].

Diagnosis

The goal of diagnosis is to classify the type of reaction, to identify the culprit insect and to explain the pathomechanism. Thus the diagnosis of HVA is based on clinical history, skin tests and measurement of specific IgE antibodies (sIgE) in serum, which has led to the publication of European and American clinical practice parameters [1-3].

However, the first comprehensive audit of the diagnosis and management of HVA patients in the UK revealed differences in current practice with respect to the European Academy of Allergy and Clinical Immunology (EAACI) Guidelines, leading to the conclusion that certain areas require greater compliance [51].

History

The patient is asked to describe his/her symptoms and the course of the sting reaction, number of stings, clues as to the type of insect involved and individual risk factors for anaphylaxis. In patients with a history of severe SR dermatological evaluation is recommended to rule out a possible diagnosis of cutaneous mastocytosis.

Uncertainty regarding the nature of the stinging insect (bee or wasp) is a common clinical conundrum except in the case of beekeepers. In patients with an unclear or suggestive psychosomatic reaction, scrutinisation of emergency room and ambulance records is recommended.

Basic Tests

As venom sensitization is found in about 10-20% of history-negative persons, only those with a history of a previous SR are in general eligible for diagnostic testing [1-3] (Table 10). In some countries diagnostic tests are also performed in some patients who have a history of LLRs solely to improve their quality of life, even though the the risk of a future SR is low [39]. Skin tests are 'gold standard' in the diagnosis and should be performed at least 2 weeks after a sting reaction in order to rule out a false negative response during the refractory period [1]. Because the duration of refractoriness may be longer, they should, if negative in the presence of a definite history of a SR, be repeated after 1–2 months. However, in some patients, sensitization is demonstrable only in the first week after the sting. Guidelines recommend stepwise incremental venom skin tests, starting with a skin-prick test (from a concentration of 10 up to 100 μg/ml) [1-3].

Table 10. Indications for diagnostic testing [Original]

Indication in:
• Patients with a history of a previous SR
No indication in:
• Subjects with a family history of a severe SR • Subjects who have undue fear of developing a sting SR arising from a news report of a fatal sting reaction • As a screening in the general population
Questionable indication in:
• Patients with a history of a previous LLR

SR: systemic reaction; LLR: large local reaction.

Even at venom concentrations of 100 μg/ml, the sensitivity of the skin prick test is lower than that of the intradermal test (0.001-1.0 μg/ml), which has to be used in order to confirm the negative result. Intradermal tests at concentrations greater than 1 μg/ml have been associated with irritant responses [39].

Skin tests with hymenoptera venoms are generally safe, even when applied in patients with mastocytosis [52]. Nevertheless, though rare, SRs can also occur in non-mastocytosis patients.

Standardised hymenoptera venom products, including lyophilized protein extract for honey bee, bumblebee, yellow jacket and *Polistes* wasp venoms, are commercially available in many countries, the latter two being mixtures of the clinically relevant species. In view of of lower cross-reactivity between venoms of the European and American species of *Polistes* [17], commercial preparations of European *Polistes dominulus* venom are now available [53]

Bumblebee venom allergy is sometimes distinct from HB venom allergy and requires specific testing. Unfortunately, there is no approved diagnostic venom for skin testing or treatment of bumblebee allergy, with the exception of Italy.

A skin prick test with aeroallergens may be useful for detecting atopic diathesis and for a better understanding of the HVs diagnostic results.

In vitro tests, such as the levels of specific IgE to hymenoptera venom, can be employed to detect sensitization. The concentration of the HV-sIgE to the causal venom increases sharply a few days or weeks after the sting due to 'boostering' in response to antigen exposure and often subsequently decreases, a pattern of this kind can help identify the culprit insect [1-3].

The most recently developed tests are usually the most sensitive. However, their sensitivity in patients with a history of systemic sting reactions is lower than that of intradermal skin tests, especially when more than a year has elapsed since the reaction [1].

If *in vitro* tests are negative in approximately 20% of positive skin tests, the converse is also true, since approximately 10% of negative skin tests yield a positive *in vitro* result. It is important to underline that the utility of laboratory tests is dependent on the reliability of the methods employed by clinical laboratories. Clinicians should familiarize themselves with variability between kits/assays and laboratories. As a standard procedure therefore, European guidelines recommend skin testing as well as evaluation of venom-specific IgE in all patients with a history of SRs [1].

There is no correlation between the severity of sting reactions and skin-test reactivity or the concentration of venom sIgE [1-3]. Indeed, the most positive skin tests occur in patients with LLRs only, while almost 25% of patients who are referred for evaluation of a sting-induced SR have a negative SPT and show a positive intradermal test only at the highest concentration (1 μg/ml), thus illustrating the importance of tests using the full panel of diagnostic venom concentrations. On the other hand, fatal sting anaphylaxis is a potential occurrence in patients without detectable venom-specific IgE in their serum.

Finally, baseline serum tryptase concentration should be checked in all patients with SRs [2,3].

Component Resolved Diagnosis (CRD)

Even though simple in itself, shortcomings in the diagnosis persist, and include the presence of IgE-negative anaphylaxis (which affects 10-20% of patients) or double positivity to both bee and *vespid* venoms in diagnostic tests in patients with a single-positive history. Negative test results can be due to the involvement of a different pathogenic mechanism, the presence of mast cell disease, the time elapsed since the last reaction, or poor test sensitivity.

Double positivity to both bee and *vespid* venoms has been observed in 25-40% of HVA patients, thus making the choice of correct venom immunotherapy prescription a difficult one. Double positivity may arise from dual sensitization, cross-reactivity between epitopes on hyaluronidase in the two venoms or more frequently to CCDs of venoms and common allergens. Since several major venom allergens have been expressed in recombinant form, some of which are now commercially available for diagnostic purposes, the so-called molecular diagnosis or CRD should also be applicable in the field of HVA. The first study published on this topic reported double IgE positivity to whole venoms in 59% of 200 venom allergic patients by CAP, but only 17% were double positive to rApi m 1 and rVes v 5 (species specific major allergens without CCDs of the honey bee and Vespula). The author concluded that double positivity to both Api m 1 and Ves v 5 indicates true double sensitization, thus suggesting immunotherapy with both venoms [54]. More recent studies [54-58] found a lower diagnostic sensitivity of CAP-FEIA rApi m 1 for the detection of HB venom allergy. However, different laboratory methods, sources of honeybee allergens as well as variations in selection criteria of patients with HB venom allergy may be the cause of these differences in sensitivity. The addition of other recombinant species-specific bee venom allergens without CCDs (Api m 3 or Api m10) would further increase diagnostic accuracy.

Implementing a similar approach might provide valid confirmation of genuine wasp venom sensitization. Because some patients with wasp venom allergy could go undiagnosed [54], the combined determination of sIgE to Ves v 1 and 5 from yellow jacket is essential [10,59]. Nevertheless, rVes v 1 and 5 failed to diagnose 8% of subjects with established allergy, thus indicating the need to add more allergens, to include Ves v 2 and probably Ves v 3 [59]. Moreover, the detection of CCD specific IgE is also possible, and different methods and carbohydrate antigens (bromelain, MUXF3, horseradish peroxidase and ascorbic acid oxidase) are used [54,60]. In the south of Europe double sensitization to either Vespula or Polistes species is more frequent than that of Vespula and honeybee. According to a recent study, the major allergens of *Polistes dominulus* and *Vespula vulgaris* venoms, namely phopholipase and antigen 5, are required to identify the probable sensitizing species in vespid-allergic patients, while Vespula hyaluronidase was shown to have no additional value as regards the specificity of the assay [61]. The importance of rPol d 1for the a CRD of Polistes venom allergy in Europe was also underlined by a recent case report [62]. One Spanish patient on immunotherapy with the American Polistes species venom mixture developed anaphylaxis following a sting challenge with *Polistes dominulus*. However, no reaction occurred with the same sting challenge when the treatment was switched to the *Polistes dominulus* extract after a more sensitive diagnosis using rPol d 1 specific IgE [62].

In conclusion, provided that the majority or all relevant venom allergens are available in recombinant form, CRD could help discrimination between genuine dual sensitization and cross-reactivity in patients with double-positive specific IgE to conventional venom extracts and enable allergists to make the correct choice of venom for immunotherapy and avoid unnecessary treatment with both insect venoms. Interestingly, CRD could also help identify patients with a positive history of Hymenoptera venom–induced anaphylaxis, who have double-negative test results to venom extracts [55]. At the present time it does not appear that CRD is able to distinguish between more and less severe systemic sting-induced reactions.

Additional Tests

Although IgE-inhibition test is helpful in distinguishing between cross-reactivity and double sensitization, it is expensive and results are sometimes difficult to interpret [1,3].

Other *in vitro* methods, such as cellular antigen stimulation test (CAST) or basophil activation test (BAT), are also expensive, labour intensive but can be used to determine immunological sensitization in 'difficult-to-diagnose' and patients with mastocytosis [52,63]; their predictive value in relation to a sting challenge has not yet been analyzed in larger studies. However, their use should be restricted to laboratories with expert technicians, bearing in mind that a positive result may also point to a non-IgE mediated mast-cell activation mechanism. Currently they have no role in the routine diagnosis of HVA [3].

Lastly, because of the risk of a severe reaction and poor negative predictive value, live insect sting challenge/s should not be used as a diagnostic tool in untreated patients to assess tolerance [1].

Preventive Measures

Based on the knowledge of living conditions and habitat of social *Aculeatae* a series of recommendations have been formulated aimed at substantially minimizing the risk of field re-sting, although as yet no evidence-based studies have been performed to support this [9,64].

Table 11 describes some of the activities and behaviours which carry a risk of receiving a Hymenoptera sting. Detailed information should be provided to subjects at risk, pertaining to where the culprit insect builds its nest, as well as the types of food, which attract it. In the case of honeybees, the stinger should be quickly removed regardless of how, since it has been demonstrated that it is the time the stinger remains embedded in the skin that determines the degree of envenomization. Patients should be instructed in person and also through booklets or pamphlets on allergen avoidance.

Untreated patients with anaphylaxis should not be given β-blockers, except when the administration of these drugs is urgently required as in the case of certain cardiac arrhythmias [2,64]. If possible, angiotensin converting enzyme inhibitors (ACEI) should also be avoided [42].

Table 11. Some activities and 'behaviours at risk' for being stung by Hymenoptera [64, modified]

• Outdoor eating and drinking
• Walking barefoot
• Gardening (especially trimming hedges, picking flowers and fruit)
• Outdoor sport (especially with scanty outfit or open mouth)
• Staying close to beehives when honey is collected, removing vespid nests from attic or windows
• Avoiding shoes and clothing while outdoors
• Wearing bright coloured clothing
• Using strong perfumes and fragrances
• Keeping uneaten food uncovered, especially outdoors
• Avoiding full protective clothing while handling bees

Emergency Treatment

Large Local Reactions

A Hymenoptera sting-induced LLR may persist for several days or more and may be accompanied by itching, pain or both. Cold compresses may help to reduce local pain and swelling; oral antihistamines and topical corticosteroids will relieve the pain and itching. In cases of very severe and protracted swelling, oral corticosteroids equivalent to 50 mg prednisone daily for a few days may be indicated. If a LLR occurs involves the mouth, the patient must be kept under close observation for possible upper airway obstruction [64].

Systemic and Anaphylactic Reactions

The most effective drugs in the treatment of systemic allergic reactions are sympathomimetics, antihistamines and corticosteroids. Injected epinephrine is the treatment of choice for cases of acute anaphylaxis [2,3,18,40,64] and immediate and prompt administration regardless of the trigger [18] is associated with better clinical outcome.

Emergency Kits

Hymenoptera venom allergic patients should carry an emergency kit for self administration at all times, especially during the insect season. Several epinephrine pre-loaded preparations for immediate self administration are commercially available. In patients subject to side effects of epinephrine (e.g. those with severe cardiovascular disease), self-administration of the drug should be reviewed by a cardiologist.

In addition, patients should receive a tablet set containing a rapidly effective oral H1-antihistamine (e.g. cetirizine 2 x 10 mg) and corticosteroids (e.g. prednisone 2 x 50 mg). In the case of re-exposure to the culprit Hymenoptera or an unidentified insect, patients who are not yet undergoing VIT should take the tablets immediately and prepare the epinephrine for self administration with the first symptoms of a systemic allergic reaction [40,64]. Patients should also be advised to adopt a supine posture with their legs raised should they develop hypotension, while seeking medical help [18]. As for paediatric HVA subjects, liaison with the school is recommended.

Self-injectable epinephrine (SIE) should be considered for all patients with a history of a SR, particularly those who have experienced 'moderate-severe' episodes or those with increased risk of future exposure to stings (beekeepers, gardners, waste management workers etc.), underlying mast cell disorders or raised baseline serum tryptase or other co-morbidities (that would further compromise cardiac and/or respiratory reserve) even if the diagnostic work-up is negative for venom specific IgE [2]. At the present time there is no consensus on the prescription of SIE in the case of mild SRs with negative testing for venom specific IgE, except for concomitant systemic mastocytosis or urticaria pigmentosa [19].

The American Guidelines [2] also provided additional discussion and guidance on the issues surrounding the prescription of epinephrine injectors and the instructions on when and when not to use them. Patients, caregivers and healthcare providers alike benefit from focused instruction and regular review of the optimal use of epinephrine in the first aid treatment of anaphylaxis.

Even in patients who have a relatively 'low risk' of severe sting-induced anaphylaxis, the decision on whether to carry injectable epinephrine can be individualized through a patient-physician discussion exploring the 'pros and cons' [2] A double dose of SIE should be prescribed in patients with previous severe anaphylactic reactions, biphasic or protracted anaphylactic reactions, those who suffer from obesity and/or do not have immediate access to emergency medical care.

Specific Immunotherapy

Venom immunotherapy is the most effective form of treatment available to physicians and patients [65], designed to reduce the risk of a subsequent SR, prevent morbidity and mortality and also improve health related quality of life (HRQL) [66].

Mechanisms of VIT

The underlying immunological mechanisms of VIT are continuously being elucidated and hymenoptera venom allergy has always played an important role in this context.

Indeed, honeybee VIT represents the best model for the study of the cellular and molecular mechanisms underlying development of immune tolerance in sensitized individuals, as well as high-dose bee venom exposure in beekeepers (BKs) through natural bee stings enables understanding of the mechanisms of T-cell tolerance to allergens in non-atopic individuals [67].

Different mechanisms involving specific cell populations, play a role in the different phases of VIT [68], which can be summarised as follows:

Peripheral T-cell tolerance represents an essential step in successful VIT, and is mainly characterized by the generation of allergen-specific T regulatory (Treg cells) [69]. In patients undergoing honeybee VIT as well as in heavily exposed BKs, the *in vitro* immune response in lymphocyte cultures following stimulation with venom proteins reveals the presence of CD4+ Treg cells which secrete IL-10, consequently inhibiting the secretion of cytokines IL-4, IL-5 and IL-13 from TH2-cells in turn down regulating specific IgE production, while venom specific IgG4 increases [68]. It is worth noting that during bee VIT, IL-10 serum levels rise from the second day of the build-up phase [70]. Also, Treg cells directly or indirectly suppress effector cells of allergic inflammation such as mast cells, basophils and eosinophils, and inhibit maturation of dendritic cells [67].

The very early effects of VIT are also associated with reduction in effector cell function. Immediately after a day 1 of an ultra rush protocol of HB VIT, histamine and leukotriene release from venom stimulated basophils is already significantly reduced [71], thus explaining the extremely precocious protection observed in HB venom allergic patients who have already reached the maintenance dose during rush or ultrarush VIT [72]. This effect during very early effective VIT may be due to the piecemeal release of mediators through the high allergen doses applied over a short period which may decrease the granule content of mediators and affect the threshold of mast-cell and basophil activation.

During VIT, specific IgG, in particular, IgG4 antibodies greatly increase within two weeks and stay elevated during the entire period of treatment, whereas skin sensitivity and specific IgE antibodies (after an initial increase) gradually fall during prolonged VIT. The result is a rapid decrease in the ratio of specific IgE to specific IgG4, and consequently the inhibition of mast cell activation through interaction of venom allergens with effector cell bound specific IgE. Blocking antibodies also inhibit IgE-facilitated allergen presentation to T cells and prevent an allergen-induced boost of memory IgE production. There is however no close correlation between the IgG titers and the clinical efficacy of VIT [9,64], while one does exist between IgG4 concentrations and the number of annual stings and years spent in beekeeping [1,9].

The role of histamine and its receptors in VIT is a new field of research [67].

Indications

Indications for VIT are based on the history of a SR, a positive venom skin test or specific IgE, knowledge of the natural history and established risk factors for a severe outcome [1,21,42]. Nevertheless, the risk of a future allergic reaction can only be expressed statistically since none of the available tests are able to accurately predict the outcome of the next sting. This makes it difficult to determine the threshold level of statistical risk at which the administration of VIT can be justified.

Recommendations for the use of VIT vary between countries. Whilst there is a strong consensus that VIT is indicated for severe systemic sting reaction/s, there is less agreement on whether adults, and especially paediatric subjects, with mild (cutaneous) reactions are suitable candidates, as the prognosis in dermal reactors *per se* is usually considered to be good [2,3,64]. Since the occurrence and severity of anaphylaxis depends on several factors, the pros and cons of not administering VIT should be thoroughly discussed on individual merits. Furthermore, even in children with mild SRs, management should also take the child's behavioural risks into consideration. The 2005 European and the more recently published British Guidelines [1,3] state that in both children and adults with a history of a systemic non-life-threatening reactions (e.g., urticaria, erythema and pruritus) other factors may influence the decision on whether or not to commence VIT including occupation and/or hobbies where there is a high risk of exposure, the culprit insect itself, concomitant cardiovascular diseases, others pathologies, such as mastocytosis or raised baseline serum tryptase and psychological factors arising from anxiety that can seriously impair patient HRQL (Table 12) [64]. Venom immunotherapy is usually not indicated in majority of children who have experienced nonlifethreatening urticaria and angioedema distant from the sting site in the absence of additional risk factors or impairment of HRQL (Table 13).

Based on limited evidence, the current consensus is that venom immunotherapy is indicated in HVA patients with mast cell diseases as the treatment can reduce SRs, *albeit* to a lesser extent than in otherwise healthy subjects with HVA [52]. Moreover, an elevated baseline serum tryptase should be included in the decision to offer the treatment [43]. According to some authors VIT should also be considered in some patients with mastocytosis with a negative allergological work up and a previous history of SR [40,73].

Even though subcutaneous VIT is effective even in LLRs [74], it is not usually recommended. However the specialist may consider it as a treatment option in highly exposed subjects such as beekeepers who need repeated short courses of corticosteroids [2,65].

Contraindications

In Europe, contraindications for VIT are the same as for inhalant specific immunotherapy (IT), with the implication that in general serious immunological diseases, cancer, chronic infections are absolute contraindications for immunotherapy in general. Indeed, in some selected venom allergic patients, the advantages of VIT may tip the balance in favour of the treatment, particularly where there is a high risk of stings, a previous history of a 'near fatal' sting reaction and perhaps in the case of mast cell diseases [65]. More multicentre studies are nevertheless required to better evaluate the effectiveness and safety of VIT in these patients.

In contrast to inhalant IT guidelines, no contraindications exist for major cardiovascular diseases as far as serious insect venom allergies are concerned. Venom immunotherapy can also be considered in the context of an elderly patient with underlying cardiac disease or patients with significant cardiac and/or pulmonary disorders where there is an increased risk of developing severe or even fatal sting reactions [46]. Also patients who developed myocardial infarction as a consequence of severe anaphylaxis could be considered for VIT [65].

Beta-blockers are not an absolute contraindication for VIT where the cardiac risk from withdrawal of treatment outweighs that of a systemic reaction during VIT [46,64]. Another strategy that warrants consideration after a cardiologist consultation is the withdrawal of beta-blocker during up-dosing and its resumption after the patient has reached the maintenance phase. In such cases, a rapid build-up phase may be considered in order to minimize the period in which the beta-blocker therapy is suspended.

Currently, there are no data to support or exclude the potentially harmful role of angiotensin-receptor blockers in VIT treated patients [65].

Table 12. EAACI Guidelines: Indications for venom immunotherapy [64]

Type of reaction	**Diagnostic tests ST and/or IgE**	**Decision regarding venom immunotherapy**
Adults / Children		
Respiratory and cardiovascular symptoms	Positive Negative	Yes No
Urticaria if risk factors or quality of life impairment present	Positive Negative	Yes No
Large local	Positive or negative	No
Unusual	Positive or negative	No

Table 13. BSACI Guidelines: Indications for venom immunotherapy [3]

Yes	Sometimes*	Not usually*	No
• Systemic reaction with hypotension ±laryngeal oedema±asthma • Must have positive venom specific IgE	• Mild asthma, moderate angio-oedema, abdominal pain, vomiting, diarrhoea, mild hypotensive symptoms (light headedness, dizziness) • In those at high risk of further stings, e.g. beekeeper/ proximity to bees, or occupational exposure, e.g. fruit farmers, gardeners, etc. • Other factors, e.g. proximity to medical help, patient preference, effect on quality of life.	Cutaneous systemic reaction, e.g. cutaneous: urticaria+/- mild angio-oedema	Local reaction Toxic reaction Any systemic reaction, independent of severity, if negative specific IgE

* Co-morbid conditions including asthma or other respiratory disease, cardiac conditions, raised baseline plasma tryptase/mastocytosis constitute 'risk factors' and should be carefully considered before making a decision for VIT.

Tricyclic antidepressants should ideally be withdrawn before commencement of VIT because of potential drug interaction (arrhythmia and hypertension) with adrenaline [3].

Venom immunotherapy should not be commenced during pregnancy, although well-tolerated maintenance VIT may be continued in order to prevent the risk of further SRs in the mother and protect the foetus [2,3,64].

Selection of Venoms

Selection is based on the positive identification of the culprit insect, the results of the diagnostic tests and venom cross-reactivity [1,2,3,64].

According to some experts it is prudent to prescribe VIT with any venom which gives positive responses for venom-specific IgE, whereas other investigators recommend treatment only with the venom of the suspected offending insect, even if skin or *in vitro* test results for other stinging insects are positive [2]. As far as vespids are concerned, the common practice in North America is to administer a mixed vespid venom preparation, containing equal parts (in general 100 µg) of each venom of yellow jacket (*Vespula* species), yellow hornet (*Dolichovespula arenaria*) and white-faced hornet (*Dolichovespula maculata*) [2]. In Europe, because of the geographical distribution of each species and the ample cross-reactivity among venoms of *Vespula*, *Dolichovespula* and *Vespa*, treatment with *Vespula* venom usually suffices in the temperate European climate [3,64]. The extracts are typically a mix of five or six species of *Vespula* (*vulgaris, germanica, maculifrons, flavopilosa, pensylvanica* and *squamosa*).

Owing to the incomplete cross-reactivity between vespinae and paper wasps (*Polistes*) in the Mediterranean, patients who test positive to both venoms should be treated with both, unless complete cross-reactivity can be demonstrated [64]. The same approach is used in the Gulf states of the USA, where *Polistes* is a common species [2,53].

The recently demonstrated weaker cross-reactivity between European and American paper wasps [17] raises the need to introduce, at least in Europe, the *P. gallicus* or *P. dominulus* extract (the latter only recently being available in some European countries) into clinical practice for diagnostic and therapeutic purposes to replace the American *Polistes* species mixture presently being used [65].

Allergic reactions to the European hornet (*V. crabro*) are rare, except in Mediterranean countries where its sting is a risk factor for severe SRs [22]. *V. crabro* venom has some antigens in common with *Vespula* venom, thought a third of *V. crabro*-allergic individuals have positive skin and sIgE tests restricted to only *V. crabro* venom [75]. As a consequence, in Italy, it is common practice to use *V. crabro* extract for both diagnostic and therapeutic purposes.

Where diagnostic tests with *Vespula* and honeybee yield dual positivity and the identity of the culprit insect is uncertain, both venoms should be used, unless complete cross-reactivity can be demonstrated [64].

Honeybee and bumblebee venoms show high cross-reactivity [1,15]. Immunotherapy with honeybee venom alone may be sufficient in non-professionally exposed bumblebee-allergic patients with bee venom primary sensitization, whose reaction is most likely due to cross-reactivity. In occupationally exposed patients, who are frequently stung by bumblebees, purified bumblebee venom for immunotherapy, when available, is recommended owing to the low or absent cross-reactivity with honeybee venom [15,64]. In the USA, no approved diagnostic or therapeutic extracts for the bumblebee or Mediterranean wasp (*P. dominulus*) are commercially available [16].

The whole-body fire ant extract used in the USA for the treatment of allergic patients [2] is not commercially available in Europe where the allergic reactions to ants are extremely rare. For this reason fire ant VIT is not described in this chapter.

Efficacy

The efficacy of subcutaneous VIT has been confirmed by both sting challenge and in-field sting in prospective controlled and uncontrolled studies - in one meta-analysis and one systematic review demonstrating that the protection rate of honeybee VIT is lower than that of vespid VIT [76-78]. The recommended maintenance dose is 100 µg of venom, both in children and adults. This dose was originally proposed because it was believed to be equivalent to the total dose of venom delivered by two stings which may not be true in the case of HB stings. The repeatedly observed difference in the success rates in honeybee and vespid venom allergic patients is not completely clear. The fact that the amount of venom delivered by a honeybee sting during a 'sting challenge' is much larger and more consistent may partially explain this difference in the reaction rate to sting challenges, which has also been observed in untreated patients [19,64]. The composition of HB venom, which is a mixture of proteins and other pharmacologically active molecules, including mellitin [1,9], may require another explanation.

The standard 100 µg dose prevents SRs in 75–95% of re-stung patients [3,64] and provides greater protection than a 50 µg dose in adults [2]. According to a recent study, a 50 µg HB maintenance dose in children provides adequate protection from future HB stings [79], almost as if the bees were able to distinguish between their adult and child victims and in consideration of such, injected the child with less venom. This study showed a SR rate of 13.6% 1 to 18 years after completion of 2 to 7 years of immunotherapy using a 50 µg maintenance dose, which was considered similar to the protection afforded by using a 100 µg maintenance dose of bee venom in adults. However, the limitations of this study are that it is retrospective, in which the young participants' accounts of the reaction type were subjective [79].

One recent study demonstrated the efficacy of a 100 µg maintenance dose of *P. dominulus* extract after a field sting [80].

It is noteworthy that when VIT is effective, it is protective immediately after the conventional maintenance dose has been reached, as demonstrated by sting challenges performed one week after reaching the maintenance dose, even after a 3-5 day rush protocol [72].

A dose of 200 µg is recommended when a SR follows an insect sting despite VIT with 100 µg and in highly exposed populations, such as beekeepers [23,81]. According to some authors, an elevated maintenance dose of usually 200 µg at the commencement of VIT should be administered to honeybee allergic patients with concomitant mastocytosis and also considered in vespid venom allergic subjects with additional risk factors [23].

Most American patients receive mixed vespid venoms, with an injectable maintenance dose of 300–400 μg, which provides approximately 98% protection [2,65].

The protection rate of 100 μg bumblebee VIT, demonstrated by sting challenge and 'in-field' stings, is estimated to be higher than 90% [15].

Some authors have demonstrated reduced efficacy of VIT in mastocytosis [52,82], and limited data thus far has not shown differences between HB and Vespid treated patients.

Table 14 presents risk factors currently known to predispose a patient to a SR at sting challenge or an 'in-field' sting during VIT.

Self-injectable epinephrine should always be prescribed until the standard protective maintenance dosage had been reached [3]. Its prescription during the maintenance phase of VIT remains a controversial question. Taking into account the known risk factors for the incomplete protection of VIT, SIE should be prescribed in cases of severe pre-VIT systemic reactions, severe HBV allergy, incomplete VIT protection, a systemic reaction during VIT and in patients with mastocytosis and elevated baseline serum tryptase [83].

Treatment Protocol

Many treatment protocols for induction phase of VIT have been designed, and vary with respect to the number of injections, doses of venom and the time needed to reach the protective dose [3,65] [Table 15]. Rush and ultra-rush protocols are particularly efficient in highly exposed subjects like BKs or in patients referred to the specialist just prior to the start of the insect season. In addition, the cost of administering ultra-rush VIT is lower than that of the slower protocols [84]. The accelerated protocols are currently employed in most, but not all, European countries and are not readily available at most American and British medical centres [2,51,53].

Table 16 shows the current rush protocol used in our Department in HB venom allergic patients [85].

The starting dose of VIT is between 0.001 and 0.1 μg (Table 15). However, in a recent report, the authors demonstrated that initiating VIT at a 1 μg dose can be safely administered in rush protocols in both adults and children [86].

If two or more venoms are required, they should be administered in separate protocols a few days apart. While the build-up phase of VIT should be performed by an allergist, in some countries, maintenance treatment is eventually continued by less expert general practitioners.

Table 14. Risk factors for treatment failure in patients on VIT (or reduced effectiveness) [65, modified]

• Honeybee venom
• Lower maintenance venom dose
• Repeated side effects during VIT
• Mastocytosis
• An elevated baseline serum tryptase concentration (vespid allergic patients)

Table 15. Some examples of treatment protocols for VIT [66]

DAY	HOUR	CONVENTIONAL*	CLUSTER*	RUSH*	ULTRARUSH*
1	0	0.01	0.001	0.01	0.1
	0.5	0.1	0.01	0.1	1
	1		0.1	1	10
	1.5				20
	2.5			2	30
					40
2	0			4	
	1			8	
				10	
				20	
3	0			40	
	1			60	
	2			80	
4	0			100	
8	0	1	1	100	
	1	2	5		
			10		
15	0	4	20	100	50
	1	8	30		
22	0	10	50		100
	1	20	50		
29		40	100	100	
36		60	100		
43		80		100	100
50		100			
57		100			
64			100		
71		100		100	100
85		100			
92			100		
99				100	100
106			100		

* Dose in μg of venom.

Further injections of the maintenance dose of 100 μg, every four weeks during the first year, every six weeks in the second.

Throughout Europe non-purified aqueous (NPA), purified aqueous (PA) extracts, and purified aluminium hydroxide adsorbed (PAHA) preparations (so-called "depot" extracts) are used to perform subcutaneous honeybee and yellow jacket VIT, though in some countries only one type of extract is available [3].

Table 16. One example of protocol of honeybee build-up rush phase [85]

Day	Dose	mL administered	μg administered	Conc. μg/mL
1	1	0.10	0.01	0.1
	2	0.10	0.1	1
	3	0.10	1	10
	4	0.20	2	10
2	5	0.30	3	10
	6	0.35	3.5	10
	7	0.35	3.5	10
3	8	0.10	10	100
	9	0.15	15	100
	10	0.15	15	100
4	11	0.20	20	100
	12	0.25	25	100
	13	0.25	25	100
5	14	0,30	30	100
	15	0.35	35	100
	16	0.35	35	100

Purified venom extracts do not contain vasoactive amines (e.g., dopamine, histamine and serotonin) and have a reduced presence of small peptides (e.g., apamine, kinins and mast-cell degranulating peptide in the final product). The efficacy of PA and depot extracts is supported by studies using both sting challenge and 'in-field' stings, and is comparable to that of non-purified preparations [87]. In the USA, neither PA nor PAHA preparations are commercially available.

The NPA and PA extracts can be used for ultrarush, rush, clustered and maintenance phases, while PAHA preparations are only administered for the conventional build-up and maintenance schedule. Many European specialists switch to depot preparations following the up-dosing phase [87].

The general consensus is that the maintenance interval should be kept at four weeks for the first year, extended to six weeks in the second year, and then to eight weeks if VIT is continued for more than five years, provided that the treatment is tolerated [2,3,64]. If a depot extract is used, extending the injection interval to eight weeks is possible without compromising the effectiveness of therapy [40].

A number of studies have shown that extending the maintenance interval up to 12 weeks may be safe and effective [88]. However, they included very few HB venom allergic patients, in which efficacy was evaluated mostly by 'in-field' stings.

Recent studies evaluating the safety and efficacy of a further prolonged interval between six-monthly injections yielded contrasting data [65].

At the present time no data are available on the optimum maintenance interval for mastocytosis patients [52,82], and presumably prolonging it may endanger the patient.

It is desirable that within the next few years, multicentre clinical trials produce results which will enable clinicians to select patients so that extending the interval between injections becomes risk free.

Table 17. Risk factors for side effects during VIT [65, modified] [63, modified]

•	Honeybee venom > vespid venom
•	Build-up phase > maintenance phase
•	Dose increase schedule (ultra-rush> rush > conventional)
•	Cardiovascular disease
•	Mastocytosis
•	An elevated baseline serum tryptase concentration (during the build-up phase)
•	Treatment with beta-blockers (?) / ACE-inhibitors (?)

Side Effects

Although highly effective, patient compliance with VIT may be impaired by LLRs and SRs [2,3,64]. With respect to inhalant IT LLRs to injections are common, especially during the incremental phase, and occur in up to 50% of patients. They are not a risk factor for a SR and do not usually necessitate a reduction in the dose of venom administered or prevent the protective dose from being reached, but they can be particularly bothersome. For SRs, from the results of multicenter studies, have shown that the proportion of patients with VIT-induced SRs is between 2 and 20%, more frequent with HB than vespid VIT [87]

A recent review of systemic reactions reported the incidence of SRs during VIT as being 25.1% for honeybee venom and 5.8% for vespid venom allergic subjects [89]. Again, in a recent multicentre European study, one of the most important factor significantly associated with severe reactions during the build-up phase of VIT was bee venom allergy [90]. The reasons why HB VIT induces SRs more frequently than vespid is not fully understood.

Presently there is no reliable test able to predict the extent of the risk. The finding that increased basophil sensitivity to allergen-specific *in vitro* stimulation is significantly associated with major side effects to VIT even in children needs to be confirmed by further studies [91]. VIT should therefore only be carried out by an allergist with experience and knowledge in this field, in centres where VIT is routinely administered to large numbers of patients and where the medical staff has expertise in treating anaphylaxis [3,65].

To reduce the incidence of VIT-induced SRs, the risk factors need to be defined. Table 17 summarizes old and new potential risk factors for side effects during VIT.

Discordant data exist on the safety profile of rapid dose increase protocols compared with conventional or cluster up-dosing regimens used mainly in vespid allergic patients [3,64,65,84], although in a large European study rapid dose increase was associated with higher rate of SRs during the build-up phase of VIT [90]. The significant variation in the reported rate of SRs between studies has been attributed at least in part to differences in patient selection criteria for VIT, premedication with antihistamine, SR classification systems and cumulative doses.

In one recent publication, 132 HB allergic subjects were administered a 3-day rush VIT using a non-purified aqueous extract resulting in 31% SRs during the maintenance phase. However, after excluding hyperreactive subjects (e.g. patients who failed to reach the maintenance dose with conventional VIT because of multiple SRs), in 85% of whom the maintenance was reached, the difference between honeybee and Vespid treated patients was not significant (23.7% versus 16%, respectively) [84]. A similar rate of SRs (27.5%) was documented using the same HB extract using a 5-day rush protocol in an Italian study, which was significantly higher than the rate of SRs (2.5%) observed with a corresponding purified aqueous extract [85].

All these data suggest that there may be a difference between honeybee and vespid venoms with respect to the tolerability of the different protocols as well as between extracts.

In any case at present, ultra-rush protocols should only be used by specialists who are experienced in managing VIT, and preferably in an emergency care setting, especially with HBV allergic patients.

Side effects during VIT are probably more frequent in mastocytosis patients, especially in those with yellow jacket venom allergy [52,82], even though risk factors for adverse reactions in these patients (e.g., type of mastocytosis and protocol) have not been extensively investigated. Moreover, BSTC correlates significantly with the frequency of severe side effects during the induction phase of VIT, probably more marked in patients undergoing vespid VIT [90].

In general, repeated anaphylactic reactions are rare, and in such cases, it should be assumed that VIT will not prevent further SRs following a sting. Moreover, treatment should be continued for approximately 6 months with the highest tolerated dose of insect venom (injection interval 1–2 weeks) and then further updosing can be attempted [40].

Table 18 shows the possible current and future strategies for reducing the risk of VIT side effects.

Pre-treatment with an H1 antihistamine has been shown to reduce the number and severity of LLRs and mild systemic reactions to VIT, such as urticaria and angioedema [92]. The finding that antihistamine pre-medication may improve the clinical efficacy of ultra-rush honey bee VIT was not confirmed in HB venom allergic subjects using the same protocol and a different antihistamine [93]. Pretreatment with a combination of H1 antihistamine and a corticosteroid have not yet been performed in honeybee and vespid VIT, except in patients with mast cell diseases [65].

As several case reports document, pretreatment with anti-IgE monoclonal antibodies has been successfully used in HB venom allergic patients, including patients with indolent systemic mastocytosis, almost all of whom experienced SRs to VIT were able to tolerate this after pretreatment with omalizumab [94]. Although fortuitous, the optimal time for the administration of the latter drug during VIT, its dosage, the long term effects and the best incremental protocol of VIT remains to be established [65]. Consequently, the use of omalizumab for this indication is currently ‘off-label’.

Sublingual immunotherapy (SLIT) using honeybee venom has been recently shown to reduce severity of LLRs to a bee sting challenge by more than 50% in 57% of active treated patients [95]. On the basis of these findings and without experimental data on the pharmacokinetics of venom SLIT, significant doubt exists regarding its clinical efficacy in the prevention of future SRs.

There is more than a theoretical basis for believing that PA and PAHA extracts, whose efficacy is comparable to that of NPA preparations, have the potential to reduce the incidence of the side effects of VIT. At present, compared with the therapy with an aqueous extract (both purified and non-purified), VIT with a depot extract is superior as regards the occurrence of LLRs and SRs, and purified extracts appear to be safer than non-purified, especially with respect to the occurrence of LLRs [87].

Table 18. Possible current and future strategies for reducing the risk of honeybee VIT-induced side effects [original]

• Premedication: Antihistamines, Omalizumab
• Purified aqueous and depot extracts
• Route of administration: Intralymphatic
• Modified allergens

A recent study compared, a PA extract and the corresponding NPA extract with identical 5-day rush protocol in HB venom allergic patients with a normal BSTC in terms of the occurrence of SRs. During the 'build-up' phase, SRs were significantly more frequent in patients treated with NPA extracts than in those treated with the corresponding PA preparations. All patients who developed a SR tolerated the depot extract and successfully reached maintenance dose [85]. Hence, if protection through VIT is to be achieved rapidly, the use of purified preparations in a 'rush schedule' and the use of depot preparations for maintenance therapy could be preferable, wherever these extracts are available [87].

VIT Monitoring

The current options for monitoring VIT include skin tests, *in vitro* tests and sting challenge tests. The level of venom-specific IgE level and skin-test sensitivity usually increase in the first months of therapy, return to baseline after 12 months and then decline steadily during maintenance VIT. This decline continues even after cessation of therapy or a sting [6,64]. Less than 20% of patients are skin-test negative after five years of VIT, but 50–60% become negative after 7–10 years [96].

Specific IgG antibodies increase and remain elevated at least as long as VIT is continued [6,64,96]. Initially, these antibodies are IgG1, and later IgG4. The ratio of venom-specific IgE to IgG4 antibodies increases at first and later decrease during VIT, although no difference in the pattern of venom-specific IgE and IgG4 was observed in patients who tolerated an 'in-field' sting compared with those who continued to experience SRs to stings despite VIT [65].

Despite the availability of new improved laboratory techniques, there are no reliable biomarkers of efficacy and data on the role of BAT are conflicting [3,91].

According to some authors, a controlled sting challenge with a single, live insect can be used in treated patients to identify unprotected subjects [40], despite its poor reproducibility and negative predictive value [97]

Duration of VIT

On the premise that the duration of VIT should be decided following a thorough patient–physician discussion of the issues involved, the present recommendations for discontinuing

VIT take into account all these findings, which are very similar in Europe [64] and America [2]. Although not a common occurrence, conversion to a negative venom skin test is an unequivocal indication that VIT should be stopped immediately. If the patient has had a very severe initial allergic reaction, an *in vitro* test should be carried out to confirm the disappearance of venom specific IgE, as only the combination of negative intradermal skin testing at 1 μg/ml with the absence of venom-specific serum IgE antibodies is associated with a strongly diminished risk of relapse [64].

Most patients with mild-to-moderate anaphylactic symptoms and positive skin tests remain protected even years after a 3–5-year course of VIT has been discontinued [64,98], which explains why a 3-5 year treatment period is usually recommended. Studies where long-term protection, up to seven years after discontinuing VIT of at least a 3-year duration, have been evaluated on the basis of 'in-field' sting/s or sting challenges, reveal more frequent relapses than those with a shorter follow-up (protection rate of ~80 vs 83–100%), and a more favourable outcome in children than in adults.

Though not entirely clear the higher risk of relapse in HB venom than in vespid venom allergic patients is well-documented, has been discussed extensively elsewhere [64].

There are no data on the outcome after more than 15 years of VIT, especially for HB VIT.

It is likely that short- and long-term results are more favourable with the much higher total dose administered in the USA than that with 100 μg used elsewhere. More European data on the discontinuation of VIT in allergic vespid patients with 100 μg maintenance dose are needed.

Owing to the small but relevant risk of a reaction from a re-sting, self-administering emergency kits, including epinephrine autoinjectors, should be discussed with every patient when discontinuing VIT [99].

A number of risk factors for the recurrence of SRs following hymenoptera stings after discontinuing VIT have since been identified and are summarized in **Table 19** [2,65]. They include insect type, old age, severity of pretreatment reactions, generalized allergic side effects to VIT injections, incomplete protection upon re-sting during VIT, mast cell diseases and an elevated baseline tryptase level.

Table 19. Risk factors for the recurrence of an SR after stopping VIT [65, modified]

•	Honeybee venom
•	Adults
•	Severe pre-treatment SR
•	SRs during VIT to treatment injection or restings
•	Mastocytosis
•	Elevated baseline serum tryptase concentration

According to the 2005 EU guidelines, longer-term treatment or life-long treatment should be considered in patients with a higher risk of 'very' severe sting reactions (e.g., older age, history of 'very' severe previous sting reactions, elevated basal serum tryptase, mastocytosis or use of beta-blockers); those who have experienced generalized allergic reactions to stings or to immunotherapy injections or during VIT; highly exposed patients, such as beekeepers and their immediate family members [64].

Regardless, some patients at a low risk of relapse prefer to pursue with long-term VIT for a sense of personal safety and improved quality of life, even though ascertaining whether or not patients experience the same improvement in HRQL after discontinuing VIT is difficult to quantify.

By contrast, in the UK as mentioned above the standard duration of VIT is 3 years. Longer or even lifelong treatment in patients with mast cell diseases or a raised baseline tryptase is not advocated in the UK since it is not considered as being evidence-based [3]. It is of note that in the UK no review has ever commissioned to assess the clinical and cost-effectiveness of Pharmalgen (which is the only marketed extract authorized in UK) in the treatment of individuals with venom SRs [99].

After discontinuing VIT, patients should continue to avoid stings. If a SR occurs after stopping VIT, allergy tests should be repeated and reinitiation of VIT should be considered.

Because of the small but real risk of re-sting reactions, self-administering emergency kits, including SIE, should be discussed with every patient when stopping VIT [1], or if the patient is in 'high risk' for the recurrence of a SR following Hymenoptera stings, when treatment was for severe honeybee allergy, in cases of severe pre-VIT reactions or systemic reactions during VIT and comorbidities such as mastocytosis, urticaria pigmentosa or raised BSTC [83,100]

In addition, continuing risk of multiple stings related to occupational activities should also be considered for prescription of SEI after discontinuation of VIT [3].

Future Perspective

The production of recombinant venom allergens will greatly enhance the accuracy of the diagnosis and undoubtedly pave way for novel future therapies.

As for diagnosis, provided that the majority of relevant HB venom allergens are available in recombinant form, CRD will enable physicians to distinguish between genuine double sensitization and cross-reactivity in patients with double-positive IgE results to conventional venom extracts, allowing optimization of patient selection for VIT.

A number of new strategies using sequences of one or more HB allergens, mostly based on genetic engineering, have been studied though only in animal models [9].

The only trial performed in humans in which the efficacy of the treatment was verified by a sting challenge used a mixture of three dominant T-cell peptides of phospholipase. Out of five patients complete protection was observed in three and partial protection in the remaining two [101], confirming that treatment with only one major allergen, even in recombinant unrefolded or point mutated form, may be insufficient.

Lastly, the therapeutic potential of phospholipase bee venom intralymphatic immunisation was analysed in sensitized mice using an anaphylaxis model, showing enhanced allergen-specific IgG and T-cell responses and a Th1-dependent subclass IgG2a production when compared with subcutaneous injections [102]. Similar studies in humans, including clinical parameters and sting challenges, are needed to assess the effectiveness of this route of allergen administration.

Clinical Cases

Case 1

A 67-year-old male patient developed anaphylaxis (facial angioedema, generalized urticaria, breathlessness, cough, hypotension) five minutes after being stung on the leg by a yellow jacket while gardening. The patient was taken to the emergency unit and intramuscular epinephrine (0.5 mg, 1 in 1,000) intravenous chlorpheniramine 10 mg and methylpredsinolone hemisuccinate (40 mg) were administered together with salbutamol nebuliser (5 mg), which slowly improved his symptoms. The patient has ischemic heart disease and had suffered with myocardial infarction in the past and was on beta-blockers (atenolol, 25 mg/d) and an angiotensin converting enzyme (ACE) inhibitor (enalapril 20 mg/d) at the time of the reaction.

The patient had been stung by single Vespids in the past with large local reactions (LLRs) and received the last sting in the previous year. An allergological evaluation was done three months after the acute episode. Skin prick tests to Vespula spp., Polistes dominulus and Apis mellifera venoms were negative (100 mcg/ml). Intradermal skin testing was positive to Vespula spp. (0.001 mcg/ml) and Polistes dominulus (0.1 mcg/ml), negative to Apis mellifera venom (1 mcg/ml). Serum specific IgE determination (CAP-system) gave positive results to Vespula germanica extract (18.5 U/ml) and Polistes venom extract (2.3 U/ml), as well as to Vespid recombinant allergens (r Ves v 5: 26.6 U/ml, r Ves v1: 12.5 U/ml; r Pol d 5: 3.2 U/ml). Serum total IgE was 112 kU/l. The baseline serum tryptase concentration was within the normal limit (4.4 mcg/L).

The final diagnosis was "anaphylactic reaction to yellow jacket venom" in a patient with ischaemic heart disease sensitized to Vespula spp. and Polistes dominulus venoms".

Autoinjectable epinephrine, antihistamine and steroids as well as specific immunotherapy (VIT) with Vespula spp. venom were prescribed.

As the patient was on ACE-inhibitor and beta-blocker, his cardiologist was consulted in order to define a shareable strategy. The ACE-inhibitor was replaced by an angiotensin-II receptor blocker (ARB - sartan) and treatment with beta-blocker was suspended during up-dosing to be resumed once the maintenance phase was reached. Before the commencement of VIT, routine ematic tests and a spirometry were performed as a matter of course.

A two-day rush immunotherapy build-up phase was carried out in our day hospital facility. The patient reached the maintenance dose of 100 mcg of Vespula spp. venom and remained symptom free throughout; the first maintenance dose was administered after one week then at 2 weeks and subsequently every four weeks. After one month treatment with beta- blocker was resumed and the patient is continuing his maintenance injections with no side effects.

Comments

1. Before experiencing his anaphylaxis, the patient was stung by single Vespids resulting in LLRs. One possible explanation is that some of the stings were from different Vespid species (e.g., Polistes dominulus). If this is not the case, as

documented by the data yielded by the limited number of studies on the natural history of LLR in fewer than 500 patients, the risk of a future systemic reaction in patients with a previous LLR is around 10% [7].

2. ACE-inhibitors are contraindicated in venom allergic patients [42]. Indeed, they appear to increase the risk for severe allergic sting reactions only in untreated patients and may be during VIT in highly selected patients. Since there are good reasons to assume that ARBs are associated with a lower anaphylactic risk than ACE inhibitors, the latter was replaced by an ARB, even though there are no current data to either support or exclude the potential harmful role of ARBs in patients treated with VIT.
3. In patients with ischemic heart disease, beta-blockers improve long term morbidity and mortality, have a preventive role by protecting against future heart attacks. In these such cases, treatment with this class of medication could be temporarily suspended during 'up-dosing' after a cardiac consultation and resumed after the maintenance dose has been reached.

Case 2

The patient in question is a 48-year-old construction worker, with a previous diagnosis of urticaria pigmentosa (1980), a history of anaphylactic shock to a Vespid sting received in 2001 (identified as *Polistes*).

In 2004, serum specific IgE (CAP-System) to *Vespula germanica, Polistes sp., Vespa crabro* and *Apis mellifera* venoms were negative. Skin tests were not performed for fear of adverse events in a patient with mast cell disease. As a result, the patient was diagnosed with "non-IgE mediated insect sting anaphylaxis in a patient with urticaria pigmentosa". Self-injectable epinephrine was prescribed and standard patient guidelines provided on how to avoid future stings. The patient was referred to us in 2006 and prick and intradermal tests with *Vespula sp., Polistes sp., Apis mellifera* venoms were negative. Baseline serum tryptase level was 27 mcg/L (normal range < 11.5 mcg/L). Since cross-reactivity between the European species of *Polistes* (*P. gallicus, P. dominulus*) is very high, but weaker between the American and European species, and the patient positively identified the stinging insect as a *Polistes*, serum specific IgE (CAP-System) to *Polistes dominulus* venom was tested and was negative. Intradermal test with *Polistes dominulus* venom was positive at a concentration of 0.1 mcg/ml. "Ultra-rush" specific immunotherapy using an acqueous *Polistes dominulus* venom extract was, therefore, performed over two mornings until a total dose of 100mcg was reached with no side effects. Presently the patient is undergoing maintenance therapy with a depot *Polistes dominulus* venom extract at 6-weekly intervals, and has suffered no side effects. One year ago he was re-stung by a Polistes with no systemic reaction.

Comments

1. Besides loss of sensitization over time and involvement of a different pathogenic mechanisms (19), poor sensitivity of current diagnostic tools should also be included among the causes of 'non-IgE-mediated' insect sting anaphylaxis.

2. Despite high cross-reactivity among the venoms of the various species of *Polistes*, the evidence of a selective specificity unique to European *Polistes* allergens [19] raises the problem of the need for *Polistes dominulus* extract both for diagnostic and therapeutic purposes, at least in Mediterranean countries. As this case demonstrates, omitting to perform skin tests for *Polistes dominulus* venom has led to the misdiagnosis of 'non-IgE-mediated' anaphylaxis, further delaying the start of specific immunotherapy.
3. Some clinicians do not perform skin testing in mastocytosis; indeed there is no evidence to suggest that the incidence of side effects is greater in these patients than non-mastocytosis venom allergic subjects [52].
4. The safest interval between injections and the duration of VIT in patients with mast cell diseases are unanswered questions [52].

Case 3

A 45-year-old female veterinary surgeon developed anaphylaxis (generalized itching, chest constriction, abdominal pain, confusion, feeling of impending disaster, incontinence and loss of consciousness) a few minutes after being stung on the neck by an unknown insect, while out cycling, though her friend stated having seen something like a stinger. Her friend called an ambulance, which responded within minutes. Intramuscular epinephrine (0.50 ml + 0.50 ml, 1 in 1,000), intravenous methylpredsinolone hemisuccinate (20 mg + 20 mg) and chlorpheniramine (10 mg) and oxygen were administered. The patient was first transported to the emergency department and then transferred to the ICU where she was intubated and discharged three days later.

The woman had received numerous stings in the past with no reaction. She developed mild urticaria to last sting from an unidentified insect six months ago. Five years ago she was diagnosed with breast cancer for which she underwent surgery and chemotherapy.

At the time of her allergological work-up, done about one month after the anaphylaxis, her cancer seemed to be in remission. Skin prick tests to Vespula spp., Polistes dominulus and Apis mellifera venoms were negative (100 mcg/ml). Intradermal skin testing was positive to *Vespula spp.* (0.1 mcg/ml), *Polistes dominulus* (1 mcg/ml), and *Apis mellifera* venom (0.1 mcg/ml). Total IgE antibodies were 154 kU/l. Serum specific IgE determination (CAP-system) was positive to *Vespula germanica* (15.6 U/ml), *Polistes* (1.2 U/ml) and *Apis mellifera* extracts (13.9 U/ml). Specific IgE to recombinant allergens gave the following results: r Ves v 5: 19.2 U/ml, r Ves v1: 5.6 U/ml; r Pol d 5: 0.87 U/ml; rApi m 1: negative; MUXF3 CCD: 12.4 U/ml. The baseline serum concentration was within the normal limit (2.5 mcg/L).

The final diagnosis was "anaphylactic shock to yellow jacket sting, in patient sensitized to Vespula spp.; cross-reactivity to CCDsIgE responsible for false positive result with honeybee venom extract".

Self-injectable epinephrine, antihistamine and steroids were prescribed.

Also, the patient was treated with *Vespula spp.* immunotherapy after a careful 'risk-benefit' analysis, taking into account the severity of the last reaction, the patient's profession and leisure risk and the time elapsed since the diagnosis of breast cancer. The patient has been receiving VIT since 2010, and to date has not been re-stung.

Comments

1. The sting site could be of significance and even though the finding that reactions to head, neck and throat stings are more severe than stings in the extremities, in fatal and non-fatal cases alike, this view is not supported by all studies [22]. Moreover, in general the risk of the recurrence of a systemic reaction is linked to the severity of the previous reaction. However, a recent study shows that a less severe preceding SR produces a booster effect which may predispose the patient to subsequent severe reactions [42].
2. Double positivity to both bee and *vespid* venoms with current diagnostic tests in patients with a single-positive history is common in clinical practice. According to the patient's friend, the culprit insect could have been a honeybee, though skin testing and specific IgE to hymenoptera extracts gave similar results for *Vespula spp.* and *Apis mellifera.* Component resolved diagnosis (CRD) enabled us to select the right venom [54,55,58], without which we would have had to prescribe two treatments, considering the severity of reaction. Another means of distinguishing between genuine dual sensitization or cross-reactivity is to use a RAST-inhibition technique, which is more expensive.
3. Malignancy, in particular 'concurrent', is considered as a contraindication for allergen immunotherapy, although this recommendation is not evidence based. There is a need for this recommendation to be discussed in cases of severe allergic reactions to Hymenoptera stings in patients with 'cancer in remission', particularly in patients with a high risk of sting exposure, a history of a 'near fatal' sting reaction or in those with mast cell diseases. In such cases the decision to administer VIT should be made on 'risk-benefit' analysis of individual cases [65].

Conclusion

Between 40% and 85% of fatal sting reaction victims had no history of previous anaphylaxis. Greater insight into the natural history and risk factors is therefore vital.

For patients with SRs, prevention of future severe allergic reactions can be achieved through improvements in emergency management by implementing techniques for prompt diagnosis and treatment of acute allergic reactions and anaphylaxis. Unfortunately, compliance with international guidelines for the treatment of anaphylaxis, even in the specific case of insect sting anaphylaxis, appears to be very low [18]. Moreover, thoroughly educating patients on allergen avoidance strategies and self-administration of 'auto-injectable epinephrine' are also essential to prevent future SRs. A prompt and accurate diagnosis identifies those patients at greatest risk for an adverse outcome and who will benefit from VIT, which remains the most effective treatment available to HVA patients.

Future VIT will probably use chemically modified and recombinant venom allergens, for both improved efficacy and safety. Patient-tailored cocktails can be prepared once all the relevant allergens of a venom are available in recombinant form.

Clinical Pearls

- Hymenoptera stings may cause systemic reactions of varying severity up to fatal anaphylaxis.
- Intramuscular injected epinephrine is regarded as the treatment of choice for acute anaphylaxis.
- Several new factors influencing the severity of hymenoptera sting reactions in untreated patients have been identified and include an elevated baseline serum tryptase level and treatment with angiotensin-converting enzyme inhibitors.
- After a systemic sting reaction, patients should be referred to an allergy specialist for evaluation and consideration of venom immunotherapy (VIT).
- Untreated patients with a history of a systemic reaction are strongly advised to carry emergency kits containing fast acting antihistamine and self-injectable epinephrine.
- Patients, caregivers and health care providers alike benefit from focused instruction and regular review of the optimal use of epinephrine in the first aid treatment of anaphylaxis.
- The standard tolls continue to play a fundamental role in the diagnosis of venom allergy.
- Component resolved diagnosis may greatly enhance the accuracy of the diagnosis, allowing physicians to optimize patient selection for immunotherapy, especially in 'double-positive' patients with a single history. However, some relevant venom allergens are not commercially available in recombinant form.
- Subcutaneous VIT is the only effective treatment for hymenoptera venom allergic patients.
- The indication and duration of VIT should be decided after a thorough patient–physician discussion of the history, consideration of individual risk factors and health related quality of life.
- Certain risk factors for reduced effectiveness of VIT have been identified; in some cases a higher protective dose can be reached.
- Some strategies for reducing the risk of side effects of VIT have been successfully implemented.
- A number of new strategies for VIT, mostly based on genetic engineering, have been described, as well as alternative routes for the administration of VIT (e.g., intralymphatic). However, the majority of them have not yet been used in humans.

References

[1] Bilò, BM; Ruëff, F; Mosbech, H; Bonifazi, F; Oude Elberink, JNG; the EAACI Interest Group on Insect Venom Hypersensitivity. Diagnosis of hymenoptera venom allergy. *Allergy*, 2005, 60(11), 1339–1349.

[2] Golden, DB; Moffitt, J; Nicklas, RA; Freeman, T; Graft, DF; Reisman, RE; Tracy, JM; Bernstein, D; Blessing-Moore, J; Cox, L; Khan, DA; Lang, DM; Oppenheimer, J; Portnoy, JM; Randolph, C; Schuller, DE; Spector, SL; Tilles, SA; Wallace, D. Joint Task Force on Practice Parameters; American Academy of Allergy, Asthma &

Immunology (AAAAI); American College of Allergy, Asthma & Immunology (ACAAI); Joint Council of Allergy, Asthma and Immunology. Stinging insect hypersensitivity: a practice parameter update 2011. *J Allergy Clin Immunol*, 2011, 127(4), 852-4.e1-23.

[3] Krishna, MT; Ewan, PW; Diwakar, L; Durham, SR; Frew, AJ; Leech, SC; Nasser, SM. British Society for Allergy and Clinical Immunology. British Society for Allergy and Clinical Immunology. Diagnosis and management of hymenoptera venomallergy: British Society for Allergy and Clinical Immunology (BSACI) guidelines. *Clin Exp Allergy*, 2011, 41(9), 1201-20.

[4] Clark, S; Long, AA; Gaeta, TJ; Camargo, CA. Jr. Multicenter study of emergency department visits for insect sting allergies. *J Allergy Clin Immunol*, 2005, 116(3), 643–9.

[5] Richter, AG; Nightingale, P; Huissoon, AP; Krishna, MT. Risk factors for systemic reactions to bee venom in British beekeepers. *Ann Allergy Asthma Immunol*, 2011, 106(2), 159-63.

[6] Müller, UR. *Insect Sting Allergy*, 1990. Gustav Fischer, Stuttgart.

[7] Bilò, BM; Bonifazi, F. Epidemiology of insect-venom anaphylaxis. Curr. Opin. *Allergy Clin. Immunol*, 2008, 8(4), 330–337.

[8] Brown, TC; Tankersley, MS. The sting of the honeybee: an allergic perspective. *Ann Allergy Asthma Immunol*, 2011, 107(6), 463-70.

[9] Müller, UR. Hymenoptera venom proteins and peptides for diagnosis and treatment of venom allergic patients. *Inflamm Allergy Drug Targets*, 2011, 10(5), 420-8.

[10] Jin, C; Focke, M; Léonard, R; Jarisch, R; Altmann, F; Hemmer, W. Reassessing the role of hyaluronidase in yellow jacket venom allergy. *J Allergy Clin Immunol*, 2010, 125(1), 184-90.

[11] Blank, S; Seismann, H; Bockisch, B; Braren, I; Cifuentes, L; McIntyre, M; Rühl, D; Ring, J; Bredehorst, R; Ollert, MW; Grunwald, T; Spillner, E. Identification, recombinant expression, and characterization of the 100 kDa high molecular weight Hymenoptera venom allergens Api m 5 and Ves v 3. *J Immunol*, 2010, 184(9), 5403-13.

[12] King, TP; Spangfort, MD. Structure and biology of stinging insect venom allergens. *Int Arch Allergy Immunol*, 2000, 123(2), 99–106.

[13] Winningham, KM; Fitch, CD; Schmidt, M; Hoffman, DR. Hymenoptera venom protease allergens. *J Allergy Clin Immunol*, 2004, 114(4), 928-33.

[14] Blank, S; Seismann, H; Michel, Y; McIntyre, M; Cifuentes, L; Braren, I; Grunwald, T; Darsow, U; Ring, J; Bredehorst, R; Ollert, M; Spillner, E. Api m 10, a genuine A. mellifera venom allergen, is clinically relevant but underrepresented in therapeutic extracts. *Allergy*, 2011, 66(10), 1322-9.

[15] de Groot, H. Allergy to bumblebees. *Curr Opin Allergy Clin Immunol*, 2006, 6(4), 294-7.

[16] Hamilton, RG. Diagnosis and treatment of allergy to hymenoptera venoms. *Curr Opin Allergy Clin Immunol*, 2010, 10(4), 323-9.

[17] Pantera, B; Hoffman, DR; Carresi, L; Cappugi, G; Turillazzi, S; Manao, G; Severino, M; Spadolini, I; Orsomando, G; Moneti, G; Pazzagli, L.Characterization of the major allergens purified from the venom of the paper wasp Polistes gallicus. *Biochim Biophys Acta*, 2003, 1623(2-3), 72-81.

[18] Simons, FE; Ardusso, LR; Bilò, MB; El-Gamal, YM; Ledford, DK; Ring, J; Sanchez-Borges, M; Senna, GE; Sheikh, A; Thong, BY. World Allergy Organization. World Allergy Organization anaphylaxis guidelines: summary. *J Allergy Clin Immunol*, 2011, 127(3), 587-93.e1-22.

[19] Ruëff, F; Dugas-Breit, S; Przybilla, B. Stinging Hymenoptera and mastocytosis. *Curr Opin Allergy Clin Immunol*, 2009, 9(4), 338-42.

[20] Sampson, HA; Muñoz-Furlong, A; Campbell, RL; Adkinson, NF; Jr; Bock, SA; Branum, A; Brown, SG; Camargo, CA; Jr; Cydulka, R; Galli, SJ; Gidudu, J; Gruchalla, RS; Harlor, AD; Jr; Hepner, DL; Lewis, LM; Lieberman, PL; Metcalfe, DD; O'Connor, R; Muraro, A; Rudman, A; Schmitt, C; Scherrer, D; Simons, FE; Thomas, S; Wood, JP; Decker, WW. Second symposium on the definition and management of anaphylaxis: summary report – Second National Institute of Allergy and Infectious Disease/Food Allergy and Anaphylaxis Network symposium. *J Allergy Clin Immunol*, 2006, 117(2), 391–7.

[21] Campbell, RL; Hagan, JB; Manivannan, V; Decker, WW; Kanthala, AR; Bellolio, MF; Smith, VD; Li JT. Evaluation of national institute of allergy and infectious diseases/food allergy and anaphylaxis network criteria for the diagnosis of anaphylaxis in emergency department patients. *J Allergy Clin Immunol.*, 2012, 129(3), 748-52.

[22] Bilò, MB; Bonifazi, F. The natural history and epidemiology of insect venom allergy: clinical implications. *Clin. Exp. Allergy*, 2009, 39(10), 1467–1476.

[23] Müller, U. Bee venom allergy in beekeepers and their family members. *Curr Opin Allergy Clin Immunol*, 2005, 5(4), 343–347.

[24] Incorvaia, C; Senna, G; Mauro, M; Bonadonna, P; Marconi, I; Asero, R; Nitti, F. Prevalence of allergic reactions to Hymenoptera stings in northern Italy. *Eur Ann Allergy Clin Immunol*, 2004, 36(10), 372–4.

[25] Navarro, LA; Pel´aez, A; de la Torre, F; Tenias Burillo, JM; Megías, J Martínez, I. Epidemiological factors on hymenoptera venom allergy in a Spanish adult population. *J Investig Allergol Clin Immunol*, 2004, 14(2), 134–41.

[26] Nittner-Marszalska, M; Liebhart, J; Liebhart, E; Dor, A; Dobek, R; Obojski, A; Medrala, W. Prevalence of Hymenoptera venom allergy and its immunological markers current in adults in Poland. *Med Sci Monit*, 2004, 10(7), 324–9.

[27] Fernandez, J; Soriano, V; Mayorga, L; Mayor, M. Natural history of Hymenoptera venom allergy in Eastern Spain. *Clin Exp Allergy*, 2005, 35(2), 179–85.

[28] Graif, Y; Romano-Zelekha, O; Livne, I; Green, MS; Shohat, T. Allergic reactions to insect stings: results from a national survey of 10 000 junior high school children in Israel. *J Allergy Clin Immunol*, 2006, 117(6), 1435–9.

[29] Onbasi, K; Onbasi, O; Eminbeyli, L; Kaynak, C. Prevalence and alternative therapy methods for bee and wasp allergy in Van. *Allergy*, 2008, 63(2), 246–7.

[30] Marques, L; Vega, A; Munoz, E; Moreno-Ancillo, A. Epidemiologic observations on Hymenoptera allergy in Spain: the alergologica-2005 study. *J Investig Allergol Clin Immunol*, 2009, 19, Suppl 2, 51–55.

[31] Yang, MS; Lee, SH; Kim, TW; Kwon, JW; Lee, SM; Kim, SH; Kwon, HS; Park, CH; Park, HW; Kim, SS; Cho, SH; Min, KU; Kim, YY; Chang, YS. Epidemiologic and clinical features of anaphylaxis in Korea. *Ann Allergy Asthma Immunol*, 2008, 100(1), 31–6.

[32] De Swert, LF; Bullens, D; Raes, M; Dermaux, AM. Anaphylaxis in referred pediatric patients: demographic and clinical features, triggers, and therapeutic approach. *Eur J Pediatr*, 2008, 167(11), 1251–61.

[33] Decker, WW; Campbell, RL; Manivannan, V; Luke, A; St Sauver, JL; Weaver, A; Bellolio, MF; Bergstralh, EJ; Stead, LG; Li, JT. The etiology and incidence of anaphylaxis in Rochester, Minnesota: a report from the Rochester Epidemiology Project. *J Allergy Clin Immunol*, 2008, 122(6), 1161–5.

[34] Tejedor Alonso, MA; Moro Moro, M; Múgica García, MV; Esteban Hernández, J; Rosado Ingelmo, A; Vila Albelda, C; Gomez Traseira, C; Cardenas Contreras, R; Sanz Sacristán, J; Hernández Merino, A. Incidence of anaphylaxis in the city of Alcorcon (Spain), a population-based study. *Clin Exp Allergy*, 2012, 42(4), 578-89.

[35] Orhan, F; Canitez, Y; Bakirtas, A; Yilmaz, O; Boz, AB; Can, D; Kuyucu, S; Harmanci, K; Tahan, F; Reisli, I; Karakas, T; Baki, A; Cokugras, H; Cakir, M; Yuksel, H. Anaphylaxis in Turkish children: a multi-centre, retrospective, case study. *Clin Exp Allergy*, 2011, 41(12), 1767-76.

[36] Sole, D; Ivancevich, JC; Borges, MS; Coelho, MA; Rosario, NA; Ardusso, LR; Bernd, LA; Latin American Anaphylaxis Working Group. Anaphylaxis in Latin America: a report of the online Latin American survey on anaphylaxis (OLASA). Clinics (Sao Paulo). 2011, 66(6), 943-7.

[37] Hompes, S; Köhli, A; Nemat, K; Scherer, K; Lange, L; Rueff, F; Rietschel, E; Reese, T; Szepfalusi, Z; Schwerk, N; Beyer, K; Hawranek, T; Niggemann, B; Worm, M. Provoking allergens and treatment of anaphylaxis in children and adolescents--data from the anaphylaxis registry of German-speaking countries. *Pediatr Allergy Immunol*, 2011, 22(6), 568-74.

[38] Tole, JW; Lieberman, P. Biphasic anaphylaxis: review of incidence, clinical predictors, and observation recommendations. *Immunol Allergy Clin North Am*, 2007, 27(2), 309–26.

[39] Tracy, JM; Khan, FS; Demain, JG. Insect anaphylaxis: where are we? The stinging facts 2012. *Curr Opin Allergy Clin Immunol*, 2012, 12(4), 400-5.

[40] Przybilla, B; Ruëff, F. Hymenoptera venom allergy. J. *Dtsch Dermatol Ges*, 2010, 8(2), 114–129.

[41] Pumphrey, RS. Fatal anaphylaxis in the UK, 1992–2001. In: Bock G; Goode J; eds. Anaphylaxis. Novartis Found Symp 257. Chichester, UK: *John Wiley and Sons*, 2004, 116–28.

[42] Ruëff, F; Przybilla, B; Biló, MB; Müller, U; Scheipl, F; Aberer, W; Birnbaum, J; Bodzenta-Lukaszyk, A; Bonifazi, F; Bucher, C; Campi, P; Darsow, U; Egger, C; Haeberli, G; Hawranek, T; Körner, M; Kucharewicz, I; Küchenhoff, H; Lang, R; Quercia, O; Reider, N; Severino, M; Sticherling, M; Sturm, GJ; Wüthrich, B. Predictors of severe systemic anaphylactic reactions in patients with Hymenoptera venom allergy: importance of baseline serum tryptase-a study of the European Academy of Allergology and Clinical Immunology Interest Group on Insect Venom Hypersensitivity. *J Allergy Clin Immunol*, 2009, 124(5), 1047-54.

[43] Stoevesandt, J; Hain, J; Kesrtan, A; Trautmann, A. Over- and underestimated parameters in severe Hymenoptera venom-induced anaphylaxis: cardiovascular medication and absence of urticaria/angioedema. *J Allergy Clin Immunol*, 2012, ahead of print.

[44] Golden, DB; Kagey-Sobotka, A; Norman, PS; Hamilton, RG; Lichtenstein, LM. Outcomes of allergy to insect stings in children, with and without venom immunotherapy. *N Engl J Med*, 2004, 351(7), 668–74.

[45] Golden, DB. Insect sting allergy and venom immunotherapy: a model and a mystery. *J Allergy Clin Immunol*, 2005, 115(3), 439–47.

[46] Mueller, UR. Cardiovascular disease and anaphylaxis. *Curr Opin Allergy Clin Immunol*, 2007, 7(4), 337–41.

[47] Bonadonna, P; Perbellini, O; Passalacqua, G; Caruso, B; Colarossi, S; Dal Fior, D; Castellani, L; Bonetto, C; Frattini, F; Dama, A; Martinelli, G; Chilosi, M; Senna, G; Pizzolo, G; Zanotti, R. Clonal mast cell disorders in patients with systemic reactions to hymenoptera stings and increased serum tryptase levels. *J. Allergy Clin. Immunol*, 2009, 123(3), 680–686.

[48] Niedoszytko, M; Bruinenberg, M; van Doormaal, JJ; de Monchy, JG; Nedoszytko, B; Koppelman, GH; Nawijn, MC; Wijmenga, C; Jassem, E; Elberink, JN. Gene expression analysis predicts insect venom anaphylaxis in indolent systemic mastocytosis. *Allergy*, 2011, 66(5), 648-57.

[49] Borer-Reinhold, M; Haeberli, G; Jandus, P; Hausmann, O; Fricker, M; Helbling, A; Müller, U. An increase in serum tryptase even below 11.4 ng/mL may indicate a mast cell-mediated hypersensitivity reaction: a prospective study in Hymenoptera venom allergic patients. *Clin Exp Allergy*, 2011, 41(12), 1777-83.

[50] Vadas, P; Gold, M; Perelman, B; Liss, GM; Lack, G; Blyth, T; Simons, FE; Simons, KJ; Cass, D; Yeung, J. Platelet-activating factor, PAF acetylhydrolase, and severe anaphylaxis. *N Engl J Med*, 2008 Jan 3, 358(1), 28-35.

[51] Diwakar, L; Noorani, S; Huissoon, AP; Frew, AJ; Krishna, MT. Practice of venom immunotherapy in the United Kingdom: a national audit and review of literature. *Clin Exp Allergy*, 2008, 38(10), 1651-8.

[52] González-de-Olano, D; Alvarez-Twose, I; Vega, A; Orfao, A; Escribano, L. Venom immunotherapy in patients with mastocytosis and hymenoptera venom anaphylaxis. *Immunotherapy*, 2011, 3(5), 637-51.

[53] Bilo`, MB; Bonifazi, F. Advances in Hymenoptera venom immunotherapy. *Curr Opin Allergy Clin Immunol*, 2007, 7(6), 567–73.

[54] Müller, UR; Johansen, N; Petersen, AB; Fromberg-Nielsen, J; Haeberli, G. Hymenoptera venom allergy: analysis of double positivity to honey bee and Vespula venom by estimation of IgE antibodies to species-specific major allergens Api m1 and Ves v5. *Allergy*, 2009, 64(4), 543-8.

[55] Hofmann, SC; Pfender, N; Weckesser, S; Huss-Marp, J; Jakob, T. Added value of IgE detection to rApi m 1 and rVes v 5 in patients with Hymenoptera venom allergy. *J Allergy Clin Immunol*, 201, 127(1), 265-7.

[56] Korošec, P; Valenta, R; Mittermann, I; Celesnik, N; Eržen, R; Zidarn, M; Košnik, M. Low sensitivity of commercially available rApi m 1 for diagnosis of honeybeevenomallergy. *J Allergy Clin Immunol*, 2011, 128(3), 671-3.

[57] Sturm, GJ; Hemmer, W; Hawranek, T; Lang, R; Ollert, M; Spillner, E; Blank, S; Bokanovic, D; Aberer, W. Detection of IgE to recombinant Api m 1 and rVes v 5 is valuable but not sufficient to distinguish bee from wasp venom allergy. *J Allergy Clin Immunol*, 2011, 128(1), 247-8.

[58] Müller, U; Schmid-Grendelmeier, P; Hausmann, O; Helbling, A. IgE to recombinant allergens Api m 1, Ves v 1, and Ves v 5 distinguish double sensitization from crossreaction in venom allergy. *Allergy*, 2012, 67(8), 1069-73.

[59] Korošec, P; Valenta, R; Mittermann, I; Celesnik, N; Silar, M; Zidarn, M; Košnik, M. High sensitivity of CAP-FEIA rVes v 5 and rVes v 1 for diagnosis of Vespula venom allergy. *J Allergy Clin Immunol*, 2012, 129(5), 1406-8.

[60] Mertens, M; Brehler, R. Suitability of different glycoproteins and test systems for detecting cross-reactive carbohydrate determinant-specific IgE in hymenoptera venom-allergic patients. *Int Arch Allergy Immunol*, 2011, 156(1), 43-50.

[61] Monsalve, RI; Vega, A; Marqués, L; Miranda, A; Fernández, J; Soriano, V; Cruz, S; Domínguez-Noche, C; Sánchez-Morillas, L; Armisen-Gil, M; Guspí, R; Barber, D. Component-resolved diagnosis of vespid venom-allergic individuals: phospholipases and antigen 5s are necessary to identify Vespula or Polistes sensitization. *Allergy*, 2012, 67(4), 528-36.

[62] Dalmau Duch, G; Gázquez García, V; Gaig Jané, P; Galán Nieto, A; Monsalve Clemente, RI. Importance of controlled sting challenge and component-resolved diagnosis in the success of venom immunotherapy. *J Investig Allergol Clin Immunol*, 2012, 22(2), 135-6

[63] Eberlein, B. Basophil activation test in the diagnosis of insect venom allergies. *Clin Exp Allergy*, 2009, 39(11), 1633-4.

[64] Bonifazi, F; Jutel, M; Bilo, BM; Birnbaum, J; Muller, U. EAACI Interest Group on Insect Venom Hypersensitivity: Prevention and treatment of hymenoptera venom allergy: guidelines for clinical practice. *Allergy*, 2005, 60(12), 1459-70.

[65] Bilò, BM; Bonifazi, F. Hymenoptera venom immunotherapy. *Immunotherapy*, 2011, 3(2), 229-4.

[66] Oude Elberink, J; de Monchy, J; van der Heide, S; Guyatt, GH; Dubois, AE. Venom immunotherapy improves health related quality of life in patients allergic to yellow jacket venom. *J Allergy Clin. Immunol*, 2002, 110(1), 174–182.

[67] Ozdemir, C; Kucuksezer, UC; Akdis, M; Akdis, CA. Mechanisms of immunotherapy to wasp and bee venom. *Clin Exp Allergy*, 2011, 41(9), 1226-34.

[68] Jutel, M Akdis, CA. T-cell regulatory mechanisms in specific immunotherapy. *Chem Immunol Allergy*, 2008, 94,158-171.

[69] Akdis, CA; Akdis, M; Blesken, T; Wymann, D; Alkan, SS; Müller, U; Blaser, K. Epitope-specific, T. cell tolerance to phospholipase A2 in bee venom immunotherapy and recovery by IL-2 and IL- 15 in vitro. *J Clin Invest*, 1996, 98(7), 1676–83.

[70] Bussmann, C; Xia, J; Allam, JP; Maintz, L; Bieber, T; Novak, N. Early markers for protective mechanisms during rush venom immunotherapy. *Allergy*, 2010, 65(12), 1558–65.

[71] Jutel, M; Müller, U; Fricker, M; Rihs, S; Pichler, WJ; Dahinden, C. Influence of bee venom immunotherapy on degranulation and leukotriene generation in human blood basophils. *Clin Exp Allergy*, 1996, 26(10), 1112-1118.

[72] Goldberg, A; Confino-Cohen, R. Bee venom immunotherapy – how early is it effective? *Allergy*, 2010, 65(3), 391-395.

[73] Koterba, AP; Greenberger, PA. Stinging insect allergy and venom immunotherapy. *Allergy Asthma Proc*, 2012, 33 Suppl 1, 12-4.

[74] Golden, DB; Kelly, D; Hamilton, RG; Craig, TJ. Venom immunotherapy reduces large local reactions to insect stings. *J Allergy Clin Immunol.*, 2009, 123(6), 1371-5.

[75] Blanca, M; Garcia, F; Miranda, A; Carmona, MJ; Garcia, J; Fernandez, J; Terrados, S; Vega, JM; Juarez, C. Determination of IgE antibodies to Polistes dominulus, Vespula germanica and Vespa crabro in sera of patients allergic to vespids. *Allergy*, 1991, 46(2), 109–114.

[76] Muller, U; Helbling, A; Berchtold, E. Immunotherapy with honeybee venom and yellow jacket venom is different regarding efficacy and safety. *J Allergy Clin Immunol*, 1992, 89(2), 529 –535.

[77] Ross, RN; Nelson, HS; Finegold, I. Effectiveness of specific immunotherapy in the treatment of hymenoptera venom hypersensitivity: a meta-analysis. *Clin Ther*, 2000, 22(3), 351–8.

[78] Watanabe, AS; Fonseca, LA; Galvao, CE; Kalil, J; Castro, FF. Specific immunotherapy using Hymenoptera venom: systematic review. *Sao Paulo Med J*, 2010, 128(1), 30–7.

[79] Houliston, L; Nolan, R; Noble, V; Pascoe, E; Hobday, J; Loh, R; Mallon, D. Honeybee venom immunotherapy in children using a 50-mg maintenance dose. *J Allergy Clin Immunol*, 2011, 127(1), 98 –99.

[80] Severino, M; Bonadonna, P; Bilò, MB; Cortellini, G; Mauro, M; Schiappoli, M; Macchia, D; Campi, P; Manfredi, M; Passalacqua, G. Safety and efficacy of immunotherapy with *Polistes dominulus* venom: results from a large Italian database. *Allergy*, 2009, 64(8), 1229–1230.

[81] Rueff, F; Wenderoth, A; Przybilla, B. Patients still reacting to a sting challenge while receiving conventional Hymenoptera venom immunotherapy are protected by increased venom doses. *J Allergy Clin Immunol*, 2001, 108(6), 1027–1032.

[82] Niedoszytko, M; de Monchy, J; van Doormaal, JJ; Jassem, E; Oude, Elberink, JN. Mastocytosis and insect venom allergy: diagnosis, safety and efficacy of venom immunotherapy. *Allergy*, 2009, 64(9), 1237–1245.

[83] Perino, A; Galimberti, M; Bilò, MB; Asero, R; Pezzuto, F; AAITO, Committee for "Use of Adrenaline in Allergy Guidelines". Use of adrenaline in allergy. *Eur Ann Allergy Clin Immunol*, 2008, 40(2), 35-52.

[84] Goldberg, A; Yogev, A; Confino-Cohen, R. Three days rush venom immunotherapy in bee allergy: safe, inexpensive and instantaneously effective. *Int Arch Allergy Immunol*, 2011, 156(1), 90-8.

[85] Bilò, MB; Cinti, B; Brianzoni, MF; Braschi, MC; Bonifazi, M; Antonicelli, L. Honeybee venom immunotherapy: a comparative study using purified and nonpurified aqueous extracts in patients with normal Basal serum tryptase concentrations. *J Allergy*, (Cairo). 2012, 2012, 869243.

[86] Roumana, A; Pitsios, C; Vartholomaios, S; 88 Kompoti, E; Kontou-Fili, K. The safety of initiating hymenoptera immunotherapy at 1 μg of venom extract. *J Allergy Clin Immunol*, 2009, 124(2), 379–381.

[87] Bilò, MB; Antonicelli, L; Bonifazi, F. Purified versus nonpurified venom immunotherapy. *Curr. Opin. Allergy Clin. Immunol*, 2010, 10(4), 330–336.

[88] Cavallucci, E; Ramondo, S; Renzetti, A; Turi, MC; Di Claudio, F; Braga, M; Incorvaia, C; Schiavone, C; Ballone, E; Di Gioacchino, M. Maintenance venom immunotherapy

administered at a 3-month interval preserves safety and efficacy and improves adherence. *J Investig Allergol Clin Immunol.*, 2010, 20(1), 63-8.

[89] Incorvaia, C; Frati, F; Dell'Albani, I; Robino, A; Cattaneo, E; Mauro, M; David, M; Qualizza, R; Pastorello, E. Safety of hymenoptera venom immunotherapy: a systematic review. *Expert Opin Pharmacother.*, 2011, 12(16), 2527-32.

[90] Ruëff, F; Przybilla, B; Biló, MB; Müller, U; Scheipl, F; Aberer, W; Birnbaum, J; Bodzenta-Lukaszyk, A; Bonifazi, F; Bucher, C; Campi, P; Darsow, U; Egger, C; Haeberli, G; Hawranek, T; Kucharewicz, I; Küchenhoff, H; Lang, R; Quercia, O; Reider, N; Severino, M; Sticherling, M; Sturm, GJ; Wüthrich, B. European Academy of Allergy and Clinical Immunology Interest Group. Predictors of side effects during the buildup phase of venom immunotherapy for Hymenoptera venom allergy: the importance of baseline serum tryptase. *J Allergy Clin Immunol*, 2010, 126(1), 105-11.

[91] Žitnik, SE; Vesel, T; Avčin, T; Šilar, M; Košnik, M; Korošec, P. Monitoring honeybee venom immunotherapy in children with the basophil activation test. *Pediatr Allergy Immunol*, 2012, 23(2), 166-72.

[92] Müller, U; Hari, Y; Berchtold, E. Premedication with antihistamines may enhance efficacy of specific-allergen immunotherapy. *J Allergy Clin Immunol*, 2001, 107(1), 81-86.

[93] Müller, UR; Jutel, M; Reimers, A; Zumkehr, J; Huber, C; Kriegel, C; Steiner, U; Haeberli, G; Akdis, M; Helbling, A; Schnyder, B; Blaser, K; Akdis, C. Clinical and immunologic effects of H1 antihistamine preventive medication during honeybee venom immunotherapy. *J Allergy Clin Immunol*, 2008, 122(5), 1001-1007.

[94] Galera, C; Soohun, N; Zankar, N; Caimmi, S; Gallen, C; Demoly, P. Severe anaphylaxis to bee venom immunotherapy: efficacy of pretreatment and concurrent treatment with omalizumab. *J Investig Allergol Clin Immunol*, 2009, 19(3), 225–229.

[95] Severino, MG; Cortellini, G; Bonadonna, P; Francescato, E; Panzini, I; Macchia, D; Campi, P; Spadolini, I; Canonica, WG; Passalacqua, G. Sublingual immunotherapy for large local reactions caused by honeybee sting: a double- blind, placebo-controlled trial. *J Allergy Clin Immunol*, 2008, 122(1), 44–48.

[96] Golden, DB; Kwiterovich, KA; Kagey-Sobotka, A; Valentine, MD; Lichtenstein, LM. Discontinuing venom immunotherapy: outcome after 5 years. *J. Allergy Clin. Immunol*, 1996, 97(2), 579–587.

[97] Ruëff, F; Przybilla, B; Müller, U; Mosbech, H. The sting challenge test in hymenoptera venom allergy. Position paper of the Subcommittee on Insect Venom Allergy of the European Academy of Allergology and Clinical Immunology. *Allergy*, 1996, 51(4), 216–225.

[98] Golden, DB. Long-term outcome after venom immunotherapy. *Curr Opin Allergy Clin Immunol*, 2010, 10(4), 337-41.

[99] Hockenhull, J; Elremeli, M; Cherry, MG; Mahon, J; Lai, M; Darroch, J; Oyee, J; Boland, A; Dickson, R; Dundar, Y; Boyle, R. A systematic review of the clinical effectiveness and costeffectiveness ofPharmalgen® for the treatment of bee and wasp venom allergy. *Health Technol Assess*, 2012, 16(12), III-IV, 1-110.

[100] Bilò, BM; Brianzoni, FM; Napoli, G; Bonifazi, F. Insect sting anoxic encephalopathy after stopping venom immunotherapy. *Allergy*, 2006, 61(2), 268–269.

[101] Müller, UR; Akdis, CA; Fricker, M; Akdis, M; Blesken, T; Bettens, F; Blaser, K. Successful immunotherapy with T cell epitope peptides of bee venom phospholipase A_2

induces specific T cell anergy in bee sting allergic patients. *J Allergy Clin Immunol*, 1998, 101(6 Pt 1), 747-754.

[102] Senti, G; Johansen, P; Kündig, TM. Intralymphatic immunotherapy. *Curr Opin Allergy Clin Immunol*, 2009, 9(6), 537-43.

In: Anaphylaxis: Principles and Practice
Editor: M. Thirumala Krishna
ISBN: 978-1-62618-688-0

Chapter X

Idiopathic Anaphylaxis

Anne Marie Ditto* and Anjeni Keswani
Division of Allergy/Immunology,
Northwestern University Feinberg School of Medicine,
Chicago, IL, US

Abstract

Idiopathic anaphylaxis is defined as recurrent episodes of anaphylaxis without a known trigger. It is a diagnosis of exclusion after triggers such as foods, medications or insect stings and diseases that mimic anaphylaxis are ruled out. The pathophysiology of idiopathic anaphylaxis is still unknown and thus, the mechanism is under investigation. Idiopathic anaphylaxis is classified according to the constellation of symptoms and frequency of episodes. It can then be treated with 'triple therapy' of epinephrine, steroids, and antihistamines for acute attacks and a regimen of remittive therapy, consisting of steroids and antihistamines, for those patients with frequent episodes. The prognosis of idiopathic anaphylaxis is favorable if it is recognized and appropriately treated.

Introduction

Idiopathic anaphylaxis (IA) is defined as an immediate, life threatening reaction without an identifiable precipitating agent, trigger or event. IA was first described in 1978, in a case series of 21 patients with severe anaphylaxis, 11 of whom had episodes without an identifiable trigger. These patients were considered to have IA and were treated with antihistamines, sympathomimetics and corticosteroids--medications successfully used in preventing anaphylactic reactions to radiocontrast media. This resulted in remission of IA or reduction in severity of attacks and/or frequency [1]. Other case reports and series have

* Corresponding author: Anne Marie Ditto, MD, 676 North St. Clair Street, Suite 1400, Chicago, IL 60611; amditto@northwestern.edu.

identified patients with IA that were responsive to treatment with prednisone and antihistamines [2, 3].

Idiopathic Anaphylaxis remains a diagnosis of exclusion. There has been significant research looking for an underlying etiology for IA and the pathogenesis continues to be studied. When IA is recognized and the appropriate treatment is instituted, the prognosis of IA is excellent.

The prevalence of IA in the United States was estimated to be 33,000 cases in 1995[4]. In a study from Florence, Italy, of patients presenting to a university hospital from 1985 to 1996 with anaphylaxis, 6% were considered to have IA [5]. In 2006, a study of 601 outpatients referred to an allergist at the University of Tennessee for anaphylaxis (excluding Hymenoptera or immunotherapy anaphylaxis), 59% were diagnosed with IA [6]. In two studies looking at all causes of anaphylaxis, the prevalence of IA as a cause of anaphylaxis was estimated at 22.4% in Singapore [7] and 11.6% in northwest England [8].

The clinical manifestations of IA are identical to those of anaphylaxis with a recognized cause. These include urticaria, angioedema, wheezing, stridor, dysphagia, tachycardia, pruritus, flushing, nausea, vomiting, abdominal pain, diarrhoea, dizziness, hypotension and loss of consciousness. In a series of 335 patients with IA, all experienced hives and angioedema with their episodes with 60% experiencing symptoms of upper airway obstruction [2]. Cardiovascular collapse can occur without other symptoms of anaphylaxis; however, from this series, all patients with IA demonstrated urticaria and/or angioedema in addition to other symptoms. Patients may experience different combinations of these symptoms, but they are usually the same manifestations with each episode of IA, similar to patients who have allergic reactions to specific foods. The time course for progression of symptoms from cutaneous reactions to life-threatening systemic symptoms can vary depending on the individual but are generally between ten minutes to several hours after the onset of the episode. It is important to distinguish IA from other forms of allergic and non-allergic disease in order to provide the appropriate treatment and counseling.

Pathophysiology

Idiopathic Anaphylaxis, like 'anaphylaxis with a known trigger', results from activation of mast cells. During an acute episode of IA, patients may have elevated levels of mast cell mediators, total serum tryptase, plasma histamine, urinary histamine and urinary methylimidazole acetic acid [9-13]. These levels are normal between anaphylactic episodes, in contrast to patients with systemic mastocytosis whose serum tryptase levels are elevated both at baseline and during acute episodes [14-16].

In the study of the pathophysiology of IA, researchers have investigated mast cell burden in skin biopsies to address if increases in mast cell number could account for IA [17]. Skin biopsies were taken from patients with "unexplained anaphylaxis/unexplained flushing", urticaria pigmentosa, systemic mastocytosis with urticaria pigmentosa, and normal subjects. Skin biopsies from patients with "unexplained anaphylaxis/unexplained flushing" contained 72 mast cells per square millimeter as compared to 38 mast cells per square millimeter in normal controls, 597 mast cells per square millimeter in lesional skin of urticaria pigmentosa, and 721 mast cells per square millimeter in urticaria pigmentosa associated with systemic mastocytosis. This is also in comparison to 168 mast cells per square millimeter in nonlesional skin of patients with urticaria pigmentosa and 184 mast cells per square millimeter in nonlesional skin of patients with systemic mastocytosis. Thus, while there is a statistically significant increase in the number of mast cells seen in skin biopsies of patients with presumed IA, it is less than that seen in patients with urticaria pigmentosa alone or with urticaria pigmentosa associated with systemic mastocytosis. Similar small increases in mast cell numbers have been observed in other skin conditions such as scleroderma, chronic urticaria and in skin after prolonged antigenic contact [17]. Additional research was aimed at determining if an increased responsiveness to mast cell-derived mediators such as histamine could explain anaphylaxis in these patients. However, a study assessing the wheal-and-flare reactions after intradermal injection of histamine did not demonstrate hyper-releasability of histamine in patients with IA as compared to normal controls and to patients with systemic mastocytosis [18]. Mast cells of patients with IA have been reported to display the same threshold response with exposure to increasing dilutions of various mediators, such as histamine, leukotriene D4, and platelet activating factor when compared to mast cells of patients with allergic rhinitis, chronic idiopathic urticaria and asthma [19]. There was no difference in *in vitro* basophil histamine release induced by anti-IgE in non-atopic patients and patients with IA [20]. These data suggest that there is no difference in mast cell burden or hyper-reactivity of mast cells in patients with IA as compared to normal controls.

Idiopathic Anaphylaxis has been associated with increased lymphocyte activation. In a small study, it was noted that patients with acute episodes of IA had a higher percentage of activated T lymphocytes in their peripheral blood as compared to patients with IA in remission, patients with acute urticaria, and normal controls. 'Active' IA patients and IA patients in remission have a higher number of activated B cells as compared to normal controls [21]. The role of the increase in activated T cells and B cells in the pathogenesis of IA has yet to be fully elucidated.

The mechanism underlying acute episodes of IA continues to be an area of active investigation. Whilst it has been shown that there is release of mast cell and basophil mediators during acute episodes of IA, the cause of this release is unknown. Glucocorticoids have not been shown to inhibit the release of mediators from human mast cells [22]. Thus, the responsiveness of IA to corticosteroid therapy suggests that steroids may be involved in stabilizing eosinophils, basophils, and mast cells in IA, similar to the pretreatment regimen of corticosteroids and antihistamines used in the prevention of anaphylactoid reactions to radiocontrast media [23-26]. In addition, steroids have immunomodulatory properties and possibly change the underlying immune reaction responsible for IA. Additionally, while corticosteroids are an effective therapy in reducing episodes, it could be potentially useful to have targeted therapy at the underlying mechanism in the future.

By definition, IA is a diagnosis of exclusion. Thus, all potential triggers for anaphylaxis such as foods, medication, or insect stings should be ruled out. Disorders that may mimic anaphylaxis such as carcinoid syndrome, pheochromocytoma, and other flushing syndromes should also be excluded (Table 1). Idiopathic Anaphylaxis should only be diagnosed when no specific trigger can be identified and the evaluation should include a complete history, physical examination, laboratory analysis and skin testing to appropriate suspected triggers. In a series by Ditto et al. of 335 cases of IA, approximately 48% of patients were atopic which may reflect a predilection of IA to develop in an atopic individual [2].

Table 1. Differential diagnosis of IA

IgE-mediated anaphylaxis	*Hereditary or acquired angioedema*
Foods, including "hidden foods" or spices	*Psychiatric conditions*
Food additives	Munchausen's syndrome
galactose-alpha-1,3-galactose hypersensitivity	Somatoform disorders
Medications	Panic attacks
Insect stings	*Miscellaneous conditions*
Latex	Severe asthma exacerbations
Exercise-induced anaphylaxis	Globus
Food-dependent exercise-induced anaphylaxis	Pheochromocytoma
Mast cell disorders	Carcinoid syndrome
Systemic mastocytosis	Scromboid toxicity
Mast cell activation syndrome	
Monoclonal mast cell activation syndrome	

Additionally, IA is responsive to pharmacologic treatment and this can help in diagnosis, in that a lack of response should prompt consideration of alternative diagnoses.

Special attention should be paid to an evaluation for food triggers, particularly "hidden" or unusual foods, as a cause for anaphylaxis in patients with suspected IA. If attacks occur within 2 hours after eating, then a food trigger should be strongly considered and any food consumed within 2 hours of the reaction should be excluded [27, 28]. Hidden food allergens or contamination with known common allergens should be sought, such as peanut or tree nuts seen in salad dressing [29]. Spices may also be a culprit in anaphylactic reactions; members of the *Apiaceae* (*Umbelliferae*) family, including fennel, coriander, and caraway, have been reported to cause anaphylaxis [30]. Food additives, such as carmine powder and psyllium, as well as foods contaminated with aeroallergens, such as "bee pollen" which may contain ragweed pollen or flour that contains mite allergen, have all been reported to cause anaphylaxis [31-34]. Investigators, through a battery of selected food-antigen skin prick tests, have demonstrated that while hypersensitivity to various foods or spices may account for anaphylactic symptoms in a minority of patients with IA, it cannot account for the majority of IA cases [35]. Twelve patients with IA, who had a potential food-related trigger due to proximity of episodes to restaurant meals and in whom no food allergen was identified, were challenged to sodium metabisulfite, a common preservative in drugs and foods often used by restaurants. There were no episodes of anaphylaxis triggered by the metabisulfite in these patients [36]. Scombroid poisoning, which can occur after histamine ingestion in poorly preserved dark meat fish such as tuna, can resemble an IgE-mediated allergic reaction and should be considered in patients who have anaphylaxis after fish ingestion but are not found to be allergic to fish on skin testing [37]. Additionally, there have been multiple cases reported, particularly in the Southeastern United States, of delayed anaphylaxis due to ingestion of beef, pork and other mammalian meat in patients who are sensitized to the carbohydrate antigen, galactose-alpha-1,3-galactose [38].

As medications are frequently associated with anaphylaxis, a search for a culprit medication is warranted prior to the diagnosis of IA. Aspirin and nonsteroidal anti-inflammatory drugs (NSAIDs) have been identified as common causes of drug hypersensitivity reactions. These medications are commonly used as over the counter pain relievers. It is important to rule out ingestion of these medications with a thorough history as patients may not recognize medications that contain these ingredients, for example, 'Alka-Seltzer' contains aspirin or that Aleve (naproxyn) is an NSAID, and thus may inadvertently consume these medications. Additionally, angiotensin converting enzyme inhibitors cause angioedema and should be considered prior to labeling a patient with IA-angioedema [39]. Mislabeled medication in a patient with drug hypersensitivity may also be a cause of anaphylaxis, as a classic paper reports that a patient experienced anaphylaxis from penicillin that was incorrectly identified as ascorbic acid [27].

Other allergic entities such as exercise-induced anaphylaxis and food-dependent exercise-induced anaphylaxis should also be considered prior to diagnosing a patient with IA[40, 41]. Latex exposure and insect bites or stings, including unusual bugs such as Triatoma, the kissing bug, should be considered [42]. Studies have investigated the role of hormonal changes, such as endogenous progesterone, in women with IA, particularly after three women improved with ovarian suppression using a luteinizing hormone-releasing hormone agonist [43]. However, further studies failed to demonstrate a correlation between progesterone peaks and episodes of IA or serum histamine levels. Progesterone and estradiol did not demonstrate an effect on the basophils from female patients with IA who were thought to have hormone-related exacerbations [44]. However, as with chronic idiopathic urticaria (CIU) and asthma, hormones may affect IA, with worsening symptoms in the premenstrual phase, usually several days prior to menses.

In addition to ruling out triggers that cause IgE-mediated and non-IgE-mediated anaphylaxis, disorders such as hereditary or acquired angioedema, systemic mastocytosis, severe asthma exacerbations, Munchausen's syndrome and other somatoform disorders should be considered. Hereditary angioedema may mimic IA-angioedema due to significant oropharyngeal edema; these patients will have a low C4 and have either low quantitative C1 esterase inhibitor levels or dysfunction of C1 esterase inhibitor. Acquired C1 esterase inhibitor deficiency should also be considered. These patients have low C1q levels due to increased consumption of the C1 inhibitor due to its destruction or to excess activation of complement. A low complement C4 level has high sensitivity in the diagnosis of hereditary and acquired angioedema and is a useful screening test.

Systemic mastocytosis is a mast cell disorder in which patients experience episodes of recurrent flushing, pruritus, urticaria, abdominal pain, and hypotension. The diagnostic criteria for systemic mastocytosis include the major criteria of multifocal dense infiltrates of mast cells in bone marrow or other extracutaneous organ(s) and the following minor criteria: (1) mast cells in bone marrow or other extracutaneous organ(s) that show an abnormal morphology; (2) 'c-kit' mutation at codon 816 in bone marrow or other extracutaneous organ(s); (3) mast cells in bone marrow that express CD2 and/or CD25; and (4) total baseline serum tryptase greater than 20 ng/ml. One major and one minor or three minor criteria must be met to establish a diagnosis of systemic mastocytosis. In adults, over 90% of patients have salmon-colored macules (urticaria pigmentosa) that urticate with light stroking known as Darier's sign. In contrast to patients with systemic mastocytosis, patients with IA do not have urticaria pigmentosa or an elevated baseline tryptase level and have normal bone marrow studies. These tests may be considered, in an appropriate clinical setting, to exclude systemic mastocytosis prior to the diagnosis of IA being made.

A severe acute asthma exacerbation may appear similar to an episode of anaphylaxis when the onset is sudden, causing severe respiratory distress, stridor, wheezing, and potentially, the inability to speak. Due to these symptoms, patients may also appear to have facial edema and erythema. There may be confusion as to whether these symptoms are caused by anaphylaxis, particularly if a patient has had previous intubations or hospitalizations for severe asthma. Once the patient has recovered, it would be prudent to pursue allergy tests to suspected foods or medications to exclude anaphylaxis as a cause of acute severe asthma.

Munchausen's syndrome and somatoform disorders may be considered when IA is suspected and does not respond to treatment. These conditions will be covered separately in this chapter. Conditions such as panic disorders causing acute dyspnea, diaphoresis, and dizziness may occur in the absence of hypotension and resolve without epinephrine. Globus which is the sensation of a "lump" in the throat may be concerning to patients; however, there are no other signs of anaphylaxis. This may be particularly difficult to distinguish from IA as some patients with IA can have isolated angioedema of the throat and airway without other signs or symptoms. Endoscopy may be beneficial in differentiating globus from IA. Carcinoid syndrome may present with episodes of flushing and diarrhoea; other findings of anaphylaxis are absent and the diagnosis can be made when urinary levels of 5-hydroxyindoleacetic acid (5-HIAA) are elevated. Pheochromocytoma can induce episodes of flushing, dyspnea, and palpitations; however, these are due to hypertension induced by catecholamine release, rather than hypotension, urticaria, and/or angioedema that are seen in anaphylaxis. In patients with pheochromocytoma who are volume depleted, orthostatic hypotension may be seen. The diagnosis of pheochromocytoma can be made when urinary concentrations of vanillylmandelic acid and catecholamines are elevated; these are normal in patients with IA.

There has been some controversy regarding the overlap of IA with mast cell activation syndrome (MCAS). Akin et al. proposed a set of diagnostic criteria for MCAS as follows: (1) absence of primary or secondary causes of mast cell activation, including mastocytosis; (2) episodic symptoms consistent with mast cell mediator release that affect 2 or more organ systems; (3) evidence of an increase in validated urinary or serum markers of mast cell activation; and (4) a decrease in severity of symptoms with anti-mediator therapy including antihistamines, leukotriene antagonists, or mast cell stabilizers [45]. With MCAS, patients may experience recurrent episodes of anaphylaxis and an increase in markers of mast cell release, in particular tryptase, during episodes, with levels being normal at baseline. A subset of patients with MCAS have evidence of a clonal mast cell disorder and bone marrow biopsy may reveal the presence of an 816 V mutation on the c-kit receptor. This is a marker for systemic mastocytosis; however, these patients do not express the full mastocytosis phenotype. Patients with clonal mast cells in conjunction with this mutation are considered to have monoclonal mast cell activation syndrome (MMCAS). In contrast, patients with IA do not demonstrate evidence of a clonal mast cell disorder on bone marrow biopsy. Patients with MCAS may have lower thresholds for mast cell degranulation, yet these thresholds are normal in IA patients as discussed above. Additionally, improvement of symptoms with medications that target mast cell mediators, such as H1- and H2-antihistamines, leukotriene antagonists, and mast cell stabilizers, are supporting evidence for a diagnosis of MCAS as above [45, 46]. However, IA is treated differently with a regimen of steroids for life-threatening symptoms with antihistamines for minor symptoms such as hives, as discussed below. Mast cells stabilizers and leukotriene antagonists have provided modest benefits for the treatment of IA compared to steroids, although they have been used successfully as steroid sparing agents[2]. Thus, IA and MCAS are considered distinct clinical entities at this time; however, there is considerable overlap in the symptoms, evaluation, and treatment modalities.

Classification

Idiopathic Anaphylaxis is classified according to symptom constellation and frequency of attacks. Patients who experience obstructive upper airway symptoms without other systemic symptoms are classified as IA-angioedema (IA-A) whereas patients who experience urticaria or angioedema accompanied by bronchospasm, cardiovascular collapse, hypotension, or gastrointestinal symptoms are described as IA-generalized (IA-G). The authors note a subset of patients with IA-G, as illustrated by case 1, whose episodes consist of an identical pattern of cutaneous and gastrointestinal symptoms. These patients initially have severe abdominal cramping followed by profuse diarrhea, hives, hypotension with or without loss of consciousness, in that order. Patients whose symptoms are controlled by prednisone but recur after prednisone is tapered below a certain dose are classified as corticosteroid dependent IA (CSD-IA). If this threshold dose of prednisone is greater than 20 mg daily or 60mg every other day, then the patient is considered to have malignant IA (M-IA).

Table 2. Classification of IA

Disease	Symptoms
IA-Angioedema-Infrequent (IA-A-I)	Urticaria or angioedema with upper airway compromise without other systemic manifestations occurring fewer than 6 times per year or fewer than once every 2 months
IA-Angioedema-Frequent (IA-A-F)	Urticaria or angioedema with upper airway compromise without other systemic manifestations occurring more than 6 times per year or more frequently than once every 2 months
IA-Generalized-Infrequent (IA-G-I)	Urticaria or angioedema with systemic manifestations of hypotension, bronchospasm, syncope, or gastrointestinal symptoms with or without upper airway obstruction occurring fewer than 6 times per year or fewer than once every 2 months
IA-Generalized-Frequent (IA-G-F)	Urticaria or angioedema with systemic manifestations of hypotension, bronchospasm, syncope, or gastrointestinal symptoms with or without upper airway obstruction occurring more than 6 times per year or more frequently than once every 2 months
IA-Questionable (IA-Q)	Patients with a presumptive diagnosis of IA for which repeated attempts to document objective findings are unsuccessful and a response to appropriate doses of prednisone does not occur, thus leading the diagnosis of IA to be uncertain.
IA-Variant (IA-V)	Symptoms and physical findings of IA vary from classic findings
Corticosteroid dependent IA (CSD-IA)	Symptoms are controlled by prednisone but patients have recurrent episodes of IA below a threshold dose of prednisone.
Malignant IA (M-IA)	High doses of prednisone (>20mg daily or 60mg on alternate days) are required to control IA.
Undifferentiated somatoform IA (US-IA)	Symptoms mimic IA but no objective findings or response to treatments occurs. Patients meet criteria for somatoform disorder as described in the DSM-IV.

There are cases that are not clearly IA-G or IA-A and thus, other characterizations such as IA-questionable (IA-Q) and IA-variant (IA-V) were established to define the uncertain status of the diagnosis. The patient in case 2 was considered to have IA-Q when she did not respond to treatment of IA and prior to her diagnosis of VCD. In some of these cases, the patient's symptoms were not of an organic origin and therefore, were classified as undifferentiated somatoform IA (US-IA) according to the criteria for somatoform disorder as described in the Diagnostic and Statistical Manual for Mental Disorders, Fourth Edition (DSM-IV).

Frequency of attacks provides an important framework in the classification and treatment of IA. Patients who experience 6 or more episodes in one year or 2 or more episodes in 2 months are classified as IA frequent (IA-F) and those patients who have fewer episodes are characterized as IA infrequent (IA-I).

This classification system (Table 2) helps to define different subsets of IA for diagnostic purposes as well as provide guidance in an algorithm for managing cases of IA.

Treatment (Figure 1)

Management of acute episodes of IA is similar to management of 'anaphylaxis with a known trigger'. Acute episodes should be treated with triple therapy as defined below and this should be readily available to all patients with IA. At the onset of symptoms of anaphylaxis, the patient should self-inject epinephrine intramuscularly into the upper lateral thigh. The dose of epinephrine is 0.3mg in patients whose weight is greater than 30 kgs. The patient should also ingest prednisone 50mg and a H1 antagonist, such as diphenhydramine 50mg or cetirizine 10mg. This regimen is known as 'triple therapy'. Once this is complete, the patient should call emergency services and proceed to the ED for monitoring and additional therapy may be required. For infrequent episodes of IA, 'triple therapy' should be available at all times and is the basis for treatment for all episodes. In patients with IA-I who have severe episodes, remittive therapy as used in IA-F should be considered especially if the risk of death and complications from a subsequent episode is high, such as in an elderly patient with hypertension and coronary artery disease (CAD) who had sustained hypotension and or increased troponins during the episode of IA. Since episodes are infrequent, it is not known if the disease course can be altered with remittive therapy but it is presumed based on treatment of IA-F that remission can be induced [2].

Patients with IA-F who have more than 6 episodes per year or greater than 2 episodes per 2 months should be started on prednisone as remittive therapy to control the disease, stop further episodes, and induce remission. IA is a corticosteroid responsive disease and with an adequate dose of prednisone, remission can be achieved in most patients. Patients should also be commenced on a daily H1 antagonist and prednisone 60mg to 100mg daily for 7 days or until symptom free for one week, followed by 60mg on alternate days for 2 weeks. The patient should then continue alternate day prednisone, the dose of which can be reduced by 5 to 10mg every 2 weeks if there are no further episodes of anaphylaxis or other indicators of active disease such as urticaria or isolated angioedema. If a life-threatening or severe episode of IA recurs following dose reduction, daily prednisone must be resumed. This should be followed by alternate-day prednisone at a higher dose with a slower reduction schedule. If symptoms are mild, such as a few isolated urticarial lesions or mild, non-life threatening angioedema, one may consider increasing H1 antihistamines prior to changing the dose of prednisone. For most patients, this regimen will induce remission of IA and prednisone can be tapered and discontinued using the above regimen. However, for a subset of patients, reducing the dose of alternate day prednisone below a certain level induces relapse. These patients have corticosteroid-dependent IA (CSD-IA). Additional medications have proven useful in controlling CSD-IA such as ketotifen 2mg two to three times daily or oral cromolyn 200mg pre-meals and at bedtime, as well as additional H1 or the addition of an H2 antagonist [47].

Pharmacologic management of pediatric cases is the same as in adults with IA; however, dosages of medications must be adjusted according to the child's body weight and age[48]. For emergency 'triple therapy', epinephrine should be administered at a dose of 0.3mg in children weighing greater than 30 kgs, 0.15mg in children weighing between 15 and 29 kgs, and at a dose of 0.01mg/kg in children weighing less than 15kgs. Children should also receive 1mg/kg of prednisone and 1mg/kg of diphenhydramine orally. For long-term management of pediatric IA-G-F, prednisone should be prescribed as 1-2mg/kg orally daily for one week or until symptoms are controlled. Patients should then be converted to alternate day prednisone at 1-2mg/kg orally with a cautious taper of 5-10mg per month if symptoms remain controlled. Anti-histamine dosages should also be adjusted for the pediatric population. Cetirizine dosing is adjusted for a child's age with recommended dosages of 2.5mg daily in children up to age 2 years, 5mg daily in children aged 2 to 5 years, and 10mg daily for children 6 years or older.

When patients are on daily prednisone with a H1 antagonist, episodes of IA should cease. It can take from 1 to 6 weeks of daily prednisone before episodes stop occurring; however, if longer courses of daily prednisone are required, then one must consider alternative diagnoses with the interim diagnosis becoming IA-Q. Alternative diagnoses such as panic disorder, prednisone non-compliance, and undifferentiated somatoform IA should all be evaluated. Additionally, a globus sensation and severe anxiety are not uncommon with prednisone use, thus some patients may mistake these symptoms for an episode of IA. Any breakthrough symptoms should be carefully evaluated prior to changing the treatment course as after initiating prednisone therapy, patients may develop GERD with globus and these symptoms may be mistaken for IA, causing an unnecessary increase or prolonging prednisone therapy. Patients with IA-F should have regular office visits to assess for steroid-related side effects and optimization of therapy. Breakthrough symptoms should be thoroughly reviewed including history and scrutinisation of emergency room records for objective signs during acute episodes, particularly when the presenting feature is isolated upper airway involvement. This may also include nasendoscopy as outlined in case scenario 2. Corticosteroid-based treatment has been successful in treatment of the disease and the risks and benefits of corticosteroids must be discussed. Establishment of a good rapport between the physician and patient is an important component in the management of IA.

A strong focus of the management is education of patients and their families regarding features of IA. It needs to be stressed that these are 'spontaneous' episodes, i.e., there is no external trigger. Patients with anaphylaxis to a known trigger, such as a particular food, may have a false sense of security that they may be able to avoid their trigger completely as a means to prevent anaphylaxis. In a study by Bock et al, 97% of patients with fatal food induced anaphylaxis had a previous allergic reaction to the food trigger [49]. Thus, avoidance was not successful. Additionally, in 90% of these patients, epinephrine was either not administered or there was a significant delay in administration [49]. Patients with IA, however, tend to be more compliant with carrying their emergency treatment probably because they do not have a known trigger for their anaphylaxis-i.e., no false sense of security that they can avoid it. In one study of compliance with emergency treatment, 91% of patients with anaphylaxis from an unknown cause carried epinephrine for self-administration as opposed to 53% of patients with an identifiable trigger [50]. Patients with IA should be offered a 'Medic Alert bracelet'. Patients with newly diagnosed IA may benefit from networking with other patients with IA, particularly those whose disease is controlled and in remission.

There are published case reports demonstrating use of omalizumab in IA. One case report of a 12 year old male patient showed reduction in IA episodes, from 4-5 per month to 0 when treated with omalizumab for severe persistent asthma. While he had had multiple oral steroid courses previously, it is unclear if he was treated according to the above algorithm with prednisone and antihistamines for IA [51].

Another case report describes a 48 year old man with IA-G-F for 15 years. He had been treated previously with daily antihistamines without significant benefit. Long-term corticosteroid treatment was successful in decreasing the frequency and severity of his episodes but led to significant morbidity. He was treated with omalizumab fortnightly with remission of IA [52]. These cases highlight potential role for omalizumab, if steroid-sparing agents are required; however, further investigation in randomized placebo controlled studies is warranted.

Outcomes and Prognosis

The goal of the treatment is to induce remission, which is defined as discontinuation of prednisone for a year with no further episodes of IA. In a study of 53 patients (age 11 to 74 years), remission was achieved in 45% using the above algorithm. Remission rates were 48% in patients with IA-G and 40% in patients with IA-A. There was also a statistically significant decrease in the number of episodes and number of ED visits in patients with IA-G-F and IA-A-F[47].

In another study of 61 patients, (age 10 to 68 years), 65% of patients with IA-I and 91% of patients with IA-F went into remission. There was a significant decrease in the number of ED visits for the three groups (IA-G-F, IA-G-I, and IA-A-I) studied. A statistically significant decrease in the number of hospitalizations occurred for the IA-G-I group and in the number of intensive care unit admissions for the IA-G-F group [53]. In a study of 335 patients with IA, 65% had achieved remission and an additional 17% of patients were without symptoms at the time of the study, less than 1 year after finishing prednisone therapy [2]. Based on this study, physicians can reassure patients that with compliance with prescribed medication, an excellent remission rate of >80% can be achieved. Most patients experience prolonged remission or infrequent, less severe episodes but a small number of patients have had recurrence of their initial symptoms [2]. In all cases patients should be adviced to always carry their emergency kit [2].

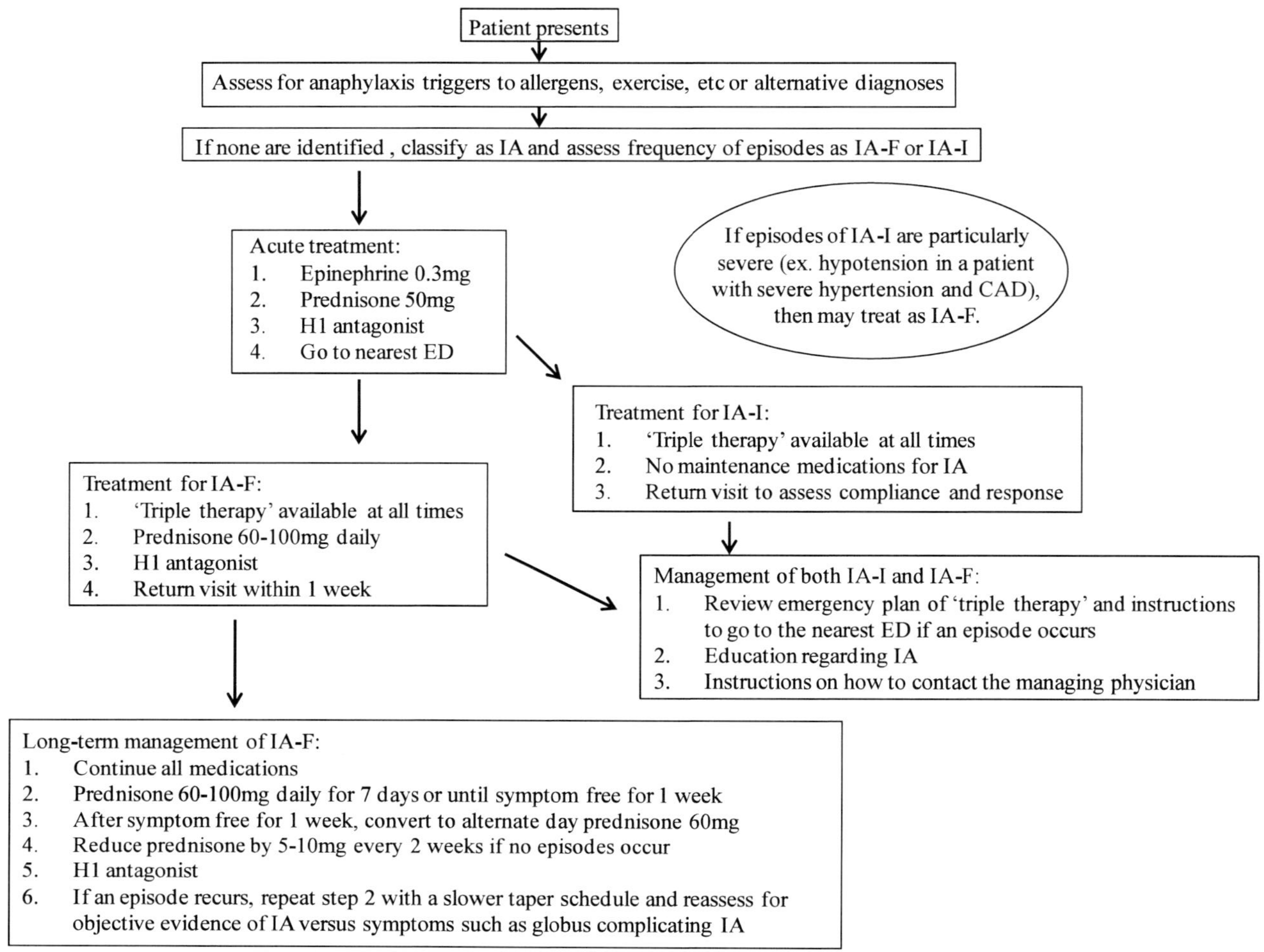

Figure 1. Algorithm for the management of idiopathic anaphylaxis.

Fatalities are rare in IA - there have been three reported fatalities. A 43 year old gentleman with asthma and a 12 year history of anaphylaxis was diagnosed with IA and aggressively treated with prednisone, hydroxyzine, and oral albuterol. At the time of his death, his regimen was prednisone 60mg on alternate days. He had an episode of anaphylaxis which consisted of acute respiratory failure while attending a friend's barbecue. Despite the use of self-administered epinephrine, he could not be resuscitated. No autopsy was performed and his final diagnosis by the ED staff was anaphylactic shock with severe bronchospasm. This is the only report of a fatality in a patient treated for IA. The patient's close friend did note that the deceased may not have been compliant with his medication regimen for IA [54]. Another fatality from IA was reported in a 52 year old man with four previous episodes of IA in a 13 year period, consisting of abdominal pain, flushing, loss of consciousness and hypotension. Four weeks after an anaphylactic episode, he had another episode of anaphylaxis with loss of consciousness. Autopsy also revealed severe coronary atherosclerosis [55]. The third reported fatality was a 25 year old woman with episodes of anaphylaxis, consisting of abdominal cramping, diarrhoea, pruritus, urticaria and angioedema, since the age of 10. The episodes occurred two to three times per year and responded to epinephrine. More intense pharmacologic therapy was refused by the patient, who thought control with epinephrine was satisfactory. She had an episode of anaphylaxis and although a family member administered epinephrine, she could not be resuscitated. Autopsy findings were consistent with acute asthma, an associated pneumothorax, and aspiration of gastric contents [55].

Special Populations

IA can occur in pediatric as well as geriatric populations. The symptoms of IA are the same, from upper airway obstruction to gastrointestinal symptoms to shock. The classification scheme and algorithm for treatment can be applied to the pediatric and geriatric populations; however, some special medical and psychosocial situations that are unique to these populations should be considered.

Pediatric Patients

Pediatric IA is currently seen with increased frequency probably due raised awareness and recognition of the condition. Patients ranging in age from 3.5 years old to 18 years old, have been reported to have IA [48]. Similar to adult patients, children respond well to treatment and are likely to have remission of their disease. Interestingly, four pediatric patients with symptoms predominantly of upper airway obstruction were successfully maintained in remission with inhaled beclamethasone dipropionate [48]. This was thought to be due to a direct anti-inflammatory effect on the upper airway.

There are concerns unique to the pediatric population regarding the treatment of IA. There may be issues of significant reservation regarding the use of prednisone in the pediatric population by parents, local physicians, and by patients themselves, particularly adolescents. Parents may not adhere strictly to the treatment plan as outlined by the treating allergist-immunologist. This may be due to numerous physician consultations prior to a diagnosis being reached, distrust of physicians, and at times, management of the symptoms by parents rather than physicians. Additionally, local physicians may not accept the diagnosis of IA and therefore, may not support the use of appropriate pharmacotherapy as recommended by the allergist-immunologist. In adolescent patients, cosmetic changes such as acne or weight gain may lead to ridicule by peers which can lead to challenging social situations at school and home. Decreased linear growth has been demonstrated with oral steroids and may be of concern to parents and children [56]. In addition, as with other forms of anaphylaxis, availability of self-injectable epinephrine may be an issue for children in school or day care. Epinephrine may not always be immediately available to a child with anaphylaxis if stored in a separate or locked area at school. School personnel or caretakers of children may not be familiar with the signs of anaphylaxis and may not recognize when treatment should be initiated. This is especially true in young children who cannot express what they are feeling or in those who do not manifest cutaneous symptoms. In a study by Sampson et al, cutaneous signs and symptoms were actually less common in fatal food-triggered anaphylaxis compared to non-fatal anaphylaxis caused by a food allergy [28]. Furthermore, some caretakers may be fearful of administering epinephrine to a child and therefore, delay treatment [57].

The unpredictable nature of IA can be particularly frightening to children and their parents, leading to a high level of anxiety. It may be helpful to parents of children with newly diagnosed IA to network with the parents of children whose disease is controlled or in remission. This may provide further reassurance that IA has a favorable prognosis and that prednisone is used to induce remission but, generally, not needed long-term. The allergist-immunologist should offer contact between families, with their consent, in order to establish a support network for patients with IA. Additionally, children with IA must always have emergency treatment available to them. All adults with patient contact (for example, teachers, day care providers, and babysitters) should be made aware of the disease and its symptoms. They should all be able to administer emergency treatment with epinephrine, prednisone, and an antihistamine and arrange for the child to be taken to the ED.

Elderly Patients

Management of IA in the elderly population can be complicated by coexisting illnesses. Patients may not tolerate anaphylaxis in the presence of underlying disease such as CAD. Concurrent CAD or cerebrovascular disease may be exacerbated during an episode of anaphylaxis, especially with hypotension, resulting in a myocardial infarction or cerebrovascular accident. It is essential that caretakers of elderly patients with IA be aware of their disease and that anaphylaxis may not be recognized as the initial precipitant for a vascular or coronary event and thus, proper treatment for anaphylaxis may not be initiated. Additionally, remittive therapy as used in frequent episodes may be needed after a single episode of IA, particularly in severe cases, as patients may not tolerate repeated episodes. Elderly patients may also take multiple medications, some of which may interfere with resuscitative efforts, in particular beta-blockers. An effort to reduce the number of medications to those that are essential to care should be undertaken in all elderly patients with IA. There may also be resistance to epinephrine in this age group. In view of serious comorbidities such as advanced CAD, elderly patients may not tolerate sustained hypotension and hence treatment with epinephrine should be administered promptly. Depending on the age of the patient, dosage of medications may need to be reduced and it may be more appropriate to prescribe pediatric doses of epinephrine to these patients as with other medications when treating geriatric patients.

Social issues are extremely important in the care of elderly patients with IA. Patients may be dependent on caretakers for transportation to multiple physician visits and for assistance in taking medications. This may require help from family members or social services. Patients living alone may require daily contact with family, friends, or neighbours. As with pediatric patients, all caretakers of elderly patients with IA should be familiar with symptoms of the disease, administration of emergency treatment, and access to emergency medical services.

Management Challenges in IA

Prednisone Fear and IA

Fear of prolonged use of prednisone, by both patients and treating physicians, can complicate the management of IA. A discussion regarding the potential side effects of corticosteroid therapy should be undertaken with all patients with IA. However, it must be strongly stressed to patients that IA is a potentially fatal disease [54, 55], and fatalities have occurred in patients not treated with remittive therapy. They should be informed that prednisone is effective in controlling IA, used according to the algorithm previously described, and is successful in inducing remission in a majority of patients. Many patients will be able to discontinue prednisone therapy within six months and for the majority of the time, patients are treated with alternate day corticosteroids, which cause fewer side effects, requiring very low doses in the last few months. Treating physicians should be aware of the potential side effects of prednisone therapy including weight gain, insomnia, osteoporosis, personality or mood changes and visual changes including glaucoma and cataracts. Weight gain can be managed by caloric restriction and exercise. For patients who gain weight on corticosteroid therapy, caloric restriction and exercise has been successful in producing weight loss after prednisone discontinuation. Patients should be screened for osteoporosis with dual-energy x-ray absorptiometry (DEXA) scans every 1 to 2 years if they require oral steroid therapy for greater than 3 months [58]. Additionally, ophthalmology consultation may prove useful in evaluating patients for visual changes. Psychiatric consultation may be useful in patients who develop significant personality or mood changes on prednisone therapy or those patients who continue to have prednisone fear despite multiple attempts at reassurance by their treating physician.

Corticosteroid-Dependent IA

In some patients with IA, prednisone controls the episodes of IA but when it is tapered below a threshold dose, there is relapse. These patients are said to have corticosteroid-dependent IA (CSD-IA). The threshold dose of prednisone varies from patient to patient and may even vary in the course of treatment of an individual patient. There is also variability in the outcomes of patients with CSD-IA. When adequate control is achieved at a certain dose of prednisone, eventual long-term remission may occur. In some patients the use of ketotifen as a steroid sparing agent may aid in achieving remission of IA symptoms and enable tapering off prednisone [59]. Other patients require increased doses of prednisone, between 60 and 80mg, for 4 to 6 weeks so that remission may occur. In some patients, there may be no alternatives to control CSD-IA. Similar to corticosteroid-dependent asthma, these patients required alternate day prednisone for control of symptoms. However CSD-IA is very uncommon and episodes of breakthrough anaphylaxis while tapering prednisone should be evaluated in detail as they may be symptoms of ‘prednisone side effects’ that mimic IA such as globus or flushing. If the symptoms are unable to be controlled on prednisone, reevaluation of the diagnosis of IA is warranted.

Malignant IA

The diagnosis of malignant (M-IA) is made when a patient’s symptoms may not be controlled with a reduction in prednisone below 60mg every other day or 20mg daily. The term “malignant” refers to the severity of the disease and difficulty involved in controlling it; it does not refer to a neoplastic process. Some patients with M-IA require doses in excess of 20mg daily or 60mg every other day and therefore, have the potential for multiple adverse effects of high dose corticosteroids. However, because IA is a potentially fatal disease, there are no proven alternatives to the use of high dose prednisone for the control of IA. A trial of ketotifen or omalizumab may be useful in patient’s with M-IA. Studies have shown that ketotifen has been beneficial in inducing remission in some patients with M-IA and CSD-IA [59]. Malignant- IA (M-IA) is an extremely rare condition and other diagnoses, such as ‘steroid side effects’ or alternative diagnoses to IA, should be considered.

Undifferentiated Somatoform Idiopathic Anaphylaxis

Undifferentiated somatoform IA (US-IA) is a diagnosis made when a patient diagnosed with IA does not respond to treatment and has no objective evidence on examination or in the medical record to corroborate the diagnosis of anaphylaxis. These patients meet criteria for a somatoform disorder, as described in the DSM-IV. Patients may describe pruritus, urticaria, swelling, symptoms of airway obstruction such as wheezing, chest tightness, stridor, dyspnea, or throat closure and dizziness [60]. Thus, it may be clinically difficult to distinguish from ‘true anaphylaxis’ leading to unnecessary intubation/s[60]. However, despite the symptoms of anaphylaxis described above, patients with US-IA do no exhibit objective findings on examination such as hypotension, oropharyngeal edema or wheezing that would be hallmarks of anaphylaxis. There may be a delay in epinephrine use without progression of symptoms. Laboratory examinations in these patients, including serum tryptase and urinary histamine levels, are not elevated. As IA is corticosteroid responsive, lack of response to prednisone based treatment regimens should alert physicians to consider US-IA, the latter being corticosteroid unresponsive.

Diagnosing US-IA can be challenging and acceptance of the diagnosis by patients is often difficult. Patients should be treated initially as IA; however, if there is no objective data and/or no response to treatment, then the patient can be placed in a category of IA-Q. A thorough evaluation for objective symptoms is needed prior to the diagnosis of US-IA. A comprehensive review of medical records for acute episodes should be undertaken, with careful attention to abnormalities on clinical examination. Patients who have symptoms of throat closure or swelling should undergo direct laryngoscopy at the time of symptoms to confirm upper airway or laryngeal edema. If patients produce loud stridorous sounds, direct laryngoscopy can demonstrate adduction of the vocal cords, or at minimum, lack of angioedema. This can be done during an episode or during a provocative challenge. Encouraging patients to cough can also eliminate stridorous noises, as early as the next inspiration. Patients who have transient desaturations to 90 percent or less due to restricted mouth breathing will respond by increasing oxygen saturation levels after being asked to take deeper breaths rapidly. Patients with US-IA may report urticaria or swelling, thus it is helpful to encourage them to produce photographic evidence from acute episodes. Patients with dermatographism may have linear wheals due to scratching rather than generalized urticaria and these may be evident in photographs. Checking blood pressure reported in medical records during symptomatic episodes is helpful as patients with US-IA do not exhibit hypotension during episodes of lightheadedness.

Once a diagnosis of US-IA is made, physicians should attempt to foster a working relationship with patients to treat it. Treatment may include frequent visits and discussion regarding the diagnosis, particularly in an attempt to avoid unnecessary ED visits. It may be helpful to reassure patients that their symptoms are not life-threatening, and in the case of pruritus or globus, can be well controlled with medication. Confrontation may lead to the patient seeking medical care at another location, leading to a cycle of office and ED visits adding to unnecessary health care costs. Anxiety, depression and stress may play a role in somatoform disorders, thus patients should be offered a psychiatric referral. However, many patients do not accept that anxiety or stress are contributing to their symptoms and may refuse psychiatric or psychological consultation. Once a diagnosis of US-IA is made, an attempt should be made to quickly taper and discontinue oral steroids. Some patients with US-IA may feel they need to be on medication for their symptoms of pruritus and dermatographism and may be managed with a daily antihistamine.

US-IA is a distinct disorder from Munchausen stridor and Munchausen anaphylaxis in that it is a somatoform disorder, not a conscious effort to produce symptoms. Munchausen stridor is a nonorganic disorder in which patients purposefully produce loud, stridorous respirations that may frighten family members and medical personnel[61]. However, Munchausen anaphylaxis is true anaphylaxis that is induced by the patient, generally by deliberate ingestion of a food or medication to which the patients is sensitized. Patients will often deny purposeful ingestion but often do so for secondary gain, resulting in many ED and hospital visits.

Globus Sensation

A globus sensation, which is described as a persistent or intermittent painless sensation of a lump or foreign body in the throat, may be mistaken for episodes of IA-A or breakthrough angioedema in patients being treated with prednisone for IA [62]. It can be distinguished from breakthrough anaphylaxis as it is typically worse with food and may last for several days. There are also no hives or angioedema as may occur with usual episodes of IA. These are differences that may help to distinguish a globus sensation from breakthrough anaphylaxis to allow for proper treatment and avoid unnecessary steroid use. The globus sensation further complicates treatment as gastroesophageal reflux disease (GERD) is a leading cause of globus and unfortunately, treatment of IA with prednisone can induce or worsen existing GERD[63, 64]. Stress and anxiety may also play a role in the globus sensation and patients may need reassurance and frequent office visits with education to distinguish between globus and breakthrough IA [65, 66]. If needed, endoscopy may be useful in diagnosing globus sensation in patients with IA. Proton pump inhibitor (PPI) therapy is useful in treating globus and response to a PPI would help corroborate the diagnosis. As globus is not uncommon, it is essential to discuss globus sensation as a potential side effect of prednisone with patients prior to the initiation of treatment.

Panic Attacks and IA

Patients with IA may be naturally frightened by the condition and after the appropriate pharmacologic treatment is initiated, some may experience panic attacks and interpret these as episodes of IA. These panic attacks may result in the use of emergency treatment, including epinephrine and visits to the ED. This may prompt the managing physicians to increase the dosage of prednisone when IA is well controlled resulting in the overuse of and increasing risk of corticosteroid-induced adverse effects. The lack of objective physical evidence should be discussed with the patient. Often, with reassurance and regular follow up visits with prednisone reduction, remission of IA and panic attacks can be achieved. Psychiatric consultation may prove useful in some patients but is rarely necessary.

Pregnancy and IA

When a diagnosis of IA is made in a woman of child-bearing age, measures should be taken to avoid pregnancy, if possible, until the IA is in a state of remission and prednisone is discontinued. Anaphylaxis in pregnancy can lead to hypoxic-ischemic encephalopathy and central nervous system damage or death of the fetus or neonate[67]. Therefore, if control of IA is required during pregnancy, treatment with prednisone and an antihistamine is indicated. Acute episodes of anaphylaxis in pregnant patients should be treated with triple therapy of intramuscular epinephrine, steroids, and an antihistamine, similar to treatment in non-pregnant patients.

Clinical Cases

Case 1

A 64 year old man with no significant past medical history presented with multiple episodes of abdominal cramping, diarrhoea, generalized urticaria and loss of consciousness approximately 30 to 90 minutes after eating. His first episode occurred 30 minutes after eating a chicken sandwich from a fast food restaurant. He developed severe abdominal cramping, diarrhoea, hives over his trunk and extremities and then fainted. He lost consciousness for approximately 10 minutes and was found to have a blood pressure of 80/40. He had used Naproxen for knee pain 1 week prior only and no NSAIDs or ASA since then. He was taken to the emergency department (ED) and given epinephrine, steroids, and antihistamines. He was discharged with epinephrine for self-administration as needed for anaphylaxis. One month later, he was watching television, eating a cheeseburger with mustard and a salad of green peppers, tomatoes, and celery. Sixty minutes later, he developed hives and pruritus for which he took cetirizine and symptoms resolved. He was not taking any non-steroidal anti-inflammatory drugs or aspirin at the time. The following week, he had another episode of abdominal cramping approximately 90 minutes after eating lunch consisting of a hot dog, carrots, and apples. He then had watery diarrhea, and while on the toilet developed hives and loss of consciousness. His wife found him on the bathroom floor, injected him with epinephrine, called emergency services and was taken to hospital.

He was then referred to an allergist and underwent skin testing to multiple foods including beef, chicken, mustard, green pepper, black pepper, celery, apples, garlic, pine nuts, carrots, corn, egg white, ginger, sesame and tomato—all foods he had eaten during episodes and avoided thereafter. Skin testing was negative. There were no medications suspected in these episodes of anaphylaxis, thus testing for medications was not undertaken.

He was commenced on pharmacotherapy with cetirizine 10mg daily and prednisone 50mg daily for 14 days. He was given an emergency pack prescription for epinephrine, prednisone, and hydroxyzine. After 2 weeks on daily prednisone with no symptoms, the patient was tapered to prednisone 50mg every other day for 14 days. He was successfully tapered to every other day prednisone by 10mg every two weeks and eventually discontinued cetirizine. His IA has remained in remission with no further episodes for 3 years after discontinuing the prednisone.

Case 2

A 42 year old woman with a history of allergic rhinitis and asthma, skin prick test positive to ragweed, presented with multiple episodes of throat swelling and stridor. She initially presented to the Emergency Department (ED) with throat swelling and shortness of breath after being commenced on ciprofloxacin for a urinary tract infection. She was treated for a presumed allergic reaction to the ciprofloxacin with steroids, diphenhydramine, and discontinuation of the culprit medication. Four days later, she presented again to the ED with throat swelling and a sensation of tongue swelling after consuming strawberries and cheese. She was again treated with steroids and diphenhydramine and was discharged with epinephrine for self-administration for potential allergic reactions in the future. She was also referred for an allergy evaluation. Skin testing to strawberry and cow's milk was negative. She was started on fexofenadine and was recommended to strictly avoid ciprofloxacin in the future. Eight days later, she presented to the ED again due to symptoms of throat closing and now with facial puffiness. She attributed her symptoms to chemical smells at her apartment and took diphenhydramine prior to going to the ED. She also described that she had used epinephrine three times in the past week for similar symptoms. She had nasopharyngeal endoscopy by otolaryngology that did not demonstrate any oropharyngeal or laryngeal edema.

The patient subsequently underwent a provocation challenge in the otolaryngology office with cleaning solutions and again developed symptoms of throat closing. She was noted to have adduction of the vocal cords with inspiration on nasendoscopy. She was diagnosed with vocal cord dysfunction (VCD) and recommended speech therapy with a VCD focus. Her fexofenadine was discontinued and her VCD remains controlled.

Conclusion

IA is a disease entity with symptoms identical to 'anaphylaxis with a known trigger'. Some physicians and patients have been reluctant to accept the diagnosis as most have not heard of IA previously and may find it difficult to understand that they can have anaphylaxis without an external trigger. However, once allergy and other systemic disorders are excluded, reassurance about the diagnosis can be offered as there are effective therapeutic algorithms that can be initiated and the prognosis is excellent. Swift diagnosis of IA can reduce medical costs through fewer ED visits and unnecessary diagnostic tests. Patients with IA should be classified according to the classification system and therapy initiated based on their specific IA disease subtype. It is important to emphasize to patients the need for corticosteroids in treatment of IA, both remittive and episodic.

With remittive therapy, once control has been established, gradual reduction in prednisone dosage can result in continued control and induction of remission, despite discontinuation of prednisone. Adjunctive medications, such as ketotifen, can be useful in helping to control IA and induce remission, having a corticosteroid sparing effect in most cases of CSD-IA and M-IA. If corticosteroids are unable to control the disease at appropriate doses, alternative diagnoses, including US-IA, globus sensation, or anxiety, should be considered. Support groups for patients with IA may be beneficial in educating patients and their families about social and emotional aspects of the disease. In the pediatric and elderly age groups, it will be prudent to ensure that personnel caring for the patient are familiar with IA, its symptoms and its treatment.

Despite the advancements in the practical aspects of classification and treatment of IA, the primary pathogenesis of the disease is still unknown. There is ongoing active investigation into the mechanisms underlying IA. As these mechanisms become clearer, there may be improved ease of diagnosis and treatment for patients with IA. It is essential to continue to study IA so that in the future, therapeutic strategies aimed at the underlying mechanisms of IA may potentially be successful.

Clinical Pearls

- IA is diagnosis of exclusion after triggers such as foods, medications or insect stings and diseases that mimic anaphylaxis have been ruled out.
- IA is a corticosteroid responsive disorder. Acute episodes should be treated with 'triple therapy' of epinephrine, corticosteroids, and antihistamines. Patients with frequent IA episodes should be treated with remittive therapy consisting of

corticosteroids and antihistamines in addition to 'triple therapy' for acute anaphylactic attacks.

- The prognosis of IA is favorable with early diagnosis and appropriate treatment.

References

[1] Bacal, E; Patterson, R; Zeiss, CR. Evaluation of severe (anaphylactic) reactions. *Clinical allergy*, 1978, 8, 295-304.

[2] Ditto, AM; Harris, KE; Krasnick, J; et al., Idiopathic anaphylaxis: a series of 335 cases. Annals of allergy, asthma & immunology: official publication of the American College of Allergy, *Asthma, & Immunology*, 1996, 77, 285-291.

[3] Boxer, MB; Greenberger, PA; Patterson, R. The impact of prednisone in life-threatening idiopathic anaphylaxis: reduction in acute episodes and medical costs. *Annals of allergy*, 1989, 62, 201-204.

[4] Patterson, R; Hogan, MB; Yarnold, PR; Harris, KE; Idiopathic, anaphylaxis. An attempt to estimate the incidence in the United States. *Archives of internal medicine*, 1995, 155, 869-871.

[5] Cianferoni, A; Novembre, E; Mugnaini, L; et al., Clinical features of acute anaphylaxis in patients admitted to a university hospital: an 11-year retrospective review (1985-1996). Annals of allergy, asthma & immunology : official publication of the American College of Allergy, *Asthma, & Immunology*, 2001, 87, 27-32.

[6] Webb, LM; Lieberman, P. Anaphylaxis: a review of 601 cases. Annals of allergy, asthma & immunology : official publication of the American College of Allergy, *Asthma, & Immunology*, 2006, 97, 39-43.

[7] Thong, BY; Cheng, YK; Leong, KP; et al., Anaphylaxis in adults referred to a clinical immunology/allergy centre in Singapore. *Singapore medical journal*, 2005, 46, 529-534.

[8] Pumphrey, RS; Stanworth, SJ. The clinical spectrum of anaphylaxis in north-west England. Clinical and experimental allergy : journal of the British Society for *Allergy and Clinical Immunology*, 1996, 26, 1364-1370.

[9] Shanmugam, G; Schwartz, LB; Khan, DA. Prolonged elevation of serum tryptase in idiopathic anaphylaxis. The *Journal of allergy and clinical immunology*, 2006, 117, 950-951.

[10] Greenberger, PA; Miller, MM. Urine histamine during episodes of anaphylaxis. *The Journal of allergy and clinical immunology*, 1994, 93, 302.

[11] Myers, G; Donlon, M; Kaliner, M. Measurement of urinary histamine: development of methodology and normal values. *The Journal of allergy and clinical immunology*, 1981, 67, 305-311.

[12] Lieberman, P; Taylor, WW; Jr., Recurrent idiopathic anaphylaxis. *Archives of internal medicine*, 1979, 139, 1032-1034.

[13] Tanus, T; Mines, D; Atkins, PC; Levinson, AI. Serum tryptase in idiopathic anaphylaxis: a case report and review of the literature. *Annals of emergency medicine*, 1994, 24, 104-107.

[14] Muller, UR. Elevated baseline serum tryptase, mastocytosis and anaphylaxis. Clinical and experimental allergy : journal of the British Society for *Allergy and Clinical Immunology*, 2009, 39, 620-622.

[15] Brockow, K; Jofer, C; Behrendt, H; Ring, J; Anaphylaxis in patients with mastocytosis: a study on history, clinical features and risk factors in 120 patients. *Allergy*, 2008, 63, 226-232.

[16] Akin, C; Scott, LM; Kocabas, CN; et al., Demonstration of an aberrant mast-cell population with clonal markers in a subset of patients with "idiopathic" anaphylaxis. *Blood*, 2007, 110, 2331-2333.

[17] Garriga, MM; Friedman, MM; Metcalfe, DD. A survey of the number and distribution of mast cells in the skin of patients with mast cell disorders. *The Journal of allergy and clinical immunology*, 1988, 82, 425-432.

[18] Keffer, JM; Bressler, RB; Wright, R; et al., Analysis of the wheal-and-flare reactions that follow the intradermal injection of histamine and morphine in adults with recurrent, unexplained anaphylaxis and systemic mastocytosis. *The Journal of allergy and clinical immunology*, 1989, 83, 595-601.

[19] Greenberger, PA; Boxer, MB; Roberts, M. Cutaneous vascular reactions to leukotriene D4, platelet activating factor, and histamine in patients with idiopathic anaphylaxis and chronic urticaria. *Clinical research*, 1986, 34, 409A.

[20] Patterson, LS; Idiopathic, R. anaphylaxis and exercise-induced “anaphylaxis”: PAR, pseudo-allergic reactions. *Involvement of Drugs and Chemicals*, 1985, 4, 45-58.

[21] Grammer, LC; Shaughnessy, MA; Harris, KE; Goolsby, CL. Lymphocyte subsets and activation markers in patients with acute episodes of idiopathic anaphylaxis. Annals of allergy, asthma & immunology : official publication of the *American College of Allergy, Asthma, & Immunology*, 2000, 85, 368-371.

[22] Cohan, VL; Undem, BJ; Fox, CC; et al., Dexamethasone does not inhibit the release of mediators from human mast cells residing in airway, intestine, or skin. *The American review of respiratory disease*, 1989, 140, 951-954.

[23] Irani, AA; Nilsson, G; Ashman, LK; Schwartz, LB. Dexamethasone inhibits the development of mast cells from dispersed human fetal liver cells cultured in the presence of recombinant human stem cell factor. *Immunology*, 1995, 84, 72-78.

[24] Finotto, S; Mekori, YA; Metcalfe, DD. Glucocorticoids decrease tissue mast cell number by reducing the production of the c-kit ligand, stem cell factor, by resident cells: in vitro and in vivo evidence in murine systems. *The Journal of clinical investigation*, 1997, 99, 1721-1728.

[25] Saavedra-Delgado, AM; Mathews, KP; Pan, PM; et al., Dose-response studies of the suppression of whole blood histamine and basophil counts by prednisone. *The Journal of allergy and clinical immunology*, 1980, 66, 464-471.

[26] Greenberger, PA; Patterson, R; Radin, RC. Two pretreatment regimens for high-risk patients receiving radiographic contrast media. *The Journal of allergy and clinical immunology*, 1984, 74, 540-543.

[27] Golbert, TM; Patterson, R; Pruzansky, JJ. Systemic allergic reactions to ingested antigens. *The Journal of allergy*, 1969, 44, 96-107.

[28] Sampson, HA; Mendelson, L; Rosen, JP. Fatal and near-fatal anaphylactic reactions to food in children and adolescents. *The New England journal of medicine*, 1992, 327, 380-384.

[29] Furlong, TJ; DeSimone, J; Sicherer, SH. Peanut and tree nut allergic reactions in restaurants and other food establishments. *The Journal of allergy and clinical immunology*, 2001, 108, 867-870.

[30] Moneret-Vautrin, DA; Morisset, M; Lemerdy, P; et al., Food allergy and IgE sensitization caused by spices: CICBAA data (based on 589 cases of food allergy). *Allergie et immunologie*, 2002, 34, 135-140.

[31] DiCello, MC; Myc, A; Baker, JR; Jr., Baldwin, JL. Anaphylaxis after ingestion of carmine colored foods: two case reports and a review of the literature. *Allergy and asthma proceedings : the official journal of regional and state allergy societies*, 1999, 20, 377-382.

[32] Khalili, B; Bardana, EJ; Jr., Yunginger, JW; Psyllium-associated anaphylaxis and death: a case report and review of the literature. Annals of allergy, asthma & immunology : official publication of the American College of Allergy, *Asthma, & Immunology*, 2003, 91, 579-584.

[33] Greenberger, PA; Flais, MJ. Bee pollen-induced anaphylactic reaction in an unknowingly sensitized subject. Annals of allergy, asthma & immunology : official publication of the *American College of Allergy, Asthma, & Immunology*, 2001, 86, 239-242.

[34] Sanchez-Borges, M; Suarez-Chacon, R; Capriles-Hulett, A; Caballero-Fonseca, F. An update on oral anaphylaxis from mite ingestion. Annals of allergy, asthma & immunology : official publication of the *American College of Allergy, Asthma, & Immunology*, 2005, 94, 216-220, quiz 220-212, 306.

[35] Stricker, WE; Anorve-Lopez, E; Reed, CE. Food skin testing in patients with idiopathic anaphylaxis. *The Journal of allergy and clinical immunology*, 1986, 77, 516-519.

[36] Sonin, L; Patterson, R. Metabisulfite challenge in patients with idiopathic anaphylaxis. *The Journal of allergy and clinical immunology*, 1985, 75, 67-69.

[37] Becker, K; Southwick, K; Reardon, J; et al., Histamine poisoning associated with eating tuna burgers. *JAMA : The journal of the American Medical Association*, 2001, 285, 1327-1330.

[38] Commins, SP; Platts-Mills, TA. Anaphylaxis syndromes related to a new mammalian cross-reactive carbohydrate determinant. *The Journal of allergy and clinical immunology*, 2009, 124, 652-657.

[39] Sondhi, D; Lippmann, M; Murali, G. Airway compromise due to angiotensin-converting enzyme inhibitor-induced angioedema: clinical experience at a large community teaching hospital. *Chest*, 2004, 126, 400-404.

[40] Castells, MC; Horan, RF; Sheffer, AL. Exercise-induced Anaphylaxis. *Current allergy and asthma reports*, 2003, 3, 15-21.

[41] Beaudouin, E; Renaudin, JM; Morisset, M; et al., Food-dependent exercise-induced anaphylaxis--update and current data. *European annals of allergy and clinical immunology*, 2006, 38, 45-51.

[42] Moffitt, JE; Venarske, D; Goddard, J; et al., Allergic reactions to Triatoma bites. Annals of allergy, asthma & immunology : official publication of the *American College of Allergy, Asthma, & Immunology*, 2003, 91, 122-128, quiz 128-130, 194.

[43] Slater, JE; Raphael, G; Cutler, GB; Jr., et al., Recurrent anaphylaxis in menstruating women: treatment with a luteinizing hormone-releasing hormone agonist--a preliminary report. *Obstetrics and gynecology*, 1987, 70, 542-546.

[44] Slater, JE; Kaliner, M. Effects of sex hormones on basophil histamine release in recurrent idiopathic anaphylaxis. *The Journal of allergy and clinical immunology*, 1987, 80, 285-290.
[45] Akin, C; Valent, P; Metcalfe, DD. Mast cell activation syndrome: Proposed diagnostic criteria. *The Journal of allergy and clinical immunology*, 2010, 126, 1099-1104 e1094.
[46] Brockow, K; Metcalfe, DD. Mastocytosis. *Chemical immunology and allergy*, 2010, 95, 110-124.
[47] Wong, S; Yarnold, PR; Yango, C; et al., Outcome of prophylactic therapy for idiopathic anaphylaxis. *Annals of internal medicine*, 1991, 114, 133-136.
[48] Ditto, AM; Krasnick, J; Greenberger, PA; et al., Pediatric idiopathic anaphylaxis: experience with 22 patients. *The Journal of allergy and clinical immunology*, 1997, 100, 320-326.
[49] Bock, SA; Munoz-Furlong, A; Sampson, HA. Fatalities due to anaphylactic reactions to foods. *The Journal of allergy and clinical immunology*, 2001, 107, 191-193.
[50] Kemp, SF; Lockey, RF; Wolf, BL; Lieberman, P. Anaphylaxis. A review of 266 cases. *Archives of internal medicine*, 1995, 155, 1749-1754.
[51] Warrier, P; Casale, TB. Omalizumab in idiopathic anaphylaxis. Annals of allergy, asthma & immunology : official publication of the American College of Allergy, *Asthma, & Immunology*, 2009, 102, 257-258.
[52] Jones, JD; Marney, SR; Jr., Fahrenholz, JM. Idiopathic anaphylaxis successfully treated with omalizumab. Annals of allergy, asthma & immunology : official publication of the American College of Allergy, Asthma, & Immunology, 2008, 101, 550-551.
[53] Krasnick, J; Patterson, R; Harris, KE. Idiopathic anaphylaxis: long-term follow-up, cost, and outlook. *Allergy*, 1996, 51, 724-731.
[54] Krasnick, J; Patterson, R; Meyers, GL. A fatality from idiopathic anaphylaxis. Annals of allergy, asthma & immunology : official publication of the American College of Allergy, *Asthma, & Immunology*, 1996, 76, 376-378.
[55] Patterson, R; Clayton, DE; Booth, BH; et al., Fatal and near fatal idiopathic anaphylaxis. *Allergy proceedings : The official journal of regional and state allergy societies*, 1995, 16, 103-108.
[56] Allen, DB. Growth suppression by glucocorticoid therapy. Endocrinology and metabolism clinics of North America, 1996, 25, 699-717.
[57] Pongracic, JA; Kim, JS. Update on epinephrine for the treatment of anaphylaxis. *Current opinion in pediatrics,* 2007, 19, 94-98.
[58] Grossman, JM; Gordon, R; Ranganath, VK; et al., American College of Rheumatology 2010 recommendations for the prevention and treatment of glucocorticoid-induced osteoporosis. *Arthritis care & research*, 2010, 62, 1515-1526.
[59] Patterson, R; Fitzsimons, EJ; Choy, AC; Harris, KE. Malignant and corticosteroid-dependent idiopathic anaphylaxis: successful responses to ketotifen. Annals of allergy, asthma & immunology : official publication of the American College of Allergy, *Asthma, & Immunology*, 1997, 79, 138-144.
[60] Choy, AC; Patterson, R; Patterson, DR; et al., Undifferentiated somatoform idiopathic anaphylaxis: nonorganic symptoms mimicking idiopathic anaphylaxis. *The Journal of allergy and clinical immunology*, 1995, 96, 893-900.
[61] Patterson, R; Schatz, M; Horton, M. Munchausen's stridor: non-organic laryngeal obstruction. *Clinical allergy*, 1974, 4, 307-310.

[62] Galmiche, JP; Clouse, RE; Balint, A; et al., Functional esophageal disorders. *Gastroenterology*, 2006, 130, 1459-1465.

[63] Woo, P; Noordzij, P; Ross, JA. Association of esophageal reflux and globus symptom: comparison of laryngoscopy and 24-hour pH manometry. Otolaryngology--head and neck surgery : official *journal of American Academy of Otolaryngology-Head and Neck Surgery*, 1996, 115, 502-507.

[64] Hill, J; Stuart, RC; Fung, HK; et al., Gastroesophageal reflux, motility disorders, and psychological profiles in the etiology of globus pharyngis. *The Laryngoscope*, 1997, 107, 1373-1377.

[65] Cook, IJ; Dent, J; Collins, SM. Upper esophageal sphincter tone and reactivity to stress in patients with a history of globus sensation. *Digestive diseases and sciences*, 1989, 34, 672-676.

[66] Deary, IJ; Smart, A; Wilson, JA. Depression and 'hassles' in globus pharyngis. The British journal of psychiatry : *The journal of mental science*, 1992, 161, 115-117.

[67] Simons, FE; Schatz, M. Anaphylaxis during pregnancy. *The Journal of allergy and clinical immunology*, 2012, 130, 597-606.

In: Anaphylaxis: Principles and Practice
Editor: M. Thirumala Krishna

ISBN: 978-1-62618-688-0

Chapter XI

Allergen Specific Immunotherapy and Systemic Reactions

Mark C. Glaum*[*] *and Richard F. Lockey
University of South Florida, Morsani College of Medicine
and James A. Haley Veterans' Hospital Tampa, FL, US

Abstract

Allergen immunotherapy is an effective, safe therapy used worldwide to treat a variety of allergic conditions. Over the last 2 decades, the sublingual route of immunotherapy administration has become more widely used in Europe and sublingual immunotherapy tablets are currently under review for approval for use in the USA. Any form of immunotherapy carries with it the risk of adverse reactions and anaphylaxis. As use of sublingual immunotherapy becomes more common worldwide, it is important to compare and contrast the safety aspects of this therapy versus allergen-specific subcutaneous immunotherapy.

There are several reports of severe systemic reactions associated with sublingual immunotherapy, but thus far no fatalities. There are various studies of systemic reactions, including those that result in death, associated with subcutaneous immunotherapy over its 100-year worldwide experience. Local reactions are common to both forms of the treatment.

Both subcutaneous and sublingual forms of immunotherapy are effective in treating allergic symptoms, while the sublingual route appears to carry a significant safety benefit. Ongoing analysis is necessary to determine how best to incorporate both forms of treatment into the management of allergic patients. Adherence to published immunotherapy treatment guidelines will reduce the likelihood of adverse reactions.

[*] Corresponding author: mglaum@health.usf.edu.

Introduction

Allergen immunotherapy (AIT) is utilized as an effective disease-modifying treatment for allergic rhinitis, allergic asthma, allergic eczema and venom hypersensitivity. Even from early comprehensive reviews of systemic allergic reactions (SAR) from subcutaneous immunotherapy (SCIT), serious and sometimes fatal reactions occurred as a result of administering such therapy. [1-9] In 1985, 13 fatalities from SCIT were reported at the annual meeting of the American Academy of Allergy Asthma and Immunology (AAAAI).[10] Stemming from the findings published in this abstract, concerns over the safety of SCIT began to build in North America and Great Britain because of two almost simultaneously published reports describing 40 and 26 fatalities associated with SCIT in the United States and Great Britain, respectively. [11,12] Based on these reports, changes took place in the United States, with the institution of SCIT practice parameters leading to a sharp decline in fatalities secondary to this form of therapy. Similarly, in Europe, restrictions on the administration of SCIT were levied by the British Committee for the Safety of Medicines resulting in a sharp decline in SCIT given in the United Kingdom over subsequent years.

As a consequence, interest in alternative routes of AIT expanded throughout the world. Two forms of AIT, SCIT and sublingual immunotherapy (SLIT), have the potential to induce localized and systemic allergic reactions (SAR). However, the latter form is much safer and less likely to cause SAR. The purpose of this chapter is to review available data and analyze the likelihood, severity and preventable causes of SAR.

Subcutaneous Immunotherapy

Traditional methods for SCIT most commonly involve two phases of allergen administration; the build-up and maintenance phases. The build-up phase begins with the subcutaneous injection of dilute concentrations of an allergen vaccine at a dose that is slowly increased over time, with subsequent injections at weekly or biweekly intervals until a maintenance dose is reached.

Once maintenance is achieved, the injection is gradually extended to monthly intervals (maintenance phase) and given for approximately 3 to 5 years, or longer, depending on the response to therapy. Other forms are also available such as rush or ultra-rush SCIT in which injections are given more frequently over a limited period of time, days to several weeks, to reach maintenance. SCIT is efficacious to treat allergic rhinitis, allergic asthma, allergic eczema as well as venom hypersensitivity but SCIT is not recommended to treat food or drug allergy or chronic urticaria.

Systemic Reactions to Subcutaneous Immunotherapy

Adverse reactions to SCIT range from local pruritus and swelling at the site of the injection to severe SAR or life-threatening anaphylaxis and even death. The likelihood of a

SAR from SCIT depends on several factors, some of which include the dosing schedule, allergen vaccine formulation, degree of allergen sensitization and the presence of asthma [13]. Other factors include the allergen dose administered, a vaccine renewed, and rate of escalation.

A review of 38 SCIT studies found an average rate of SAR to range from 0.05 to 3.2% with fewer reactions occurring during the maintenance versus build-up phase.[14] A retrospective study of SAR of 4600 SCIT patients over two 10-year periods demonstrates a reaction rate of 5.2% over the first versus fewer reactions over the second decade. No fatalities were reported over the 20-year span [15]. The SAR rate was one in 47 patients in a prospective study of 4578 patients receiving SCIT for over one year, all of whom were receiving high-dose maintenance SCIT.

The rate of reactions was significantly higher during the build-up phase increasing to one in 32 with approximately 30% of said reactions occurring more than 30 min after the SCIT injection [16]. In another prospective study, 419 subjects received standardized grass or dust mite allergen vaccines by a conventional dosing schedule. SAR occurred in 4.8% of patients, many of whom had asthma. In these patients, reactions occurred in a significantly higher proportion during the build-up phase of SCIT as compared to the maintenance phase [17]. Over the past 15 years, the approximate rate of SAR to SCIT is estimated to be 0.2%. [18].

Fatalities Secondary to Subcutaneous Immunotherapy

Serious reactions to SCIT include severe SAR or anaphylaxis, some of which are fatal. A committee of the AAAAI, beginning in 1984, collected information on deaths from SCIT and skin testing from 1945 to 1984. Of the 46 deaths reported during this time interval, 30 had sufficient information for a complete analysis. Six deaths were attributable to skin testing and 24 were caused by SCIT. The mean age was 34 years, with no gender difference. Errors in administration of the vaccine were suspected in 3 or possibly 4 of the cases. In 9 of 24 (38%) of the cases, fatal reactions occurred during the build-up phase and in 7 of 24 (29%), death occurred in the maintenance phase.

Signs and symptoms of anaphylaxis appeared in less than 20 minutes in 20 subjects, in 20-30 minutes in two subjects and in 30 or more minutes in 3 subjects (5 were unknown or not reported) [19]. A second survey by the AAAAI administered between 1985 and 1989 found evidence for 17 fatalities from SCIT but none from skin testing.[20] Another study of fatal reactions from SCIT and skin testing performed by the same committee from 1990 to 2001[21] reported that over the 12 years of the survey, of those who responded to the short questionnaire, 41 fatal reactions were reported (21 directly reported and 20 indirectly reported cases by local physicians) with an estimated mean of once per 6.85 million injections (average 3.4 deaths per year). One of these fatal reactions was confirmed after skin testing with multiple food allergens. Of those responding to the long questionnaire, 17 fatalities were reported with 15 of 17 fatalities (88%) diagnosed with asthma. Initial signs and symptoms of anaphylaxis appeared within 30 minutes of the immunotherapy injection in 10 of 13 (77%) respondents. In 3 patients, reactions began 30 or more minutes after the SCIT injection.

These findings were similar to the results of the original survey published by Lockey et al. in 1987. [11] In all three studies, asthma was considered a major risk factor for a systemic allergic reaction and death secondary to a SCIT injection [19-21]. An extension of this survey focused on near-fatal reactions associated with hypotension and/or severe respiratory compromise requiring epinephrine therapy. It found that 46% of reactions were attributable to dosing errors and that 58% of near fatal reactions occurred with a maintenance dose during the peak of the allergy season [22].

With a further extension of this same survey, the AAAAI and the American College of Allergy Asthma and Immunology (ACAAI) collaborated in establishing a national surveillance database for adverse reactions to SCIT and allergen skin testing. Although 6 fatalities from SCIT were documented between 2001 and 2007, no fatalities have been directly or indirectly reported from SCIT during the first 3 years of the surveillance project (2008 –2010) [23], and through 2012, no fatalities have been reported. There are 3 unsubstantiated, unconfirmed reports of fatalities (2008-2012). (Personal communication with David Bernstein.) While these observations are preliminary, a longer surveillance project is underway to verify that the annual fatalities from SCIT in the U.S.A. will continue to decline in comparison with previous findings.

Based on these observations, the AAAAI and ACAAI Practice Parameters on allergen immunotherapy recommend that SCIT injections be given in a physician's office and under the supervision of a physician, qualified physician extender (nurse practitioner or physician assistant) or both appropriately trained in emergency treatment of SARs [24].

Sublingual Immunotherapy

SLIT is a form of immunotherapy in which drops or soluble allergen-containing tablets are administered under the tongue, held there for 1-2 minutes, and then swallowed. Although SLIT is used in many parts of Europe and other parts of the world for routine care, the USA Federal Drug Administration (FDA) has not yet approved such therapy. Studies of SLIT are currently ongoing in the U.S.A.

Localized Reactions to Sublingual Immunotherapy

The most commonly reported reactions from SLIT are localized oral reactions including irritation and itching of the mouth. Such reactions to SLIT occur in up to 100% of patients, however, most of these reactions remit within a week or so with ongoing administration of vaccine [25].

In a controlled study of efficacy of grass pollen vaccine SLIT in 127 subjects with allergic rhinitis, local reactions, including mouth and throat irritation, occurred in 69% of the treated group versus 40% of those on placebo. However no SARs were reported.[26] A study of 77 subjects enrolled in a phase I safety and dosing study of SLIT demonstrated that, during an 8 week course of treatment, 91% of all adverse effects were localized to the eyes, nose, mouth/throat, gut, or ear with no reported SARs [27].

Table 1. World Allergy Organization Immunotherapy Systemic Reaction Grading System

Grade 1	Grade 2	Grade 3	Grade 4	Grade 5
Symptom(s)/sign(s) of 1 organ system present*	Symptom(s)/sign(s) of more than 1 organ system present or	Lower respiratory Asthma (eg, 40% PEF or FEV1 drop NOT responding to an inhaled bronchodilator)	Lower or upper respiratory Respiratory failure with or without loss of consciousness	Death
Cutaneous Generalized pruritus, urticaria, flushing, or sensation of heat or warmth or Angioedema (not laryngeal, tongue or uvular)	Lower respiratory Asthma: cough, wheezing, shortness of breath (eg, less than 40% PEF or FEV1 drop, responding to an inhaled bronchodilator)	or Upper respiratory laryngeal, uvula, or tongue edema with or without stridor	or Cardiovascular Hypotension with or without loss of consciousness	
or Upper respiratory Rhinitis - (eg, sneezing, rhinorrhea, nasal pruritus and/ or nasal congestion)	or Gastrointestinal Abdominal cramps, vomiting, or diarrhea or Other Uterine cramps			
or Throat-clearing (itchy throat)				
or Cough perceived to originate in the upper airway, not the lung, larynx, or trachea				
or Conjunctival Erythema, pruritus or tearing				
Other Nausea, metallic taste, or headache				

Systemic Reactions to Sublingual Immunotherapy

No life-threatening reactions were reported in 4378 subjects receiving SLIT in a 2006 review of 66 studies [28]. Adverse reactions were reported in 12% of subjects giving a rate of 2.7 reactions per 1000 doses administered. In a placebo-controlled trial of SLIT and SCIT in birch-induced rhinoconjunctivitis, mild SARs were observed in subjects receiving SCIT, SLIT and placebo, while more serious SARs were observed in those receiving SCIT but not SLIT [29].

A placebo-controlled double-blinded trial utilizing a soluble grass allergen tablet was performed in 55 centers in 8 countries. Foregoing a traditional build-up phase, subjects were immediately started on a once daily maintenance dose and given therapy for 8 weeks prior to the grass pollen season. Adverse events likely related to the drug were reported in 66% of subjects on treatment versus 26% on placebo. Twenty-three of 26 subjects that withdrew due to adverse events were on study drug.[30] In a related follow-up study 634 subjects were randomized to receive either grass tablets at a once daily maintenance dose 16 weeks prior to and throughout the grass season.[31] Of treated subjects, 46% experienced oral pruritus compared to 4% on placebo. Four percent of subjects on active drug withdrew from the study.

A third study reported on 351 of these same subjects treated for an average period of 22 months.[32] The adverse event profile was similar between placebo and treatment arms during the second year of the study and unlike the first year, there was no increased incidence of local reactions reported. A different 3-month study was designed to examine the safety of single dose compared to multiple dose SLIT in a group of 159 subjects. Adverse events related to SLIT were similar in those receiving single vs. multiple dose therapy.[33]

Table 2. Safety measures to reduce the likelihood of an adverse reaction to immunotherapy

Proper patient selection
Special consideration given to asthmatics, particularly those who are highly sensitized
Assessment of clinical status on treatment days
Check for new medication usage, particularly beta blockers
Check dosing – double check right patient, right dose
Dose adjustment during allergy season
Compliance with treatment schedules
Dose adjustments for freshly made vaccines
Early recognition and treatment of adverse reactions
Discontinuation of therapy in patients who repeatedly have SARs
Vigilance: Reactions can occur after years of maintenance therapy and well after the 30 minute waiting period

Cases of Severe Reactions to Sublingual Immunotherapy

A report in the European literature describes an 11 year-old female with allergic rhinitis and asthma receiving 2 SLIT vaccines; one in the morning and one in the evening. Three minutes following administration of the evening pollen vaccine, the patient experienced lip swelling, chest pain and abdominal pain. She was treated and released from the emergency room [34]. A case of a severe SAR from SLIT is reported in a 31 year-old female with asthma and allergic rhinitis who was self-administering a mixed vaccine containing pollens, cat, dog and *Alternaria*. Within minutes of administering the mixed vaccine under her tongue, she experienced generalized pruritus, wheezing, dyspnea, and angioedema. She self-administered albuterol by inhalation, an oral glucocorticosteroid and antihistamine with good response and did not seek further medical care. The patient subsequently discontinued SLIT. [35] A 16-year old patient with asthma and allergic rhinitis experienced a near-fatal reaction after taking 6 times the normal dose of her SLIT allergen vaccine and experienced urticaria, pruritus and flushing within minutes of administration. The patient subsequently experienced respiratory and cardiovascular collapse after being transferred to an emergency room where she was pulseless. She was treated in the intensive care unit and recovered. [36] A review of 11 published SLIT case reports of non-fatal anaphylaxis graded the severity of SAR according to World Allergy Organization (WAO) criteria (Table 1). The authors found that all 11 cases reported met the WAO criteria for a SAR. Skin /mucosal symptoms and respiratory symptoms predominated in these cases. Six of the 11 cases had hypotension and shock but no deaths were reported. The authors concluded that given the excellent safety profile of SLIT and the very low incidence of SARs in the European experience, home administration of maintenance doses of SLIT should be considered. However, no formal recommendations on providing self-injectable epinephrine to SLIT patients currently exist. Given the fact that severe, life-threatening reactions to SLIT are reported, consideration should be given to providing epinephrine for self-administration for SLIT patients administering doses outside a medical facility.[37]

Prevention of AIT Reactions

Careful adherence to AIT treatment guidelines is crucial to minimize the likelihood of an adverse SAR (Table 2). International and U.S.A. guidelines for AIT have been continually updated over the past decade or two with the goal of enhancing its safety and effectiveness. Highly allergic and unstable asthmatic patients are generally at highest risk for serious SAR and the recommendations indicate that such patients considered for SCIT should have stable asthma. [24] In an AAAAI survey of SAR from 1990-2001, respiratory failure occurred primarily in asthmatic patients, and 4 (57%) of 7 asthmatic patients had a baseline FEV1 of less than 70% of predicted value when they received their SCIT injection.[22] Patients should be evaluated for use of certain medications such as beta-blockers, which can potentially make anaphylaxis more difficult to treat. With any type of injection, a process should be established so that physicians and other healthcare professionals administering such therapy appropriately identify the patient, not only to assure that they receive the appropriate vaccine, but the appropriate dose. Doses on newly formulated vaccines, where appropriate, should be decreased to levels to account for the potential loss of potency from the previous vaccine. Clinic and nursing staff should be trained to recognize the early signs and symptoms of a SAR and how and when to initiate treatment, realizing that a SAR can occur at any time even after years of stable maintenance therapy. Patients on such therapy should remain in the clinic for at least 30 minutes following a SCIT injection and discontinuation of such therapy should be considered in patients with repeated life-threatening reactions. When a SAR occurs later than 30 minutes, after the patient has left the treatment facility, a longer wait period may be instituted and consideration should be given to provide the patient with epinephrine for self-administration. While these recommendations are primarily made for SCIT, some of these same principles may apply to self-administered SLIT vaccines. One particular concern is the risk of SLIT vaccine overdose.

One study of allergic children in Italy on SLIT found that a significant majority (85%) used more than 75% of their annual SLIT vaccine over 3 vs. a 12-month period suggesting that patients were not compliant with the prescribed dosing schedule [38].

Clinical Cases

Case 1

A 48 year-old female presents with 3 year history of worsening asthma symptoms. She reports symptoms of wheezing, coughing and chest tightness that wakes her from sleep 3 nights per week and requires use of albuterol every day. Approximately 4 years ago a cat was brought into the home. The patient had prick-puncture skin test that revealed significant sensitivity to cat, dust mites and several seasonal aeroallergens. Spirometry revealed an FEV1 of 70% predicted with 15% reversibility with a bronchodilator. The patient has had 2 visits to the emergency room and 4 systemic corticosteroid bursts for asthma exacerbations in the past year despite the regular use of high-dose inhaled corticosteroids and long-acting bronchodilator combination therapy. The patient is interested in starting on SCIT for better long-term control of her asthma symptoms.

This patient with allergic asthma would likely benefit from immunotherapy for better control of her symptoms. However, several factors place her at higher risk of SARs. The first factor that puts her at higher risk is uncontrolled asthma manifested by the fact that she has break-through symptoms in spite of reasonable medical therapy. A second factor that places her at higher risk is a decreased FEV1 at 70% predicted. A low FEV1 is associated with a higher incidence of SARs from SCIT. Better pharmacologic control of asthma would be recommended in this patient before initiating such therapy.

Case 2

A 29 year-old male who lived in the Northeastern United States experiences symptoms of itchy, watery eyes, sneezing, nasal congestion and post-nasal drip every year for the past 3 years only during the grass pollen season with no other significant symptoms. He works as a pharmaceutical representative and travels regionally. Prick-puncture skin test reveals significant sensitivity to Northern grasses, (timothy and others), several molds, dust mites and dog. Medications used to treat these symptoms have been largely ineffective. The patient is interested in starting immunotherapy but cannot consistently travel to the allergy clinic during injection hours due to his work schedule.

This patient has seasonal allergic rhinitis with skin test reactivity to Northern grasses [subfamily Pooideae (brome, meadow fescue, perennial ryegrass, timothy, sweet vernal, redtop, Kentucky bluegrass, western wheatgrass)] as well as several perennial allergens but only clinically relevant sensitivity to the grass pollen season. Although both SCIT and SLIT would be reasonable options for this patient, self-administration of Northern grass pollen SLIT would be a practical treatment option for him. Treatment is not necessary with the other allergens to which he is sensitive since he has no clinical symptoms when exposed to these allergens. The patient is likely to experience local oral pruritus when initiating SLIT. He can be reassured that these local symptoms typically improve within the first few weeks of therapy.

Conclusion

The use of AIT to treat allergic diseases over the past 100 years has enabled physicians and other health care professionals to identify the risk/benefit and type of allergic reactions caused by such therapy. Opportunities exist to characterize the true risk of a reaction with SLIT as this form of AIT becomes more widespread. It may even be equally effective as SCIT. Data suggest that SLIT carries a significant safety advantage compared to SCIT, illustrated by the fact that most patients are able to receive SLIT at home.[39]

Clinical Pearls

- Serious adverse reactions including deaths from anaphylaxis have been reported with SCIT.
- Infrequent reports of anaphylaxis without any fatalities have also been reported from SLIT.
- Risk factors for anaphylaxis with AIT include: uncontrolled asthma, "Rush" immunotherapy build-up schedules, dosing errors and history of previous SARs. A 30-minute wait in a medical facility is mandated for SCIT.
- Self-injectable epinephrine should be considered for patients who have had SARs after this wait period. Systemic allergic reactions from SLIT are much less common in SCIT. Self-injectable epinephrine continues to be an option for such patients.

Key Take Home Messages:

- AIT is a safe, effective treatment for certain allergic conditions when prescribed and administered in accordance with established immunotherapy treatment guidelines
- Any form of immunotherapy carries a risk of causing anaphylaxis. Clinicians prescribing and administering such therapy should be aware and take precautions to minimize these risks

References

[1] Lamson, RW. So-called fatal anaphylaxis in man. *JAMA*, 1929, 93, 1776
[2] Waldbott GL. The prevention of anaphylactic shock. *JAMA*, 1932, 98, 446.
[3] Vaughan, WT; Black, JH. *Practice of allergy*. St. Louis: The CV Mosby Co, 1939.
[4] Vance, BM; Strassmann, G. Sudden death following injection of foreign protein. *Arch Pathol*, 1942, 34, 849.
[5] James, LP; Austin, KF. Fatal systemic anaphylaxis in man. *N Engl J Med*, 1964, 270, 597.
[6] Rands, DA. Anaphylactic reaction to desensitization for allergic rhinitis and asthma. *Br Med J*, 1980, 281, 854.
[7] Pollard, RCH. Anaphylactic reaction to desensitization [Letter]. *Br Med J*, 1980, 281, 854.
[8] Van Arsdel, PP; Sherman, WB. Risk of inducing constitutional reactions in allergic patients. *J Allergy*, 1957, 28, 251-261.
[9] Cooke, RA; Veer, AV. Human sensitization. *J Immunol*, 1916, 1, 201-305.
[10] Lockey, RF; Benedict, LM; Turkeltaub, P. Fatalities from immunotherapy and skin testing. *J Allergy Clin Immunol*, 1985, 1, 246.
[11] Lockey, RF; Benedict, LM; Turkeltaub, PC; Bukantz, SC. Fatalities from immunotherapy (IT) and skin testing (ST). *J Allergy Clin Immunol*, 1987, 79, 660-677.
[12] CSM Update: Desensitizing vaccines. *Br Med J.*, 1986, 293, 948.
[13] Windom, HH; Lockey, RF. An Update on the Safety of Specific Immunotherapy. *Curr Opin Allergy Clin Immunol*, 2008, 8, 571-576.
[14] Stewart, GE; Lockey, RF. Systemic reactions from allergen immunotherapy. *J Allergy Clin Immunol*, 1992, 90, 567-578.
[15] Ragusa, VF; Massolo, A. Non-fatal systemic reactions to subcutaneous immunotherapy: a 20-year experience comparison of two 10-year periods. *Eur Ann Allergy Clin Immunol*, 2004, 36, 52-55.
[16] Tinkleman, DG; Cole, WQ; Tunno, J. Immunotherapy: A one-year prospective study to evaluate risk factors of systemic reactions. *J Allergy Clin Immunol*, 1995, 95, 8-14.
[17] Tabar, AI; Garcia, BE; Rodriguez, A; et. al. A prospective safety-monitoring study of immunotherapy with biologically standardized extracts. *Allergy*, 1993, 48, 450-453.
[18] Cox, L; Larenas-Linnemann, D; Lockey, RF; Passalacqua, G. Speaking the Same Language: the World Allergy Organization Subcutaneous Immunotherapy Systemic Reaction Grading System. *J Allergy Clin Immunol*, 2010, 125, 569-574.
[19] Lockey, RF; Benedict, LM; Turkeltaub, PC; Bukantz, SC. Fatalities from immunotherapy(IT) and skin testing (ST). *J Allergy Clin Immunol*, 1987, 79, 660-677.
[20] Reid, MJ; Lockey, RF; Turkeltaub, PC; et al. Survey of fatalities from skin testing and immunotherapy 1985-1989. *J Allergy Clin Immunol*, 1993, 92, 6-15.
[21] Bernstein, DI; Wanner, M; Borish, L; Liss GM. Twelve year survey of fatal reactions to allergen injections and skin testing: 1990-2001. *J Allergy Clin Immunol*, 2004, 113(6), 1129-1136.
[22] Amin, HS Liss, G; Bernstein, DI. Evaluation of near-fatal reactions to allergen-immunotherapy injections. *J Allergy Clin Immunol*, 2006, 117, 169-175.

[23] Epstein, TG; Liss, GM; Murphy-Berendts, K; Bernstein, DI. Immediate and delayed-onset systemic reactions after subcutaneous immunotherapy injections: ACAAI/AAAAI surveillance study of subcutaneous immunotherapy: year 2. *Ann Allergy Asthma Immunol*, 2011, 107(5), 426-431.

[24] Cox, L; Nelson, H; Lockey, R; et al. Allergen Immunotherapy Practice Parameter: a third update. *J Allergy Clin Immunol*, 2011, 127(1 Suppl), S1-55.

[25] Didier, A; Malling, HJ; Worm, M; et al. Optimal dose, efficacy and safety of once-daily sublingual immunotherapy with a 5-grass pollen tablet for seasonal allergic rhinitis. *J Allergy Clin Immunol*, 2007, 120, 1338-1345.

[26] de Blay, F; Barnig, C; Kanny, G; et al. Sublingual-swallow immunotherapy with standardized 3-grass pollen extract: a double-blind, placebo-controlled study. *Ann Allergy Asthma Immunol*, 2007, 99, 453-461.

[27] Esch, RE; Bush, RK; Peden, D; Lockey, RF. Sublingual-oral administration of standardized allergenic extracts: phase 1 safety and dosing results. *Annals Allergy*, 2008, 100(5), 475-81.

[28] Cox, LS; Linnemann, DL; Nolte, H; et al. Sublingual immunotherapy: a comprehensive review. *J Allergy Clin Immunol*, 2006, 117, 1021-1035.

[29] Khinchi, MS; Poulsen, LK; Carat, F; et. al. Clinical efficacy of sublingual and subcutaneous birch pollen allergen-specific immunotherapy: a randomized, placebo-controlled, double blind, double dummy study. *Allergy*, 2004, 59, 45-53.

[30] Durham, SR; Yang, W; Pedersen, MR; *et al.* Sublingual immunotherapy with once-daily grass allergen tablets: a randomized controlled trial in seasonal allergic rhinoconjunctivitis. *J Allergy Clin Immunol*, 2006, 117, 802–809.

[31] Dahl, R; Kapp, A; Colombo, G; *et al.* Efficacy and safety of sublingual immunotherapy with grass allergen tablets for seasonal allergic rhinoconjunctivitis. *J Allergy Clin Immunol*, 2006, 118, 434–440.

[32] Dahl, R; Kapp, A; Colombo, G; et al. Sublingual grass allergen tablet immunotherapy provides sustained clinical benefit with progressive immunologic changes over 2 years. *J Allergy Clin Immunol*, 2008, 121, 512–518.

[33] Lombardi, C; Gargioni, S; Cottini, M; et al. The safety of sublingual immunotherapy with one or more allergens in adults. *Allergy*, 2008, 63, 375–376.

[34] Eifan, AO; Keles, S; Bahceciler, NN; Barlan, IB. Anaphylaxis to multiple pollen allergen sublingual immunotherapy. *Allergy*, 2007, 62, 567–568.

[35] Dunsky, EH; Goldstein, MF; Dvorin, DJ; Belecanech, GA. Anaphylaxis to sublingual immunotherapy. *Allergy*, 2006, 61, 1235.

[36] Blazowski, L. Anaphylactic shock because of sublingual immunotherapy overdose during third year of maintenance dose. *Allergy*, 2008, 63, 374.

[37] Calderón, MA; Simons, FE; Malling, HJ; Lockey, RF; Moingeon, P; Demoly, P. Sublingual allergen immunotherapy: mode of action and its relationship with the safety profile. *Allergy*, 2012, 67(3), 302-11.

[38] Passalacqua, G; Musarra, A; Pecora, S; et al. Quantitative assessment of the compliance with once-daily sublingual immunotherapy in children (EASY Project: evaluation of a novel SLIT formulation during a year) *Pediatr Allergy Immunol*, 2007, 18, 58-62.

[39] Di Bona, D; Plaia, A; Leto-Barone, MS; La Piana, S; Di Lorenzo, G. Efficacy of subcutaneous and sublingual immunotherapy with grass allergens for seasonal allergic

rhinitis: A meta-analysis-based comparison. *J Allergy Clin Immunol*, 2012, 130(5), 1097-1107.

In: Anaphylaxis: Principles and Practice
Editor: M. Thirumala Krishna
ISBN: 978-1-62618-688-0

Chapter XII

Primary Mast Cell Disorders and Anaphylaxis

Jasper J. van Doormaal**, *Joanne N. G. Oude Elberink* and *Jan G. R. de Monchy
Department of Allergology, University Medical Center Groningen,
University of Groningen, Groningen, The Netherlands

Abstract

Primary mast cell disorders that may underlie anaphylaxis are characterised by clonal proliferation of pathological mast cells. These disorders are divided into mastocytosis and the less frequently occurring and less well understood monoclonal mast cell activation syndrome. Cutaneous mastocytosis (CM) with its typical skin lesions in the absence of the pathological mast cells in extra-cutaneous tissues is predominantly present in children. Spontaneous resolution is common, usually before the onset of puberty. Systemic mastocytosis (SM) is defined by the presence of the abnormal mast cells outside the skin. Nearly all adults have SM, mostly the indolent form (ISM). ISM progresses slowly, is stable or can decline in activity. Other SM subtypes are rare. The ISM prevalence is probably >13.0 cases per 100.000 inhabitants aged ≥15 years. It increases with age. About 4% of the patients with a history of Hymenoptera sting anaphylaxis have CM or SM.

The etiology of mastocytosis is largely unknown. The clonal mast cell population shows somatic mutations, in particular in the tyrosine kinase *KIT*, mostly the D816V mutation, and in genes, regulating mast cell activity. Mast cell accumulation is predominantly due to a decrease in apoptosis.

Symptoms in mastocytosis are caused by mediator release or by mast cell infiltration in tissues. Histamine and other mediators can induce circulatory, gastro-intestinal, skeletal, dermal and neuro-psychological manifestations. Patients are more susceptible to anaphylaxis if also specific IgE is produced, particularly in response to Hymenoptera stings. Other important eliciting factors of anaphylaxis are nonsteroidal anti-

* Corresponding author: j.j.van.doormaal@home.nl.

inflammatory drugs (NSAIDs), opioids, radiocontrast media, general anaesthetics and muscle relaxants used in anaesthesia. About half of the ISM patients, especially men aged <50 years develop osteoporosis and/or osteoporotic fractures. Mast cell infiltration can lead to typical skin lesions, enlargement of liver, spleen and lymph nodes, local osteolysis and cytopenias.

Screening by dermatological investigations and measurement of serum basal tryptase and urinary histamine metabolites should be considered in patients with anaphylaxis or with unexplained osteoporosis. If SM is considered, a bone marrow biopsy and smear, and flow cytometry and *KIT* mutation analysis of bone marrow aspirate should be done.

Treatment is symptomatic by histamine H1 and H2 receptor antagonists, with addition of oral cromoglycate and/or NSAIDs, if needed. Osteoporotic manifestations are treated with calcium and vitamin D supplementation and bisphosphonates. Cytoreductive therapy is not indicated in ISM. Besides the known elicitor(s) in the individual patient, other well-known elicitors of anaphylaxis should be avoided. Immunotherapy (life-long so far) should be offered to patients with a history of Hymenoptera sting anaphylaxis. To protect the skeleton, calcium and vitamin D supplementation should be considered in all SM patients.

Abbreviations

ASM	aggressive systemic mastocytosis
BAT	basophylic activation test
CM	cutaneous mastocytosis
ISM	indolent systemic mastocytosis
KIT	c-kit proto-oncogene
MCL	mast cell leukemia
MH	N tau-methylhistamine
MIMA	N tau-methylimidazoleacetic acid
MIS	mastocytosis in the skin
MMAS	monoclonal mast cell activation syndrome
NSAID	non-steroidal anti-inflammatory drug
SM	systemic mastocytosis
SM-AHNMD	systemic mastocytosis with a clonal hematological non-mast cell lineage disease
SSM	smoldering systemic mastocytosis
UP	urticaria pigmentosa
WHO	World Health Organization

Introduction

Signs and symptoms of mast cell activation range from nausea to abdominal cramping and diarrhea, from mild itching to anaphylaxis and life threatening hypotension, and from tachycardia or unexplained arrhythmias to neurological or even psychiatric symptoms. Anaphylaxis is one of the most feared features of systemic mast cell activation. Anaphylactic reactions can develop within minutes to life threatening events, sometimes resulting in permanent disability, or even death. The following three criteria should be met to diagnose systemic mast cell activation: (1) typical clinical signs and symptoms; (2) substantial and transient increase in one or more mast cell derived mediators in biological fluids; and (3) an objective major response of clinical symptoms to agents that attenuate the production or activity of mast cell derived mediators (Table 1) [1].

Symptoms of mast cell activation are manifestations of mast cell disorders. These mast cell disorders can be classified in three types: primary, secondary, and idiopathic (Table 2) [1]. Primary mast cell disorders are characterised by a clonal proliferation of pathological mast cells, as evidenced by the abnormal expression of proteins and the presence of a "gain of function" mutation (mostly the D816V mutation) of the c-kit proto-oncogene (*KIT*). This gene contains the code of the transmembrane receptor KIT for the stem cell factor, which is critical for mast cell growth and differentiation from hematopoietic progenitors, as well as mast cell survival and chemotaxis. Secondary mast cell disorders are conditions in which mast cells are normal in quantity and function and are responding to an external stimulus such as an allergen, autoantibody, drug, or products of complement activation. Idiopathic mast cell disorders are conditions in which there is no identifiable cause of mast cell activation.

Table 1. Three criteria for the diagnosis of systemic mast cell activation

1. Typical clinical signs and symptoms (flushing, pruritus, urticaria, angioedema, nasal congestion, nasal pruritus, wheezing, throat swelling, headache, hypotension and diarrhea)
2. Increase in serum total tryptase by ≥20% above baseline level* plus 2 μg/l during or within 4 hours after a symptomatic period
3. Response of clinical symptoms to histamine receptor 1 and/or 2 blockers or mast cell targeting agents (e.g. cromoglycate)

* Baseline level is defined as the level before the acute event or ≥24 hours after all clinical signs and symptoms have completely resolved after the acute event.

Table 2. Classification of mast cell disorders associated with mast cell activation

Primary mast cell disorders Mastocytosis Monoclonal mast cell disorder*
Secondary mast cell disorders Allergic disorders Mast cell activation associated with chronic inflammatory or neoplastic disorders Physical urticarias Drug induced mast cell activation (e.g. non-steroidal anti-inflammatory drugs) Chronic autoimmune urticaria
Idiopathic mast cell disorders Idiopathic anaphylaxis Idiopathic urticaria Idiopathic angioedema (some subtypes) Mast cell activation syndrome

*Also known as monoclonal mast cell activation syndrome or clonal systemic mast cell activation syndrome.

It is important to recognize that anaphylaxis can be the first symptom of an underlying primary mast cell disorder. Mastocytosis is the most prevailing disease between the two forms of primary mast cell disorders. Clinically, two subtypes of mastocytosis are recognized. Cutaneous mastocytosis (CM) is characterized by typical skin lesions caused by the invasion of an enhanced number of the abnormal and aggregates forming mast cells in the dermis, while the presence of the abnormal mast cells in extra-cutaneous tissues is lacking. In contrast, systemic mastocytosis (SM) is defined by the presence of the abnormal mast cells outside of the skin. The typical skin lesions of mastocytosis are not always present in SM. In SM patients with a history of anaphylaxis to a sting of a wasp or bee, only a minority have skin lesions [2].

The monoclonal mast cell activation syndrome (MMAS), also known as clonal systemic mast cell activation syndrome, is the other form of primary mast cell disorder. This syndrome has recently been recognized as a distinct mast cell disorder. MMAS differs from SM by the fact, that MMAS patients do not fulfill the diagnostic criteria of SM. MMAS patients have similar symptoms as SM patients, but do not have the typical skin lesions of mastocytosis. In patients with MMAS, the *KIT* point mutations and the expression of the aberrant protein CD25 (alpha chain of the high affinity IL-2 receptor) may be only detectable in a bone marrow sample enriched for mast cells rather than in unfractionated bone marrow samples, or when highly sensitive diagnostic assays (such as those based on mutation specific primers) are employed [1].

Mastocytosis

Classification

Typical skin lesions in the absence of detectable abnormal mast cells in extra-cutaneous tissues characterize CM, notwithstanding a thorough and adequate examination of the bone marrow. In contrast, SM is defined by the presence of the abnormal mast cells outside the skin. Especially in the bone marrow, the abnormal mast cells can be demonstrated, but also other organs, e.g. liver, spleen, lymphoid tissues and the gastro-intestinal tract can be invaded by the abnormal mast cells. "Mastocytosis in the skin" (MIS) is a condition defined by the presence of the typical skin lesions without proven presence of the abnormal mast cells in extra-cutaneous tissue while a thorough and adequate examination of the bone marrow has not (yet) been performed[3].

SM is subdivided according to the extent of mast cell infiltration in various tissues and organs and the effect of this infiltration on their functioning. Using B- and C-findings (Table 3), SM patients can be classified into the following four subtypes: indolent SM (ISM), smoldering SM (SSM), aggressive SM (ASM) and mast cell leukemia (MCL). SM is sometimes present in combination with a clonal hematologic non-mast cell lineage disease (SM-AHNMD) (Table 4) [4]. In ISM, the mast cell burden is low and skin lesions are frequently present. The variant with no skin lesion is also known as bone marrow mastocytosis.

Table 3. B- and C-findings

B-findings
Bone marrow biopsy showing >30% infiltration by mast cells (focal, dense aggregates) and/or serum total tryptase level >200 μg/l
Signs of dysplasia or myeloproliferation, in non-mast cell lineage(s), but insufficient criteria for definitive diagnosis of a hematopoietic neoplasm (AHNMD), with normal or only slightly abnormal blood cell counts
Hepatomegaly without impairment of liver function, and/or palpable splenomegaly without hypersplenism, and/or lymphadenopathy on palpation or imaging
C-findings
Bone marrow dysfunction manifested by one or more cytopenia (absolute neutrophil count <1.0x10^9/l, Hb <6.2 mmol/l (10 g/dl), or platelets <100x10^9/l), but no obvious non-mast cell hematopoietic malignancy
Palpable hepatomegaly with impairment of liver function, ascites and/or portal hypertension
Skeletal involvement with large osteolytic lesions and/or pathological fractures
Palpable splenomegaly with hypersplenism
Malabsorption with weight loss due to gastro-intestinal mast cell infiltrates

Table 4. Subtypes of systemic mastocytosis

Indolent systemic mastocytosis (ISM) Meets criteria for SM. No B- or C findings. No evidence of an associated non-mast cell lineage clonal hematological malignancy/disorder.
Smoldering systemic mastocytosis (SSM) As ISM, but with 2 or more B-findings but no C-findings
Aggressive systemic mastocytosis (ASM) Meets criteria for SM. One or more C-findings. No evidence of mast cell leukemia. Usually without skin lesions.
Mast cell leukemia (MCL) Meets criteria for SM. Bone marrow biopsy shows a diffuse infiltration, usually compact, by atypical, immature mast cells. Bone marrow aspirate smears show ≥20% mast cells. In typical MCL, mast cells account for ≥10% of peripheral white blood cells. Usually without skin lesions.
Systemic mastocytosis with associated clonal hematological non-mast cell lineage disease (SM-AHNMD) Meets criteria for SM and criteria for an associated, clonal hematological non-mast cell lineage disorder (e.g. myelodysplastic syndrome, myeloproliferative neoplasm, acute myeloid leukemia, lymphoma, or other hematological neoplasm that meets the criteria for a distinct entity in the WHO classification)

The above-mentioned classification has prognostic relevance. The life-expectancy of ISM patients is (near) normal, whereas the life-expectancy of ASM and MCL is considerably shorter. The associated hematological disease determines the prognosis of SM-AHNMD. The prognosis of SSM patients is unknown, but probably not substantially worse than that of ISM patients as long as no transition to aggressive forms of SM or hematologic malignancies occurs. In ISM and SSM patients such transition rarely occurs [5-7]

Epidemiology

In children, 60-80% of the cases with MIS appear during the first year of life. Studies on bone marrow examinations to diagnose SM are scarce. In the majority of cases the disease seems to be limited to the skin. Most eventually improve or resolve completely by adolescence [8].

In adults, SM is the most prevalent type of mastocytosis. The indolent form is by far the most prevailing subtype. Although the activity of ISM can decline [9], complete remissions were not reported so far. Mastocytosis affects males and females in equal ratios [5, 7].

Mastocytosis, in all its forms, is a rare disorder. The incidence of UP in the general population was estimated to amount to one new case per 150.000 persons per year[10]. Data on the exact prevalence were unknown till very recently. In a Dutch region the prevalence of ISM was at least 13.0 cases per 100,000 inhabitants aged ≥15 years. ISM prevalence increased with age. The number of referred patients in this study steeply increased from 1998 to 2010, very likely because of an increase in the experience of the local mastocytosis team and the continuing educational activities of the team to general practitioners and medical specialists during these years [11].

Pathogenesis

The aetiology of mastocytosis is largely unknown. The clonal mast cell populations show somatic mutations, in particular mutations in the tyrosine kinase *KIT* and in enzyme and receptor genes with crucial involvement in the regulation of mast cell activity [12]. In almost all patients with CM or ISM *KIT* mutations have been found, especially the D816V mutation [13]. In the majority of patients, these mutations are limited to derivatives of hematopoietic stem cells. The mutations convert *KIT* into a constitutively active, deregulated stem cell factor independent tyrosine kinase, driving aberrant mediator production/release [12]. Associations between SM and polymorphisms in various genes have been reported. Rarely, familial cases have been reported. Mast cell accumulation is predominantly due to a decrease in mast cell apoptosis as well as on a limited scale to an increase in cell proliferation [12].

Symptomatology

a. Overview

Symptoms and signs are caused by release of mast cell mediators and local accumulation of mast cells. Mast cells produce and release a large number of different mediators, e.g. histamine, prostaglandin D2, platelet activating factor, proinflammatory cytokines, leukotriene C4 and D4, chemokines and tryptase. Histamine and prostaglandin D2 are thought to be clinically the most important ones [1]. Manifestations vary strongly in nature and severity. Many patients have no mediator related complaints at all. An overview of the manifestations resulting from release of mast cell mediators is given in Table 5. Symptoms arising from mast cell infiltration are shown in Table 6.

Table 5. Manifestations resulting from release of mast cell mediators

Manifestations
Circulatory manifestations
Anaphylaxis
Flushing
Hypotension
Arrhythmias
Gastro-intestinal manifestations
Abdominal cramping
Diarrhea
Vomiting
Gastritis, duodenitis
Peptic ulcer disease
Skeletal manifestations
Osteoporosis
Osteosclerosis (diffuse or localized)
Osteolytic lesions
Dermal manifestations
Itching
Neuro-psychological manifestations
Tiredness
Cognitive impairment
Depression

Table 6. Manifestations resulting from mast cell infiltration

Manifestations
Skin lesions
Urticaria pigmentosa
Mastocytoma
Diffuse cutaneous mastocytosis
Hepatic enlargement
Portal hypertension (C-finding)
Ascites (C-finding)
Splenic enlargement
Hypersplenism (C-finding)
Lymph node enlargement
Gastro-intestinal tract infiltration
Malabsorption
Colonic polyps
Bone marrow infiltration
Osteolytic lesions and/or pathological fractures (C-finding)
Cytopenias (C-finding)

b. Anaphylaxis

Anaphylaxis is the most feared manifestation of mastocytosis. Anaphylactic reactions can within minutes develop to life threatening events, sometimes resulting in permanent disability [14]. Several cases with a fatal outcome have been described following Hymenoptera stings [15][16], consumption of peanuts[17], in perioperative period[18] and of unknown cause in children and adults[19]. Symptoms in adults with mastocytosis are primarily cardiovascular in nature with dizziness, tachycardia, hypotension and shock. Biphasic anaphylaxis rarely occurs. A lot of eliciting factors are known (Table 7). The most common elicitors for severe anaphylactic reactions are Hymenoptera stings, whereas foods and medications most often lead to milder systemic reactions. A substantial percentage of reactions were supposed to have occurred only after a combination of several factors, notably alcohol and food[20]. Systemic reactions due to Hymenoptera stings are very likely IgE mediated, whereas systemic reactions due to drugs are mostly not.

The prevalence of atopic disorders in patients with CM and SM appears to be similar to that of the general population (i.e. between 20 and 30% in westernized nations)[21][22], but patients are more susceptible to anaphylaxis if also specific IgE is produced, particularly in response to Hymenoptera stings [20]. To discriminate between an IgE-dependent and IgE-independent mechanism by a certain eliciting factor, establishment of sensitization by routine tests should be performed. However, skin prick testing should be performed with caution [3]. Routine tests may fail, especially in case of low total IgE levels, as often found in mastocytosis and thought to possibly be due to binding to an increased number of mast cells [22]. Sensitization may only be diagnosed by basophilic histamine release tests or basophilic activation tests (BAT) [23, 24]. However, a recent study showed that BAT did not add valuable information, because it was invariably negative when standard diagnostic tests were negative in SM patients with Hymenoptera sting reactions [25]. The hypothesis that in such patients insect venom directly induces mediator release from the abundant mast cell mass ("pseudo-allergy") is unlikely because of the following arguments. If this hypothesis were to be true, virtually all patients with mastocytosis should uniformly experience systemic reactions after a sting from any member of the order Hymenoptera and the reaction should be most prominent in those patients presenting with a high mast cell burden in SM. In fact, not all patients with SM develop anaphylactic sting reactions and in many patients with CM or SM and simultaneous Hymenoptera venom anaphylaxis react only to stings of one genus while tolerating stings of other. Furthermore, the natural course is not in line with the pseudo-allergy hypothesis. Patients were sometimes initially found to tolerate stings whereas later hypersensitivity reactions occurred [23].

Table 7. Eliciting factors of anaphylactic reactions in mastocytosis

Hymenoptera sting
Alcoholic beverages
Drugs (aspirin, non-steroidal anti-inflammatory drugs, opioids)
Contrast media
General anaesthetics
Muscle relaxants used in anaesthesia
Exercise
Unexplained

Adults with CM have a lower prevalence of anaphylaxis than adults with ISM[20]. Only a few cases of anaphylaxis in aggressive forms of SM were reported[14]. The prevalence of anaphylaxis in children with mastocytosis is low. Increased basal serum tryptase levels in association with extensive cutaneous involvement identifies children with mastocytosis at risk for severe mast cell activation events [26]. In children, Hymenoptera stings seem to play no major part in eliciting anaphylaxis [20]. Data on the frequency of anaphylaxis in adult patients with mastocytosis are affected by referral and selection bias and different definitions on anaphylaxis. An overview of the data on adult ISM populations in various centres is given in Table 8a. To assess the influence of referral and selection bias, the frequency of urticaria pigmentosa (UP), which is the typical skin lesion in adults, is also included. The higher the percentage of UP in the ISM population the lower is the percentage of patients with anaphylaxis. Some studies suggest that the risk of Hymenoptera venom anaphylaxis in mastocytosis increases with rising levels of basal serum tryptase levels[27][28][29][30]. However, a recent study showed that the risk declined with a further increase in the higher range of the mast cell load parameters basal serum tryptase and urinary histamine metabolites, and was near nil at very high levels. The risk was maximal at a basal serum tryptase level of about 28 µg/l[31].

A small number of studies have been reported on the frequency of mastocytosis in patients with a history of anaphylactic reaction to a Hymenoptera sting. Between these studies, the selection procedures for bone marrow sampling to establish the diagnosis of SM were markedly different. Ruëff et al., studying Hymenoptera allergic patients, performed further examinations in case of a basal serum tryptase level >11.4 µg/l or when UP was suspected [23]. In an initial study, Bonadonna et al. performed bone marrow examinations in patients with a grade IV reaction combined with a basal serum tryptase level >11.4 µg/l, selected from a total of 552 patients [2]. In a second study of the same population Bonadonna et al. selected from a total of 379 patients with a history of systemic reaction to a Hymenoptera sting those with a basal tryptase >11.4 µg/l[36]. Oude Elberink et al. selected patients with UP or a combination of a basal serum tryptase level ≥10.0 µg/l and an elevated level of urinary methylhistamine (≥176 µmol/mol creatinine) and/or methylimidazoleacetic acid (≥2.0 mmol/mol creatinine) [unpublished data]. Urinary histamine metabolites have previously been shown to be a sensitive and specific method to detect ISM patients in the absence of UP [32]. The calculated frequency of ISM in the three studies combined (Ruëff, second study of Bonadonna, Oude Elberink) is ranging from 2.7 % (proven ISM) to 4.0% (proven ISM plus high ISM risk) (Table 8b). From these calculations, an earlier report from our center was omitted, because at that time tryptase measurements were not yet performed and the WHO-criteria to diagnose SM were not yet established [37]. In ISM patients with a history of Hymenoptera sting anaphylaxis, the risk of anaphylaxis when re-stung is almost 100% [38]. This is in contrast to Hymenoptera allergic patients not suffering from SM, where the risk is not higher than 20-50% [39].

c. Other Mediator Related Symptoms

In all types of mastocytosis, attacks of flushing may occur. Attacks of flushing vary in frequency from several times a day to sporadic, in duration from minutes to hours, sometimes lasting for a few days, and in severity from only noticed by spouses to disabling conditions with hypotension, vomiting, abdominal cramping, diarrhea, fever and/or arrhythmias. Changes in frequency, duration and severity can occur in time, also without concomitant changes in parameters of mast cell burden in the same direction. Flushing attacks differ from postmenopausal hot flushes by duration (mostly >5 minutes), perspiration (mostly slight to mild) and lack of beneficial effect of hormonal replacement therapy.

Table 8a. Prevalence of anaphylaxis in indolent systemic mastocytosis populations of various centres

Author[ref]	adult ISM patients evaluated (n)	Patients with UP (n; %)	Patients with any anaphylaxis (n; %)	Patients with Hymenoptera venom anaphylaxis (n; %)
Van Doormaal[32]	53	0	36 (68%)	30 (57%)
Rossini[33]	79	35 (44%)	54 (68%)	n.a.
Van Anrooij[31]	232	151 (65%)	n.a.	72 (31%)
Van Anrooij[31]	152[a]	109 (72%)	n.a.	72 (47%)
Escribano[7]	145	131 (90%)	33 (22%)	n.a.
Florian[34]	25	24 (96%)	7 (28%)	7 (28%)
Barete[35]	75	72 (96%)	15 (20%)[b]	n.a.
Brockow[20]	61[c]	n.a.	34 (56%)	n.a.
Wimazal[14]	74	n.a.	32 (43%)[d]	n.a.

ISM: indolent systemic mastocytosis;
UP: urticaria pigmentosa;
n.a.: not available;
[a]: only patients with a history of Hymenoptera sting in adult life;
[b]: anaphylactic shock;
[c]: including one patient with smoldering systemic mastocytosis and one with systemic mastocytosis with associated clonal hematological non-mast cell lineage disease;
[d] : anaphylactic shock in 13 (18%) patients.

Table 8b. Frequency of mastocytosis in patients with a history of Hymenoptera venom anaphylaxis

Author[ref]	Adult patients evaluated (n)	Patients with elevated basal tryptase level[a] (n; %)	Patients with UP (n; %)	Patients with CM (n; %)	Patients with high ISM risk[b] (n; %)	Patients with ISM (n; %)
Ruëff [23]	1102	106 (9.6%)	21 (1.9%)	13 (1.2%) [c]	8 (0.7%)	8 (0.7%)
Bonadonna [2]	552	33 (6.0%)[d]	2 (1.6%)	0	n.a.	15 (2.7%) [e]
Bonadonna [36]	379	44 (11.6%)	4 (1.1%)	0	11 (2.9%)	21 (5.5%) [f]
Oude Elberink[g]	389	37 (9.5%)	1 (0.3%)	0	5 (1.3%)	6 (1.5%)

See Table 8a for abbreviations
[a]: Ruëff: >11.4 μg/l; Bonadonna: >11.4 μg/l; Oude Elberink: ≥10.0 μg/l;
[b]: high risk defined as having elevated basal tryptase level without adequate bone marrow examinations performed;
[c]: bone marrow examinations were not possible in 8 patients;
[d]: tryptase only measured in the 121 patients with a grade IV reaction;
[e]: one patient known with the diagnosis of systemic mastocytosis before was excluded from the calculations;
[f]: bone marrow examinations adequately performed in 33 of the 44 patients with an elevated tryptase;
[g]: unpublished data.

Some patients have chronic complaints of abdominal cramping and diarrhea without abnormal findings by endoscopy and histological examinations of biopsies from the gastro-intestinal tract. Often, the complaints decline remarkably or disappear by treatment with histamine H1 and H2 receptor blocking agents. This response can be helpful to differentiate between complaints caused by mastocytosis versus complaints from other origin.

Osteoporosis and/or osteoporotic fractures occur in about half of the ISM patients, especially in men below the age of 50 years [35, 40]. This may be related to the production and release of mast cell mediators, e.g. histamine and heparin. Both substances are known to have deleterious effects on bone metabolism [41, 42]. In addition, activated mast cells release the proinflammatory cytokines IL-1, IL-6, and TNF-a [43], which are important regulators of bone resorption [41]. Increased plasma levels of IL-6 have been observed in patients with ISM [44, 45].

Cognitive impairment and depression are recently recognized as neuro-psychological effects of mastocytosis [46, 47]. Whether neuro-psychological symptoms in mastocytosis are caused by specific mediators or are in response to a chronic disease is unknown but strikingly depression seems to improve by treatment with the protein kinase inhibitor masitinib, as recently shown in an open label study [47].

d. Skin Lesions

Skin lesions in mastocytosis are divided in three types: (a) UP; (b) solitary mastocytoma(s); and (c) diffuse CM (notably: the term CM is in fact wrongly used, as far as extra-cutaneous involvement has not yet been excluded). UP, also called maculopapular CM (notably: see before) is the most common type in children and is the only occurring type in adults. The UP lesions are red to brown to yellow, measure a few millimetres to 1-2 cm in diameter and present as multiple lesions in the form of maculae, plaques or nodules (Figure 1 and 2). The affected areas include the trunk and extremities. Less affected are the palms, soles, scalp and face as well as sun-exposed body areas. The number of lesions can range from a few to countless. Meticulous history taking can help to differentiate from other skin lesions. In almost all patients, lesions become reddish and develop slight swelling after exposure to heat (warm bath or shower, sunbathing), cold wind or rubbing clothes. Sometimes these lesional changes are accompanied by localized itching. Wheal and flare formation after rubbing of one or several lesions (positive Darier's sign) strengthens the suspicion on UP. UP is diagnosed by the typical exanthema (major criterion) and one or two of the following minor criteria: (a) monomorphic mast cell infiltration that either consist of large aggregates of tryptase-positive mast cells (>15 cell/cluster) or scattered mast cells exceeding 20 cells per microscopic high power field (x40); and (b) detection of a *KIT* gene mutation at codon 816 in lesional skin [3]. In children, lesions tend to resolve by the age of 10 years [8].

Solitary mastocytoma(s) are typically identified in infants and young children (Figure 3). Most cases resolve by puberty. Diffuse CM is rare, and can appear at birth or in infancy. It can involve the entire skin with the central region and scalp mostly affected (Figure 4). Bullous forms have been reported [8].

e. Other Signs of Mast Cell Accumulations

A slight enlargement of liver, spleen and (retroperitoneal) lymph nodes can be found in ISM cases with a high mast cell load. In patients with SSM, enlargement is more prominent

(B-finding) and in ASM cases, by definition, organomegaly is associated with functional impairment (C-finding). Enlargement can be caused by localized or generalized mast cell accumulations. Also, osteosclerotic and osteolytic bone lesions with nearly no progression in time can occasionally be found in ISM patients.

Diagnosis

To diagnose CM and SM bone marrow examinations are needed. To avoid unnecessary examinations by these invasive and unpleasant procedures various screening methods are used to assess the risk of detectable primary mast cell disorders.

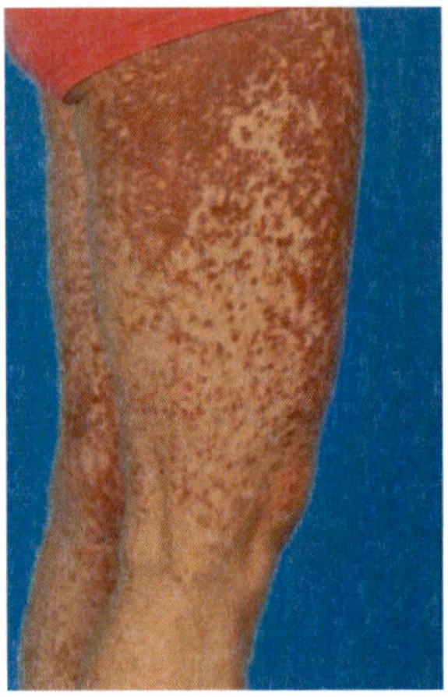

Figure 1. Prominent urticaria pigmentosa lesions in an adult female with indolent systemic mastocytosis.

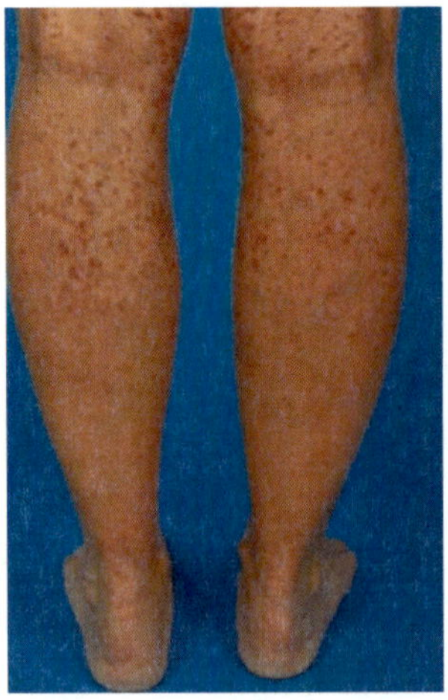

Figure 2. Less prominent urticaria pigmentosa lesions in another adult female with indolent systemic mastocytosis.

a. Screening Methods

Dermatological investigations are the first step for the risk assessment, since the Year-2005 Working Conference of leading international experts in the field of mastocytosis recommends bone marrow investigation in all adults with UP to diagnose SM, irrespective of serum tryptase level (see below) [3]. Meticulous history taking and skin inspection, preferably by an experienced dermatologist may reveal suspected skin lesions of mastocytosis, in adults (nearly) always UP. A skin biopsy is needed for confirmation of the diagnosis. If the exanthema is atypical it is important to know that histological mast cell hyperplasia might be seen as a secondary phenomenon in other inflammatory and neoplastic conditions of the skin such as dermatofibromas, psoriasis, and atopic dermatitis. In a small study of adult patients with UP immunoreactivity for CD25 in cutaneous mast cells appeared to be predictive of SM [48]. Therefore, CD25 immunohistochemistry might also be valuable in differentiating from secondary mast cell hyperplasia in skin biopsies.

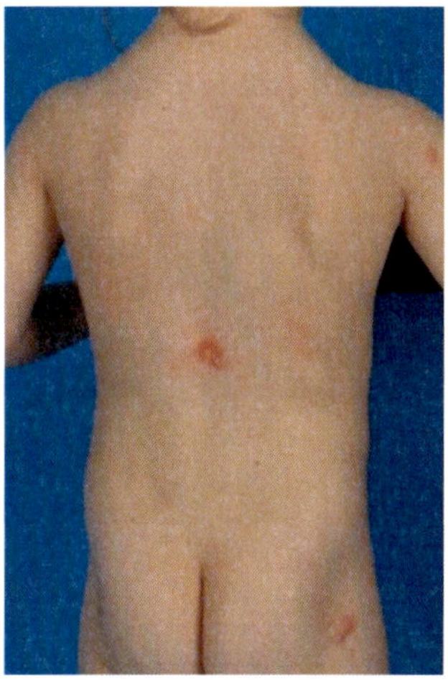

Figure 3. Mastocytomas in a three year old girl.

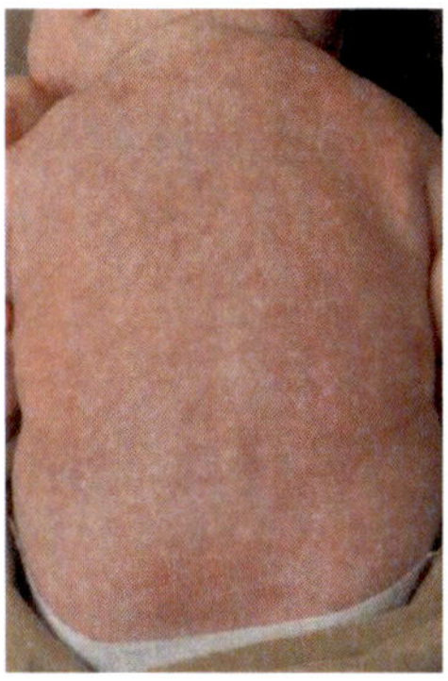

Figure 4. Diffuse cutaneous mastocytosis in a one year old girl.

Measurement of the baseline total tryptase in serum is the recommended laboratory test to employ in the diagnostic work-up in suspected cases [3]. Tryptase is a protease produced predominantly in mast cells, although a small amount is made by basophils and myeloid precursors as well. Total tryptase can be measured in serum with a commercially available assay [ImmunoCAP Tryptase®, Thermo Fisher Scientific Inc. (previously Phadia), Uppsala, Sweden], which is recently adapted to prevent false positive concentrations by interference of heterophilic antibodies. The assay is performed at many laboratories. By this method, mature, active forms of tryptase, as well as immature, inactive forms (protryptases) are measured. Baseline total tryptase is made up of immature (pro) tryptases that are constitutively secreted outside of the mast cell. Mature tryptase is stored in mast cell granules and is elevated in serum as a consequence of mast cell activation. Mature tryptase levels >1 μg/l, total tryptase levels >11 μg/l, and a ratio of total to mature of <10 in serum are each consistent with systemic anaphylaxis [49]. However, measurement of mature tryptase in serum is at the moment not widely available. Total tryptase levels may also rise during anaphylaxis, and a rise in total tryptase levels above baseline may be at least as sensitive as a single mature tryptase level. Serum or plasma for tryptase should be obtained ideally within the second to third hour after anaphylaxis. An additional sample to serve as a baseline sample should be collected at least 24 hours, preferably several days after all signs and symptoms have resolved. Total tryptase level can temporarily decrease after the anaphylactic event to a level below baseline level, probably as a consequence of a phase of refilling of depots before secretion restarts. The minimal elevation of the acute total tryptase level that is considered to be clinically significant is suggested to be ≥20% above baseline level (baseline level is defined as the level before the acute event or ≥24 hours after all clinical signs and symptoms have completely resolved after the acute event) plus 2 μg/l during or within 4 hours after a symptomatic period [1].

Reference values of total tryptase (hereafter shortly tryptase) in serum for healthy individuals are reported by the manufacturer, showing a geometric mean level of 3.8 μg/l and an upper 95th percentile of 11.4 μg/l. Therefore, many laboratories use the value of 11.4 μg/l as the upper normal level. However, the upper 95th percentile was reported to be somewhat lower in other studies and tryptase levels appeared to be elevated by obesity, older age and decreased kidney function [50,51, 52, 53]. Serum tryptase level decreases gradually during pregnancy up to about 25% on average (unpublished data), probably by distension of the plasma compartment.

The differential diagnosis of an elevated tryptase also includes myeloid non-mast cell lineage neoplasms such as acute or chronic myeloid leukemia, myeloproliferative disorders, and myeloid dysplastic syndromes. In these patients, serum tryptase levels may be elevated in the absence of a coexisting SM [3].

Histamine is released from mast cells and to a lesser extend from basophils. Blood histamine levels, however, show variability among healthy individuals, even when the same method of detection is used. Standardization of the assays has proven to be difficult. Elevated levels of histamine in urine can be found in SM patients. Local synthesis of histamine by bacteria in the urinary tract may result in false elevations. Measurement of the histamine metabolites N tau-methylhistamine (MH) and N tau-methylimidazoleacetic acid (MIMA) in urine are the preferred indirect method of assessment of baseline histamine levels in patients [54, 55]. The techniques for the determination of these urinary histamine metabolites [56, 57, 58, 59] are widely available on laboratories that have a chromatography section. The amount of MH and MIMA produced and subsequently excreted does not solely depend on histamine synthesis and subsequent release, but also to some extent on the contribution of exogenous histamine from food and drinks [60, 61], and on the activity of the enzymes histamine N tau-methyltransferase and diamine oxidase, which break down histamine into MH, MIMA and imidazoleacetic acid [61]. The latter metabolite is also a degradation product of histidine and therefore measurement of this metabolite is irrelevant. Genetic polymorphisms [62], alcohol [61,63,64], drugs [61] and pregnancy [65] can influence these enzyme activities, potentially leading to changes in the distribution of the three excreted metabolites. During pregnancy excretion of MH decreases with about 50%, while that of MIMA does not change (unpublished data). Comparing 24-hour urine and morning urine samples no significant differences in MH and MIMA excretion were found, provided that the subjects were on a histamine-poor diet for at least 24 hours [66]. To measure MH and MIMA, we are used to ask patients to collect urine samples after an overnight fast, discarding the first voiding after wakening and to refrain from histamine rich foods and drinks, such as cheese, sauerkraut, canned fish, yoghurt, and wine for the last 24 hours. To avoid formation of MH and MIMA by bacterial contamination, proper storage of the urine sample or adding a small amount of chlorhexidine to the sample is advised.

The 24-hour MIMA excretion appears to correlate with the mast cell burden in patients with mastocytosis [55]. Although one study on a small number of patients found serum tryptase levels to be a more sensitive indicator of limited disease [67], we found a higher diagnostic accuracy of MIMA to assess the risk on ISM compared to tryptase in subjects >50 years with BMI>25 kg/m^2, while this was comparable in subjects <50 years and/or with BMI <25 kg/m^2 (unpublished data). Because basophils also contain histamine, hematologic disorders presenting with basophilia, such as some myeloproliferative disorders, can also cause elevated levels of histamine or its metabolites [68]. Other surrogate markers of mastocytosis are 11-β-prostaglandin F_2 α in urine as metabolite of prostaglandin D_2, and soluble CD25 and CD117 in plasma. Their role in diagnostics and assessment of disease extent has to be further evaluated [68].

Using the above mentioned screening methods the following indications for performing bone marrow examinations in suspected patients has been put forward: (a) all adult patients with UP, and in the absence of UP: (b) all adult patients with tryptase >10 μg/l and a high urinary excretion of MH (≥176 μmol/mol creatinine) or MIMA (≥2.0 mmol/mol creatinine) [32], and (c) all adult patients with symptoms of mast cell activation and a REMA score ≥2 [69, 70]. The REMA score consists of the assignment of positive or negative points, as depicted in Table 9, under the condition that all variables are measured. Since the clinical symptoms in this scoring system have not been reported in detail, the scoring system might be difficult to apply in clinical practice. Occasionally, it is prudent to apply the indications not too strictly (Table 10). In children with MIS bone marrow examinations are generally not indicated. They should only be considered in cases with suspected hematologic disease (abnormal peripheral blood cell counts, organomegaly, lymphadenopathy) or suspicion on SM by severe recurrent systemic mast cell mediator-related symptoms or clinical changes suggestive of SM [8, 71]. Only serum tryptase levels that are clearly elevated (>20 μg/l) are not enough to undertake investigations of bone marrow [71].

b. Bone Marrow Examinations

Bone marrow examinations should contain a thorough histological and immunohistochemical examination of a bone marrow biopsy, cytological examination of bone marrow aspirate and investigation of bone marrow aspirate by flow cytometry and *KIT* mutation analysis. The trephine bone biopsy should be of at a least 2 cm in length and immunohistochemical stained with antibodies against tryptase, CD117 and CD25 [72]. Metachromatic stains such as Giemsa or toluidine blue may fail to stain mast cells in the bone marrow core sections, as fixation and decalcification of the specimen can interfere with these stains. In addition, degranulated mast cells may loose their metachromatic staining properties. Bone marrow aspirate should be examined for morphologically abnormal mast cells with both a Wright-Giemsa and toluidine blue staining. To perform flow cytometry, bone marrow aspirates should recovered in EDTA or heparin. Cells should be processed within 24 hours. They may be kept at 4°C up to room temperature in EDTA. With heparinized samples, storage at 4°C is recommended. The minimum standard panel recommended includes CD2, CD25, CD45, and CD117 [3]. Mast cells from SM patients express, unlike normal and reactive mast cells, the surface markers CD2 and/or CD25. All suspected patients should undergo a mutational analysis of *KIT*, particularly for the presence of the D816V mutation. This analysis can be performed on bone marrow cells or cells from other tissues. However, bone marrow tissue yields the most sensitive results. Analysis of peripheral blood cells is the least sensitive, as the mutation generally becomes detectable in peripheral blood in advanced forms of disease with multilineage involvement. When appropriate tissues are analyzed, the D816V *KIT* mutation is identified in more than 90% of the SM patients. The D816V *KIT* mutational analysis of bone marrow aspirates is commercially available in the United States. If the D816V mutation cannot be detected, other rare *KIT* mutants can be present [3].

Table 9. REMA score to predict systemic mastocytosis and monoclonal mast cell activation syndrome in patients who present with systemic mast cell mediator release symptoms in the absence of urticaria pigmentosa

Variable	Score
Gender	
Male	+1
Female	-1
Clinical symptoms	
Absence of urticaria, pruritus and angioedema	+1
Urticaria, pruritus and/or angioedema	-1
Presyncope and/or syncope	+3
Baseline serum tryptase	
<15 μg/l	-1
>25 μg/l	+2

Highly sensitive diagnostic methods including multiparameter flow cytometry immunophenotyping and the *KIT* mutation analysis for mast cell identification to frequencies as low as $<10^{-4}$ to 10^{-5} bone marrow cells should be applied in suspected patients, especially those without the typical skin lesions of mastocytosis[13]. In patients with leukocytosis, eosinophilia, or both, examination for *BCR/ABL*, *JAK2* mutations and *FIP1L1-PDGFRA* fusion genes, as well as routine karyotyping, should be performed to detect certain subtypes of SM-AHNMD [73].

Table 10. Indications for performing bone marrow examinations in adult patients suspected to have systemic mastocytosis

Indication	Remarks
UP	Low SM risk if tryptase <5 μg/l (own observations)
No UP, baseline serum tryptase >10 μg/l, with: • normal MH and MIMA excretion • elevated MH and/or MIMA excretion	No bone marrow examinations unless high normal levels of tryptase, MH and/or MIMA in males and in case of insect venom anaphylaxis[32] or longstanding symptoms[13]
No UP, systemic symptoms of mast cell activation with REMA score ≥2	Can also be used to detect patients with MMAS

UP: urticaria pigmentosa;
SM: systemic mastocytosis;
MH: N tau-methylhistamine;
MIMA: N tau methylimidazoleacetic acid;
MMAS: monoclonal mast cell activation syndrome

Table 11. Diagnostic criteria for systemic mastocytosis

Major criterion
Multifocal, dense infiltrates of mast cells (≥15 mast cells in aggregates) detected in section of bone marrow and/or other extra-cutaneous organ(s)
Minor criteria
(1) In biopsy sections of bone marrow or other extra-cutaneous organs, >25% of the mast cells in the infiltrate are spindle-shaped or have atypical morphology or, of all mast cells in bone marrow aspirate smears, >25% are immature or atypical
(2) Detection of an activating point mutation at codon 816 of *KIT* in bone marrow, blood or another extra-cutaneous organ
(3) Mast cells in bone marrow, blood or other extracutaneous organs express CD2 and/or CD25 in addition to normal mast cell markers
(4) Serum total tryptase level persistently exceeds 20 μg/l (unless there is an associated clonal myeloid disorder, in which case this parameter is not valid)

According to the World Health Organization's (WHO) diagnostic criteria, the definitive diagnosis of SM requires either the presence of one major and one minor criterion or three out of four minor criteria (Table 11) [4]. Bone marrow biopsy showing >30% infiltration by mast cells (focal, dense aggregates) is a B-finding (Table 3) and suspect of SSM. In MCL, bone marrow biopsy shows a diffuse, usually compact infiltration by atypical, immature mast cells, and bone marrow aspirate smears show ≥20% mast cells.

c. Other Investigations

If the diagnosis of SM has been established further investigations are warranted (Table 12). They are needed to determine the subtype of SM and to detect osteopenia, osteoporosis and asymptomatic osteoporotic vertebral fractures in an early phase. Endoscopy in the absence of gastro-intestinal symptoms is not indicated.

Table 12. Further investigations if systemic mastocytosis has been diagnosed

Peripheral blood cell counts
Liver enzymes
LDH
Alkaline phosphatase
Abdominal ultrasonography (liver, spleen, lymph nodes)
Bone mineral density measurement of lumbar spine and hip
Vertebral fracture assessment or X-ray of the thoracolumbar spine

Treatment

a. Symptomatic Treatment

Except for cases with the more aggressive subtypes of mastocytosis, the primary objective of disease management is to inhibit the release of mast cell mediators and to block their effects in order to control the symptoms and signs of the disease. Treatment regimens are based on experiences in daily practise and not on randomized double blind placebo controlled trials.

Regarding skin lesions of mastocytosis triggering factors of local or generalised dermal mast cell activation should be avoided in the individual patient, if symptoms of mast cell activation are disturbing. The most common triggering factors are physical stimuli, such as changes of environmental temperature, extreme temperatures in bath/shower, swimming pool or air conditioning, dryness of skin, and rubbing. If symptoms remain disturbing notwithstanding the avoidance of triggering factors, histamine H1 receptor antagonists alone or combined with histamine H2 receptor antagonists and/or topical cromoglycate can be effective. Pruritus is preferably treated by histamine H1 receptor antagonists and in case of insufficient effect, combined with histamine H2 receptor antagonists and/or leukotriene receptor antagonists [3]. Cosmetically favorable effects can be achieved by sunbathing, ultraviolet irradiation or photochemotherapy by oral psoralen plus ultraviolet A irradiation. However, skin lesions usually recur after stopping this therapy and long-term use is associated with an increased risk of skin cancer.

Treatment of the sequels of an acute mast cell mediator release, such as anaphylaxis does not differ from that in patients without mastocytosis. Epinephrine is the primary treatment. Patients should have at least two doses of epinephrine in a self-injectable form available at all times for treatment of possible anaphylaxis, since a single dose may be inadequate to counteract the massive release of mediators that can occur in mastocytosis[3]. If avoidance of eliciting factor(s) (if known) fails or is impossible, maintenance anti-mediator treatment can be considered, thereby taking the frequency and severity of the acute attacks into account.

In most patients, maintenance anti-mediator therapy by the combination of histamine H1 and H2 receptor antagonists is effective to treat recurrent or chronic cardiovascular, gastro-intestinal and neurological symptoms. In some resistant cases, additional drug treatment is needed despite high doses of antihistamines: non-steroidal anti-inflammatory drugs (NSAIDs) in case of cardiovascular symptoms, proton pump inhibitors to treat peptic ulcer disease and oral cromoglycate in case of other gastro-intestinal symptoms. Leukotriene receptor antagonists can be considered in case of gastro-intestinal complaints, although experience with that type of drug treatment in mastocytosis is limited. In an acute exacerbation of symptoms short-term treatment glucocorticoids can give relief [3]. Cytoreductive agents are not recommended for treatment of mediator-related events.

Osteoporosis and low energy trauma (osteoporotic) fractures are indications for treatment with supplementation with calcium and vitamin D combined with oral or intravenous bisphosphonates. In a recently published study of SM patients, this therapeutic regimen resulted in a significant increase of the bone mineral density of the lumbar spine of 2% per year, which is slightly higher than that observed in patients treated for postmenopausal or corticosteroid-induced osteoporosis [35].

Table 13. Agents that should be avoided in patients with mastocytosis, unless exposure happened without mast cell activation after the beginning of the mastocytosis process

NSAIDs, aspirin
Opioids
Vancomycin
Radiocontrast agents
Certain muscle relaxants
Certain general anaesthetics

Series with other anti-osteoporotic regimens, as parathormone analogues, strontium ranelate and denosumab are not reported so far. We recommend an intake of 1200 mg of calcium (total of diet and supplement) and 20 μg (800 I.U.) of vitamin D daily, as is advised for patients with established osteoporosis [74]. Monitoring of the efficacy of vitamin D supplementation by measurement of serum/plasma 25 OH vitamin D (notably: 25 OH vitamin D = 25 OH vitamin D2 plus 25 OH vitamin D3) is advisable. The level of 75 nmol/l (30 μg/l) is suggested as the best point estimate for an optimal threshold for fracture prevention [75].

In patients with normal absorptive capacity, for every 2.5 μg (100 I.U.) of added vitamin D3, serum 25 OH vitamin D concentrations increase by approximately 1.75 to 2.5 nmol/l, with larger increments in patients with lower baseline 25 OH vitamin D levels[76].

Only in ASM and MCL, cytoreductive treatment is indicated. The most commonly administered therapies are interferon alpha 2b, interferon alpha 2b plus glucocorticoids, cladribine, glucocorticoids alone, the investigational tyrosine kinase inhibitors masitinib or midostaurin, and hydroxyurea [77].

b. Preventive Measures

Anaphylactic events can be life threatening in mastocytosis. Therefore, it is of utmost importance to find out the eliciting factor or combination of eliciting factors to avoid exposure to this factor again. Apart from avoidance of the known eliciting factor(s) in the individual patient with mastocytosis, it is standard to instruct all patients to avoid agents and situations that might precipitate a reaction. Theoretically, all substances that can induce histamine release from mast cells are potential elicitors. The most common agents that should be avoided are listed in Table 13. Despite the potential for problems with these medications listed, the majority of patients do tolerate these drugs. If (thoughtless) exposure happened after the beginning of the first symptoms or signs of mastocytosis without a systemic reaction, re-exposure is supposed to be safe. If use of a NSAID or opioid is needed we are used to offer the patient to test the tolerability by administrating the drug in the hospital under strict surveillance. Many agents used in anaesthesia can trigger mast cell degranulation. Therefore, patients with mastocytosis are high-risk patients when undergoing anaesthesia. For induction of general anaesthesia propofol, etomidate, ketamine (a fentanyl-type opioid), cis-atracurium or pancuronium are recommended. Anaesthesia can be maintained either by a total intravenous technique or with a volatile anaesthetic such as sevoflurane [78]. Premedication with antihistamines and a glucocorticoid is recommended for patients undergoing anaesthesia or administration of radiocontrast agents. The optimal regimen for prevention of mast cell degranulation in mastocytosis patients has not been formally studied. We suggest the scheme, as shown in Table 14.

Table 14. Premedication scheme (oral and intravenous administration) applicable to patients undergoing anaesthesia or administration of radiocontrast agents

Time	Drug	Dose
Oral administration		
- 17 hours	Prednisolone	30 mg
- 7 hours	Prednisolone Levocetirizine	30 mg 5 mg
- 2 hours	Prednisolone Levocetirizine	30 mg 5 mg
0	Procedure	
Intravenous administration		
- 17 hours	Prednisolone	30 mg
- 7 hours	Prednisolone Clemastine	30 mg 2 mg
- 1 hours	Prednisolone Clemastine	30 mg 2 mg
0	Procedure	

If severe attacks of mediator release appeared to be caused by sensitization to a certain allergen and re-exposure cannot be fully avoided with certainty, specific immunotherapy should be considered. So far, only data on immunotherapy with Hymenoptera venom are available. The risk/benefit ratio favors this immunotherapy, since patients with mastocytosis can suffer severe anaphylaxis in response to an insect sting, and fatalities have been reported in SM patients who were stung by Hymenoptera, despite self-treatment with epinephrine [15]. Series on a total of 138 patients were reported so far. The overall protection rate (sting challenge and field sting together) is about 70%, while the mean rate of side effects during treatment is about 25% [79, 80]. Both are less favorable compared to immunotherapy in the general population of patients with a history of Hymenoptera sting anaphylaxis. Sometimes, systemic side effects require epinephrine administration [79]. Patients should be counseled about these data when giving consents to receive immunotherapy. Most experts agree that the duration of the venom immunotherapy should be life-long [79, 81]. Immunotherapy should be performed according to the normal schedule with the same maintenance dose as in the non-mastocytosis population. Whether a higher maintenance dose (e.g. 200 μg instead of 100 μg), as suggested by some authors [82] induces a higher protection rate is unknown. Special precautions should be taken into account notably during the build up phase of the therapy. Immunotherapy should be performed in (semi-) intensive care conditions with intravenous device and continuous observation. Safety measures during administration of immunotherapy include starting with a less concentrated venom preparation (i.e., 0.01 to 0.1 micrograms/ml) and premedication with histamine H1 receptor antagonist on the day of each injection. There are case reports that in cases with recurrent severe side-effects premedication with omalizumab might be helpful [83].

SM patients run a high risk of osteoporosis and osteoporotic fractures. To protect the skeleton against bone loss as much as possible, supplementation with calcium and vitamin D should be considered early on in all SM patients. The optimal dose of calcium and vitamin D is uncertain. In SM patients who have not (yet) developed osteoporotic manifestations, we recommend 1200 mg of calcium (total of diet and supplement) and 20 μg (800 I.U.) of vitamin D daily[74], like advised for SM patients with osteoporotic manifestations. The Recommended Dietary Allowance of elemental calcium for postmenopausal women is 1200 mg daily. A recently published meta-analysis showed that supplementation with ≥20 μg vitamin D was somewhat favorable in the prevention of hip fracture and any non-vertebral fracture in persons 65 years of age or older [75]. Patients should exercise (prudently) for at least 30 minutes three times per week, as exercise has been associated with a reduced risk of hip fracture in older women [84]. Smoking cessation is strongly recommended because smoking cigarettes accelerates bone loss. Smoking one pack per day throughout adult life was associated with a 5 to 10% reduction in bone density [85]. Since osteoporotic manifestations (osteoporotic fractures and/or bone mineral density T-score <-2.5 SD) in ISM patients was found to be independently related to the histamine metabolite MH excretion [40], it might be possible that treatment with histamine receptor antagonists would be beneficial to prevent (further) bone loss.

c. Counselling, Diet and Life Style

As in many chronic diseases patients with mastocytosis may feel handicapped and suffer depression [47]. Usually this is most outspoken at the onset of the disease [86]. ISM patients may worry that they are suffering from a form of cancer or that their symptoms with time will steadily worsen. Notably, young woman with UP will seek cosmetic help. Moreover, having gone through anaphylaxis is a frightening experience. It is important that doctors treating mastocytosis patients understand and address these feelings. Many patients wonder if life style or keeping a diet will improve symptoms but in fact there is very little support for this idea [87]. When doctors fail to communicate well with chronically ill patients they may turn to alternative healers and self help medication which could clearly worsen the prognosis of SM patients. It is important to inform patients as early as possible and in understandable language about their diagnosis and prognosis [88].

Natural Course (Figure 5)

The prognosis of the skin lesions of mastocytosis is related to the age at presentation. It is excellent for children who have the onset of skin lesions within the first two years of life, because spontaneous resolution is common after several years (usually before the onset of puberty). Mastocytomas in children usually involute spontaneously after several years. UP in children resolve during adolescence in over 50% of patients, with fading or improvement of the lesions in most of the remaining patients [89, 90]. The children with remaining lesions may have persistent CM or may progress to SM. Skin lesions that develop after the age of two years or in adulthood tends to persist. Approximately 90% of adult patients with skin lesions have evidence of SM at the time of diagnosis, with the majority belonging to the category of ISM.

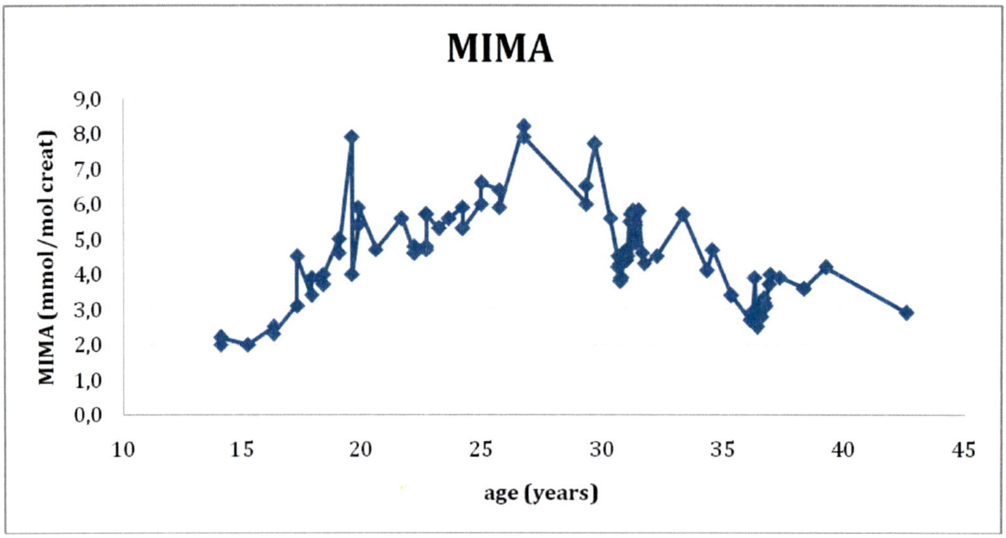

Figure 5. Natural course of indolent systemic mastocytosis as reflected by the urinary excretion of N tau-methylimidazoleacetic acid (MIMA), in a female patient with urticaria pigmentosa and indolent systemic mastocytosis from the age of 14 years. Upper normal level of MIMA excretion is 1.9 mmol/mol creatinine in urine.

Serum tryptase and urinary histamine metabolite levels progress slowly or not at all and can even substantially decline, especially in older patients [9], suggesting parallel changes in mast cell mass. A typical example of the natural course of ISM is depicted in Figure 5. Irrespective of the course of mast cell mass, mediator related symptoms may increase, remain constant, diminish or disappear over the years, as shown by case scenarios 1 and 3. The life-expectance of ISM patients is (near) normal [5, 7]. However, severe disability and death have been reported from anaphylactic episodes. Approximately 1 to 5% of patients with an initial diagnosis of ISM will progress to a more severe form of SM, including ASM, MCL or SM-AHNMD. Progression may occur within months to years from the initial diagnosis as demonstrated in a large prospective study of 145 consecutive patients with ISM, followed for a median of 9 years. In this study, increased serum levels of beta-2-microglobulin, combined with the presence of D816 *KIT* mutation in all hematopoietic cell lines, identified patients at higher risk for progression [7]. About 10% of the adult patients with ISM and UP may experience a regression of UP lesions [91]. Notwithstanding disappearance of skin lesions with normalization of serum tryptase levels ISM may persist, as recently was found in a case at our institute. The life-expectance of ASM and MCL is considerably shorter. The associated hematological disease determines the prognosis of SM-AHNMD. The prognosis of SSM patients is unknown, but probably not substantially worse than that of ISM patients as long as no transition to aggressive forms of SM or hematologic malignancies occurs [7].

Monoclonal Mast Cell Activation Syndrome

MMAS, also known as clonal systemic mast cell activation syndrome, has recently been recognized as a distinct mast cell disorder. MMAS differs from SM by the fact, that MMAS patients do not fulfill the diagnostic criteria of SM. MMAS patients have similar symptoms as SM patients, but do not have the typical skin lesions of mastocytosis. In patients with MMAS the *KIT* point mutations and the aberrant expression of the protein CD25 may be only detectable in a bone marrow sample enriched for mast cells rather than in unfractionated bone marrow samples, or when highly sensitive diagnostic assays (such as those based on mutation specific primers) are employed. It is unknown whether MMAS is an incipient phase in the development of ISM [72]. In patients with anaphylaxis SM is much more commonly diagnosed than MMAS [36, 69, 70].

Clinical Cases

Case 1. Mr. N.

Mr. N. was first seen in our department at the age of 51 years. He was referred from a hospital elsewhere because of attacks of flushing with itching hands and feet and dyspnoea. Several times a low blood pressure had been documented during these attacks. At one occasion he developed a coma and was admitted to an emergency department where he had to be reanimated because of an asystole. Subsequently, an ICD was implanted, since a primary heart disease was considered. Later the ICD had to be removed because of a myocardial perforation.

His symptoms had started about 20 years earlier and had steadily increased in severity and frequency. Originally, he only suffered from attacks of flushing, a sense of blocked nose, itching hand palms and palpitations. Sometimes the attacks were also accompanied by diarrhea. He felt tired and run down. Skin inspection revealed no lesions, suggestive of UP. Since the symptoms of flushing, itch, tachycardia and hypotension were suggestive of histamine overproduction a urine sample was tested for MH and MIMA. Both values were elevated and subsequently, a bone marrow biopsy was performed in a hospital elsewhere showing a slight increase in elongated mast cells, but no 'mast cell infiltrates' of >15 mast cells. However, revision of the biopsy at our institute showed at least 2 'mast cell aggregates' of >15 mast cells and an atypical morphology of >25% of the mast cells, retrospectively confirming the diagnosis of ISM based on the major and one minor criterion according to the WHO definition. At that moment detection of the D816V *KIT* mutation was not yet possible. Serum tryptase level appeared to be elevated with a value of 44 μg/l. There was no evidence of osteoporosis or enlargement of liver, spleen or lymph nodes. The patient was advised to use maintenance treatment with histamine H 1 and H 2 receptor blocking drugs and epinephrine for self-administration.

In the following years the attacks became less frequent but nevertheless he had to use his auto-injector on several occasions with good results. After a follow up period of 13 years he could stop the antihistaminic medication without recurrence of flushing or hypotensive attacks. The levels of serum tryptase and histamine metabolites were more or less stable over the years.

This case illustrates that the diagnosis of mastocytosis is still often overlooked which can have fatal results. The characteristic history combined with elevated levels of serum tryptase and/or urinary histamine metabolites found both during and outside the attacks is suggestive of ISM. A bone marrow biopsy with adequate staining and immunohistochemistry nowadays facilitates the diagnosis. It is interesting to note that attacks of flushing, tachycardia and hypotension may be transient without evident decrease of mast cell load parameters.

Case 2. Mrs. H.

Mrs. H., a 50-year old patient, was referred to our department because of UP. She had discovered red-brownish marks on her skin about 15 years earlier. Her skin lesions had been asymptomatic. Only after showering the skin was sometimes red. She did not suffer from flushing, tachycardia or hypotensive attacks. In the past she had collapsed several times, but these attacks were probably vasovagal reactions as they always occurred in relation to experienced pain or fear. She had no history of gastro-intestinal complaints, allergy, or bone fractures. She had been stung by a wasp in the past without developing any systemic symptoms. Upon inspection she showed multiple brown-reddish maculae three to five millimetres in diameter on the upper half of the body, but the Darrier sign was negative. Serum level of tryptase was 52 μg/l. Urinary level of MH was 124 umol/mol creatinine (normal value <176 μmol/mol creatinine) and that of MIMA was 2.6 mmol/creatinine (normal value <2.0 mmol/mol creatinine). Bone marrow examination showed a normal hematopoiesis and at least 2 'mast cell aggregates' of >15 mast cells and an atypical morphology of >25% of the mast cells, confirming the diagnosis of ISM based on the major and one minor criterion according to the WHO definition. In the bone marrow aspirate, the D816V mutation of *KIT* was detectable and mast cells expressed CD25. Ultrasound examination of the upper abdomen showed an enlarged caudal part of the liver, a normal spleen and no enlarged lymph nodes. There was no evidence of osteoporosis.

In the 8 years follow up period she developed some minor attacks of flushing, and liver ultrasound examinations showed no increase in liver size. Serum tryptase levels remained constant around 50 to 60 μg/l. She used no antihistamines and was not given an epinephrine auto-injector as she never suffered from anaphylaxis or other severe systemic symptoms. In the summer of 2012, she was stung by a wasp. Only a large local reaction developed. Eight weeks later she was stung again. Within 2 minutes she felt light-headedness, developed difficulty with breathing and collapsed within 4 minutes. Within 7 minutes an ambulance arrived and she was treated with epinephrine (several injections first subcutaneously, later on intravenously), fluid infusion, antihistamines and corticosteroids intravenously, but she remained deeply hypotensive. Initial intubation proved difficult because of swelling of the tongue, but succeeded after 15 minutes. Notwithstanding massive amounts of epinephrine and full reanimation she did not regain consciousness. Four days later an infaust neurological outcome was diagnosed and the treatment was stopped.

In retrospect serum was determined from three years earlier showing no sensitization to wasp venom. Serum from the day she was stung showed a low level IgE against wasp venom (0.51 KU/l; normal value <0.35 KU/l). However, IgE against recombinant wasp venom Ves-v-5 showed 2.31 KU/l. Two days later this value had increased to 4.77 KU/l.

This tragic case shows that a patient initially diagnosed as UP was suffering from ISM although she had during many years only minimal symptoms. Wasp stings in the past did not cause any systemic anaphylaxis, but only after having received two wasp stings within a relatively short period she developed a therapy-resistant anaphylactic shock and died. This reaction could have been labelled as a non-allergic anaphylaxis due to the very low levels of IgE to wasp venom in a routine assay. However, determination of IgE against one of the recombinant wasp venom antigens showed clear-cut sensitization. This case also suggests that all mastocytosis patients should be prescribed epinephrine auto-injectors even if they have tolerated wasp stings in the past. The question remains however whether prompt self-administration of epinephrine would have saved this patient's life.

Case 3. Mr. H

Mr. H, 44 years old hobby sportsman developed low back pain during a simple trampoline exercise. X-ray examinations showed a vertebral compression fracture of T12. He reported that he had difficulty to regain his former condition after this event. He also indicated that lately his defecation pattern had changed, with now frequent diarrhea. Hot showers and sunbaths cause itching and red marks on his skin. He felt depressed and tired. His body weight had increased to 98 kg with a length of 184 cm (used to be 186.5 cm). The skin showed subtle lesions, which were dubiously suspect for UP. Laboratory evaluation showed normal values for hemoglobin and blood cell counts, normal electrolytes, kidney and liver tests, and normal values of serum calcium, phosphate, PTH, TSH and testosterone. There was no evidence of malabsorption or coeliac disease. A normal value for cortisol excretion, but a strongly elevated MH level (374 μmol/mol creatinine, normal value <176 μmol/mol creatinine) and MIMA level (5 mmol/mol creatinine, normal value <2.0 mmol/mol creatinine) in urine were found. Serum tryptase in this patient was slightly elevated with values around 25 μg/l. Bone mineral density showed low values for radius (Z-score -3.6 SD, T-score -4.0 SD), lumbar spine (Z-score -4.1 SD, T-score -4.4 SD) and proximal femur (Z-score -1.1 SD, T-score -1.4 SD). A skin biopsy of a red macula on the chest showed no abnormalities. Bone marrow biopsy showed normal hematopoietic cell lines but multiple infiltrates of abnormal mast cells and eosinophilic granulocytes. The bone structure showed evident osteoporosis. ISM was diagnosed and the patient was prescribed the bisphosphonate Risedronate and supplementation of calcium and vitamin D. Later histamine H 1 and H 2 receptor blockers were added because of persistent itch. However, the effect was incomplete. For this reason a controlled introduction of acetylsalicylic acid was performed. The patient responded well to this treatment and felt also much less tired. Two years later he experienced a high-energy trauma in a car accident, which resulted in a vertebral fracture of T6. During his stay in hospital he was treated with opioids without any evidence of increased mast cell degranulation. After 5 years of treatment Risedronate was briefly changed to the PTH analogue Teriparatide, and later changed back again to Risedronate. The patient was stung several times by a wasp without any complications and without developing IgE to wasp venom.

The follow up of bone mineral density 8 years after the initial diagnosis showed more or less constant bone mineral density values for radius (Z-score of -2.5 SD, T-score -3.1 SD), lumbar spine (Z-score -3.1 SD, T-score -3.6 SD) and for proximal femur (Z-score -1.1 SD, T-score -1.5 SD). He had no further fractures. The symptoms of flushing, the abdominal complaints and the extreme tiredness disappeared and remained absent after discontinuation of antihistamines and acetylsalicylic acid. When last seen he was doing well, his body length was 183 cm. The levels of serum tryptase and urinary histamine metabolites were more or less stable over the years.

This case shows that osteoporosis in a young male should rise suspicion of SM, even if there are no or minimal skin lesions or signs of mast cell activation. This case also illustrates that adequate treatment may halt the progress of osteoporosis in these patients and again that symptoms of mast cell activation may spontaneously subside with time without a decrease in mast cell load parameters.

None of the 3 cases showed progression to a smoldering or aggressive form of SM; anaphylaxis and osteoporosis being the major threat to these patients. Moreover although all three patients demonstrated here suffered from ISM, their clinical picture and laboratory parameters varied markedly, illustrating the broad spectrum of the disease.

Conclusion

Anaphylaxis can be the presenting symptom of mastocytosis, which is a disease characterised by a clonal proliferation of abnormally functioning mast cells. Detection of this disease is important since about half of the patients develop osteoporosis and/or osteoporotic fractures. Moreover, patients should be identified in order to advise them on how to deal with the risk of life threatening anaphylaxis.

Clinical Pearls

- Mastocytosis is characterised by a clonal proliferation of abnormal mast cells, which accumulate in bone marrow, liver, spleen, lymphoid tissue and gastro-intestinal tract (systemic mastocytosis; SM), and/or (only) in the skin (cutaneous mastocytosis).
- In about 4% of adult patients presenting with Hymenoptera sting anaphylaxis, mastocytosis is the underlying disease.
- About half of the patients with SM develop osteoporosis and/or osteoporotic fractures.

- All patients presenting with anaphylaxis should be screened for mastocytosis by skin inspection and determination of serum tryptase level. In case of dubious results determination of urinary histamine metabolites may be helpful.
- Bone marrow investigations to establish the diagnosis of SM should include histological examination with immunohistochemical staining (CD117, tryptase, CD25), bone marrow smear, flow cytometry (CD2, CD25) and D816V *KIT* mutation analysis.
- All SM patients with a history of Hymenoptera sting anaphylaxis should be offered venom immunotherapy (life-long so far)
- Even SM patients without a history of anaphylaxis should be counseled on the use of an auto-injector with epinephrine in case of an impending anaphylaxis.
- In all patients with SM calcium and vitamin D supplementation should be considered to protect the skeleton.
- Mast cell mass in indolent SM does not progress in all cases, but can even decline. Irrespective of the course of mast cell mass, mediator related symptoms may increase, remain constant, diminish or disappear over the years.
- Compared to indolent SM, the so-called monoclonal mast cell activation syndrome and other, more aggressive forms of SM occur far less frequently.

References

[1] Valent, P; Akin, C; Arock, M; Brockow, K; Butterfield, JH; Carter, MC; et al. Definitions, criteria and global classification of mast cell disorders with special reference to mast cell activation syndromes: a consensus proposal. *Int Arch Allergy Immunol*, 2012, 157, 215-225.

[2] Bonadonna, P; Zanotti, R; Caruso, B; Castellani, L; Perbellini, O; Colarossi, S; et al. Allergen specific immunotherapy is safe and effective in patients with systemic mastocytosis and Hymenoptera allergy. *J Allergy Clin Immunol*, 2008, 121, 256-257.

[3] Valent, P; Akin, C; Escribano, L; Fodinger, M; Hartmann, K; Brockow, K; et al. Standards and standardization in mastocytosis: consensus statements on diagnostics, treatment recommendations and response criteria. *Eur J Clin Invest*, 2007, 37, 435-453.

[4] Horny, HP; Metcalfe, DD; Bennet, JM; Escribano, L; Bennett, JM; Valent, P; et al. Mastocytosis. In: Swerdlow SH; Campo E; Harris NL (eds), *WHO classification of tumours of haematopoietic and lymphoid tissues, 4th ed.* Lyon, France: IARC, 2008.

[5] Lim, KH; Tefferi, A; Lasho, TL; Finke, C; Patnaik, M; Butterfield, JH; et al. Systemic mastocytosis in 342 consecutive adults: survival studies and prognostic factors. *Blood*, 2009, 113, 5727-5736.

[6] Pardanani, A; Lim, KH; Lasho, TL; Finke, CM; McClure, RF; Li, CY; et al. WHO subvariants of indolent mastocytosis: clinical details and prognostic evaluation in 159 consecutive adults. *Blood*, 2010, 115, 150-151.

[7] Escribano, L; Alvarez-Twose, I; Sanchez-Munoz, L; Garcia-Montero, A; Nunez, R; Almeida, J; et al. Prognosis in adult indolent systemic mastocytosis: a long-term study of the Spanish Network on Mastocytosis in a series of 145 patients. *J Allergy Clin Immunol*, 2009, 124, 514-521.

[8] Castells, M; Metcalfe, DD; Escribano, L. Diagnosis and treatment of cutaneous mastocytosis in children: practical recommendations. *Am J Clin Dermatol*, 2011, 12, 259-270.

[9] Kors, JW; Van Doormaal, JJ; Breukelman, H; Van Voorst Vader, PC; De Monchy, JG. Long-term follow-up of indolent mastocytosis in adults. *J Intern Med*, 1996, 239, 157-164.

[10] Rosbotham, JL; Malik, NM; Syrris, P; Jeffery, S; Bedlow, A; Gharraie, S; et al. Lack of c-kit mutation in familial urticaria pigmentosa. *Br J Dermatol*, 1999, 140, 849-852.

[11] van Doormaal, JJ; Arends, S; Brunekreeft, KL; van der Wal, VB; Sietsma, J; van Voorst Vader, PC; et al. Prevalence of indolent systemic mastocytosis in a Dutch region. *J Allergy Clin Immunol*, in press.

[12] Haenisch, B; Nothen, MM; Molderings, GJ. Systemic mast cell activation disease: the role of molecular genetic alterations in pathogenesis, heritability and diagnostics. *Immunology*, 2012, 137, 197-205.

[13] Alvarez-Twose, I; Matito, A; Sanchez-Munoz, L; Morgado, JM; Orfao, A; Escribano, L; et al. Contribution of highly sensitive diagnostic methods to the diagnosis of systemic mastocytosis in the absence of skin lesions. *Allergy*, 2012, 67, 1190-1191.

[14] Wimazal, F; Geissler, P; Shnawa, P; Sperr, WR; Valent, P. Severe life-threatening or disabling anaphylaxis in patients with systemic mastocytosis: a single-center experience. *Int Arch Allergy Immunol*, 2012, 157, 399-405.

[15] Oude Elberink, JN; de Monchy, JG; Kors, JW; van Doormaal, JJ; Dubois, AE. Fatal anaphylaxis after a yellow jacket sting, despite venom immunotherapy, in two patients with mastocytosis. *J Allergy Clin Immunol*, 1997, 99, 153-154.

[16] Pumphrey, RS. Lessons for management of anaphylaxis from a study of fatal reactions. *Clin Exp Allergy*, 2000, 30, 1144-1150.

[17] Wehner, F; Wehner, HD; Fritz, P; Benz, D; Schulz, MM. Sudden death in the presence of systemic mastocytosis and urticaria pigmentosa. *Arch Kriminol*, 2008, 222, 187-194.

[18] Vaughan, ST; Jones, GN. Systemic mastocytosis presenting as profound cardiovascular collapse during anaesthesia. *Anaesthesia*, 1998, 53, 804-807.

[19] Murphy, M; Walsh, D; Drumm, B; Watson, R. Bullous mastocytosis: a fatal outcome. *Pediatr Dermatol*, 1999, 16, 452-455.

[20] Brockow, K; Jofer, C; Behrendt, H; Ring, J. Anaphylaxis in patients with mastocytosis: a study on history, clinical features and risk factors in 120 patients. *Allergy*, 2008, 63, 226-232.

[21] Gonzalez de Olano, D; de la Hoz Caballer, B; Nunez Lopez, R; Sanchez Munoz, L; Cuevas Agustin, M; Dieguez, MC; et al. Prevalence of allergy and anaphylactic symptoms in 210 adult and pediatric patients with mastocytosis in Spain: a study of the Spanish network on mastocytosis (REMA). *Clin Exp Allergy*, 2007, 37, 1547-1555.

[22] Muller, U; Helbling, A; Hunziker, T; Wuthrich, B; Pecoud, A; Gilardi, S; et al. Mastocytosis and atopy: a study of 33 patients with urticaria pigmentosa. *Allergy*, 1990, 45, 597-603.

[23] Ruëff, F; Placzek, M; Przybilla, B. Mastocytosis and Hymenoptera venom allergy. *Curr Opin Allergy Clin Immunol*, 2006, 6, 284-288.

[24] Gonzalez-de-Olano, D; Alvarez-Twose, I; Morgado, JM; Esteban Lopez, MI; Vega Castro, A; Diaz de Durana, MD; et al. Evaluation of basophil activation in mastocytosis with Hymenoptera venom anaphylaxis. *Cytometry B Clin Cytom*, 2011, 80, 167-175.

[25] Bonadonna, P; Zanotti, R; Melioli, G; Antonini, F; Romano, I; Lenzi, L; et al. The role of basophil activation test in special populations with mastocytosis and reactions to hymenoptera sting. *Allergy*, 2012, 67, 962-965.

[26] Alvarez-Twose, I; Vano-Galvan, S; Sanchez-Munoz, L; Morgado, JM; Matito, A; Torrelo, A; et al. Increased serum baseline tryptase levels and extensive skin involvement are predictors for the severity of mast cell activation episodes in children with mastocytosis. *Allergy*, 2012, 67, 813-821.

[27] Ludolph-Hauser, D; Rueff, F; Fries, C; Schopf, P; Przybilla, B. Constitutively raised serum concentrations of mast-cell tryptase and severe anaphylactic reactions to Hymenoptera stings. *Lancet*, 2001, 357, 361-362.

[28] Rueff, F; Przybilla, B; Bilo, MB; Muller, U; Scheipl, F; Aberer, W; et al. Predictors of severe systemic anaphylactic reactions in patients with Hymenoptera venom allergy: importance of baseline serum tryptase-a study of the European Academy of Allergology and Clinical Immunology Interest Group on Insect Venom Hypersensitivity. *J Allergy Clin Immunol*, 2009, 124, 1047-1054.

[29] Guenova, E; Volz, T; Eichner, M; Hoetzenecker, W; Caroli, U; Griesinger, G; et al. Basal serum tryptase as risk assessment for severe Hymenoptera sting reactions in elderly. *Allergy*, 2010, 65, 919-923.

[30] Stoevesandt, J; Hain, J; Kerstan, A; Trautmann, A. Over- and underestimated parameters in severe Hymenoptera venom-induced anaphylaxis: cardiovascular medication and absence of urticaria/angioedema. *J Allergy Clin Immunol*, 2012, 130, 698-704.

[31] van Anrooij, B; van der Veer, E; de Monchy, JGR; van der Heide, S; Kluin-Nelemans, JC; van Voorst Vader, PC; et al. Higher mast cell load lowers risk of Hymenoptera venom anaphylaxis in mastocytosis. *J Allergy Clin Immunol*, in press.

[32] van Doormaal, JJ; van der Veer, E; van Voorst Vader, PC; Kluin, PM; Mulder, AB; van der Heide, S; et al. Tryptase and histamine metabolites as diagnostic indicators of indolent systemic mastocytosis without skin lesions. *Allergy*, 2012, 67, 683-690.

[33] Rossini, M; Zanotti, R; Bonadonna, P; Artuso, A; Caruso, B; Schena, D; et al. Bone mineral density, bone turnover markers and fractures in patients with indolent systemic mastocytosis. *Bone*, 2011, 49, 880-885.

[34] Florian, S; Krauth, MT; Simonitsch-Klupp, I; Sperr, WR; Fritsche-Polanz, R; Sonneck, K; et al. Indolent systemic mastocytosis with elevated serum tryptase, absence of skin lesions, and recurrent severe anaphylactoid episodes. *Int Arch Allergy Immunol*, 2005, 136, 273-280.

[35] Barete, S; Assous, N; de Gennes, C; Grandpeix, C; Feger, F; Palmerini, F; et al. Systemic mastocytosis and bone involvement in a cohort of 75 patients. *Ann Rheum Dis*, 2010, 69, 1838-1841.

[36] Bonadonna, P; Perbellini, O; Passalacqua, G; Caruso, B; Colarossi, S; Dal Fior, D; et al. Clonal mast cell disorders in patients with systemic reactions to Hymenoptera stings and increased serum tryptase levels. *J Allergy Clin Immunol*, 2009, 123, 680-686.

[37] Dubois, AE. Mastocytosis and Hymenoptera allergy. *Curr Opin Allergy Clin Immunol*, 2004, 4, 291-295.

[38] Luiting, J; Rouwendal, I; van Doormaal, J; Niedoszytko, M; de Monchy, J; Kluin-Nelemans, H; et al. The epidemiology and natural history of insect venom allergy in

patients with indolent systemic mastocytosis not treated with VIT. *Allergy*, 2010, 65 (Suppl. 92):99.

[39] Muller, UR. Hymenoptera venom hypersensitivity: an update. *Clin Exp Allergy*, 1998, 28, 4-6.

[40] van der Veer, E; van der Goot, W; de Monchy, JG; Kluin-Nelemans, HC; van Doormaal, JJ. High prevalence of fractures and osteoporosis in patients with indolent systemic mastocytosis. *Allergy*, 2012, 67, 431-438.

[41] Chiappetta, N; Gruber, B. The role of mast cells in osteoporosis. *Semin Arthritis Rheum*, 2006, 36, 32-36.

[42] Rajgopal, R; Bear, M; Butcher, MK; Shaughnessy, SG. The effects of heparin and low molecular weight heparins on bone. *Thromb Res*, 2008, 122, 293-298.

[43] Theoharides, TC; Alysandratos, KD; Angelidou, A; Delivanis, DA; Sismanopoulos, N; Zhang, B; et al. Mast cells and inflammation. *Biochim Biophys Acta*, 2012, 1822, 21-33.

[44] Theoharides, TC; Boucher, W; Spear, K. Serum interleukin-6 reflects disease severity and osteoporosis in mastocytosis patients. *Int Arch Allergy Immunol*, 2002, 128, 344-350.

[45] Brockow, K; Akin, C; Huber, M; Metcalfe, DD. IL-6 levels predict disease variant and extent of organ involvement in patients with mastocytosis. *Clin Immunol*, 2005, 115, 216-223.

[46] Moura, DS; Sultan, S; Georgin-Lavialle, S; Barete, S; Lortholary, O; Gaillard, R; et al. Evidence for cognitive impairment in mastocytosis: prevalence, features and correlations to depression. *PLoS One*, 2012, 7, e39468.

[47] Moura, DS; Sultan, S; Georgin-Lavialle, S; Pillet, N; Montestruc, F; Gineste, P; et al. Depression in patients with mastocytosis: prevalence, features and effects of masitinib therapy. *PLoS One*, 2011, 6, e26375.

[48] Hollmann, TJ; Brenn, T; Hornick, JL. CD25 expression on cutaneous mast cells from adult patients presenting with urticaria pigmentosa is predictive of systemic mastocytosis. *Am J Surg Pathol*, 2008, 32, 139-145.

[49] Schwartz, LB. Diagnostic value of tryptase in anaphylaxis and mastocytosis. *Immunol Allergy Clin North Am*, 2006, 26, 451-463.

[50] Gonzalez-Quintela, A; Vizcaino, L; Gude, F; Rey, J; Meijide, L; Fernandez-Merino, C; et al. Factors influencing serum total tryptase concentrations in a general adult population. *Clin Chem Lab Med*, 2010, 48, 701-706.

[51] Fenger, RV; Linneberg, A; Vidal, C; Vizcaino, L; Husemoen, LL; Aadahl, M; et al. Determinants of serum tryptase in a general population: the relationship of serum tryptase to obesity and asthma. *Int Arch Allergy Immunol*, 2012, 157, 151-158.

[52] Schliemann, S; Seyfarth, F; Hipler, UC; Elsner, P. Impact of age and heterophilic interference on the Basal serum tryptase, a risk indication for anaphylaxis, in 1, 092 dermatology patients. *Acta Derm Venereol*, 2012, 92, 484-489.

[53] Sirvent, AE; Gonzalez, C; Enriquez, R; Fernandez, J; Millan, I; Barber, X; et al. Serum tryptase levels and markers of renal dysfunction in a population with chronic kidney disease. *J Nephrol*, 2010, 23, 282-290.

[54] Keyzer, JJ; de Monchy, JG; van Doormaal, JJ; van Voorst Vader, PC. Improved diagnosis of mastocytosis by measurement of urinary histamine metabolites. *N Engl J Med*, 1983, 309, 1603-1605.

[55] Granerus, G; Olafsson, JH; Roupe, G. Studies on histamine metabolism in mastocytosis. *J Invest Dermatol*, 1983, 80, 410-416.

[56] Keyzer, JJ; Wolthers, BG; Muskiet, FA; Kauffman, HF; Groen, A. Determination of N tau-methylhistamine in plasma and urine by isotope dilution mass fragmentography. *Clin Chim Acta*, 1981, 113, 165-173.

[57] Keyzer, JJ; Wolthers, BG; Breukelman, H; van der Slik, W. Determination of N tau-methylhistamine in urine by gas chromatography using nitrogen-phosphorus detection. *J Chromatogr*, 1983, 275, 261-269.

[58] Oosting, E; Keyzer, JJ. Measurement of urinary N tau-methylhistamine excretion: correlation of a newly developed radioimmunoassay (RIA) with gas chromatography mass spectrometry (GCMS). *Agents Actions*, 1991, 33, 215-217.

[59] Keyzer, JJ; Wolthers, BG; Breukelman, H; Kauffman, HF; de Monchy, JG. Determination of N tau-methylimidazoleacetic acid (a histamine metabolite) in urine by gas chromatography using nitrogen-phosphorus detection. *Clin Chim Acta*, 1982, 121, 379-387.

[60] Keyzer, JJ; Breukelman, H; Wolthers, BG; van den Heuvel, M; Kromme, N; Berg, WC. Urinary excretion of histamine and some of its metabolites in man: influence of the diet. *Agents Actions*, 1984, 15, 189-194.

[61] Maintz, L; Novak, N. Histamine and histamine intolerance. *Am J Clin Nutr*, 2007, 85, 1185-1196.

[62] Garcia-Martin, E; Ayuso, P; Martinez, C; Blanca, M; Agundez, JA. Histamine pharmacogenomics. *Pharmacogenomics*, 2009, 10, 867-883.

[63] Chrostek, L; Cylwik, B; Szmitkowski, M. Interactions between ethanol and histamine. *Pol Merkur Lekarski*, 2007, 23, 225-230.

[64] Zimatkin, SM; Anichtchik, OV. Alcohol-histamine interactions. *Alcohol Alcohol*, 1999, 34, 141-147.

[65] Maintz, L; Schwarzer, V; Bieber, T; van der Ven, K; Novak, N. Effects of histamine and diamine oxidase activities on pregnancy: a critical review. *Hum Reprod Update*, 2008, 14, 485-495.

[66] Oosting, E; Keyzer, JJ; Wolthers, BG. Correlation between urinary levels of histamine metabolites in 24-hour urine and morning urine samples of man: influence of histamine-rich food. *Agents Actions*, 1989, 27, 205-207.

[67] Granerus, G; Lonnqvist, B; Nystrand, J; Roupe, G. Serum tryptase measured with B12 and G5 antibody-based immunoassays in mastocytosis patients and its relation to histamine turnover. *Br J Dermatol*, 1998, 139, 858-861.

[68] Akin, C; Metcalfe, DD. Surrogate markers of disease in mastocytosis. *Int Arch Allergy Immunol*, 2002, 127, 133-136.

[69] Alvarez-Twose, I; Gonzalez de Olano, D; Sanchez-Munoz, L; Matito, A; Esteban-Lopez, MI; Vega, A; et al. Clinical, biological, and molecular characteristics of clonal mast cell disorders presenting with systemic mast cell activation symptoms. *J Allergy Clin Immunol*, 2010, 125, 1269-1278.

[70] Alvarez-Twose, I; Gonzalez-de-Olano, D; Sanchez-Munoz, L; Matito, A; Jara-Acevedo, M; Teodosio, C; et al. Validation of the REMA score for predicting mast cell clonality and systemic mastocytosis in patients with systemic mast cell activation symptoms. *Int Arch Allergy Immunol*, 2012, 157, 275-280.

[71] Heide, R; Beishuizen, A; De Groot, H; Den Hollander, JC; Van Doormaal, JJ; De Monchy, JG; et al. Mastocytosis in children: a protocol for management. *Pediatr Dermatol*, 2008, 25, 493-500.

[72] Horny, HP; Sotlar, K; Valent, P. Evaluation of mast cell activation syndromes: impact of pathology and immunohistology. *Int Arch Allergy Immunol*, 2012, 159, 1-5.

[73] Valent, P; Sperr, WR; Schwartz, LB; Horny, HP. Diagnosis and classification of mast cell proliferative disorders: delineation from immunologic diseases and non-mast cell hematopoietic neoplasms. *J Allergy Clin Immunol*, 2004, 114, 3-11.

[74] Verbrugge, FH; Gielen, E; Milisen, K; Boonen, S. Who should receive calcium and vitamin D supplementation? *Age Ageing*, 2012, 41, 576-580.

[75] Bischoff-Ferrari, HA; Willett, WC; Orav, EJ; Lips, P; Meunier, PJ; Lyons, RA; et al. A pooled analysis of vitamin D dose requirements for fracture prevention. *N Engl J Med*, 2012, 367, 40-49.

[76] Heaney, RP; Davies, KM; Chen, TC; Holick, MF; Barger-Lux, MJ. Human serum 25-hydroxycholecalciferol response to extended oral dosing with cholecalciferol. *Am J Clin Nutr*, 2003, 77, 204-210.

[77] Lim, KH; Pardanani, A; Butterfield, JH; Li, CY; Tefferi, A. Cytoreductive therapy in 108 adults with systemic mastocytosis: Outcome analysis and response prediction during treatment with interferon-alpha, hydroxyurea, imatinib mesylate or 2-chlorodeoxyadenosine. *Am J Hematol*, 2009, 84, 790-794.

[78] Konrad, FM; Unertl, KE; Schroeder, TH. Mastocytosis. A challenge in anaesthesiology. *Anaesthesist*, 2009, 58, 1239-1243.

[79] Niedoszytko, M; de Monchy, J; van Doormaal, JJ; Jassem, E; Oude Elberink, JN. Mastocytosis and insect venom allergy: diagnosis, safety and efficacy of venom immunotherapy. *Allergy*, 2009, 64, 1237-1245.

[80] Gonzalez de Olano, D; Alvarez-Twose, I; Esteban-Lopez, MI; Sanchez-Munoz, L; de Durana, MD; Vega, A; et al. Safety and effectiveness of immunotherapy in patients with indolent systemic mastocytosis presenting with Hymenoptera venom anaphylaxis. *J Allergy Clin Immunol*, 2008, 121, 519-526.

[81] Gonzalez-de-Olano, D; Alvarez-Twose, I; Vega, A; Orfao, A; Escribano, L. Venom immunotherapy in patients with mastocytosis and hymenoptera venom anaphylaxis. *Immunotherapy*, 2011, 3, 637-651.

[82] Rueff, F; Wenderoth, A; Przybilla, B. Patients still reacting to a sting challenge while receiving conventional Hymenoptera venom immunotherapy are protected by increased venom doses. *J Allergy Clin Immunol*, 2001, 108, 1027-1032.

[83] Bonadonna, P; Zanotti, R; Muller, U. Mastocytosis and insect venom allergy. *Curr Opin Allergy Clin Immunol*, 2010, 10, 347-353.

[84] Feskanich, D; Willett, W; Colditz, G. Walking and leisure-time activity and risk of hip fracture in postmenopausal women. *JAMA*, 2002, 288, 2300-2306.

[85] Hopper, JL; Seeman, E. The bone density of female twins discordant for tobacco use. *N Engl J Med*, 1994, 330, 387-392.

[86] Cassileth, BR; Lusk, EJ; Strouse, TB; Miller, DS; Brown, LL; Cross, PA; et al. Psychosocial status in chronic illness. A comparative analysis of six diagnostic groups. *N Engl J Med*, 1984, 311, 506-511.

[87] Vlieg-Boerstra, BJ; van der Heide, S; Oude Elberink, JN; Kluin-Nelemans, JC; Dubois, AE. Mastocytosis and adverse reactions to biogenic amines and histamine-releasing foods: what is the evidence? *Neth J Med*, 2005, 63, 244-249.

[88] Huyard, C. What, if anything, is specific about having a rare disorder? Patients' judgements on being ill and being rare. *Health Expect*, 2009, 12, 361-370.

[89] Kiszewski, AE; Duran-Mckinster, C; Orozco-Covarrubias, L; Gutierrez-Castrellon, P; Ruiz-Maldonado, R. Cutaneous mastocytosis in children: a clinical analysis of 71 cases. *J Eur Acad Dermatol Venereol*, 2004, 18, 285-290.

[90] Ben-Amitai, D; Metzker, A; Cohen, HA. Pediatric cutaneous mastocytosis: a review of 180 patients. *Isr Med Assoc J*, 2005, 7, 320-322.

[91] Brockow, K; Scott, LM; Worobec, AS; Kirshenbaum, A; Akin, C; Huber, MM; et al. Regression of urticaria pigmentosa in adult patients with systemic mastocytosis: correlation with clinical patterns of disease. *Arch Dermatol*, 2002, 138, 785-790.

Index

#

9alpha, 11beta-PGF2, 53

A

abuse, 36
access, 9, 69, 73, 74, 76, 126, 170, 199, 240
acetaminophen, 156, 165, 171, 173, 174
acetic acid, 37, 41, 164, 166, 228
acetylcholine, 140
acid, 3, 37, 52, 64, 88, 126, 164, 165, 166, 175, 182, 184, 185, 232, 264, 273, 277, 279, 285, 288, 293
acne, 239
Aculeatae, 182, 197
acute asthma, 30, 74, 121, 170, 232, 238
acute infection, 4, 77
acute myeloid leukemia, 267
additives, 92, 230
adduction, 38, 242, 245
adjunctive therapy, 97
adolescents, 12, 20, 26, 38, 42, 46, 67, 79, 87, 98, 108, 109, 112, 113, 174, 190, 220, 238, 247
adrenaline, 8, 30, 33, 34, 35, 38, 41, 60, 61, 71, 156, 203, 223
adulthood, 284
adults, 1, 7, 12, 16, 17, 20, 22, 24, 31, 34, 43, 73, 74, 76, 78, 86, 87, 88, 90, 96, 107, 111, 119, 120, 137, 145, 152, 173, 188, 190, 191, 192, 193, 201, 204, 205, 211, 219, 231, 235, 239, 246, 247, 261, 263, 268, 269, 270, 274, 275, 290, 294
adverse effects, 38, 102, 164, 171, 241, 243, 254
adverse event, 136, 139, 214, 256
aetiology, 119, 191, 268
aggressiveness, 188
agonist, 70, 75, 103, 106, 123, 152, 231, 248
airways, 32, 64, 70, 127, 152
alcohol, 33, 37, 41, 87, 88, 93, 94, 125, 126, 127, 130, 131, 270, 277, 294
alfentanil, 151
algorithm, 11, 234, 236, 238, 240
alkaloids, 70
allergic asthma, 12, 169, 252, 258
allergic inflammation, 52, 168, 200
allergic rhinitis, 9, 107, 124, 171, 229, 244, 252, 254, 256, 259, 260, 261, 262
allergist, 5, 148, 151, 152, 179, 205, 208, 228, 238, 239, 244
allergy testing, 60, 89, 136, 148
alpha blocker, 33
American Psychiatric Association, 36
amine(s), 37, 146, 183, 207, 295
amino acid(s), 184, 185
ammonium, 140
amniotic fluid embolism, 35, 44, 45
analgesic, 172, 174
anaphylactic shock, 23, 46, 65, 80, 92, 95, 117, 146, 214, 215, 238, 260, 271, 287
anaphylactoid, 3
anesthetics, 146, 158
angina, 37, 46, 70
angioedema, 3, 22, 31, 32, 35, 36, 40, 50, 51, 53, 54, 65, 91, 92, 116, 127, 130, 139, 146, 152, 156, 167, 168, 169, 170, 175, 187, 192, 201, 209, 213, 220, 228, 230, 231, 232, 233, 234, 238, 242, 248, 255, 257, 265, 279, 292
angiotensin, 16, 33, 53, 63
angiotensin converting enzyme, 11, 52, 53, 87, 88, 198, 213, 231
angiotensin II, 52
anisakis, 39, 46, 47
anorexia nervosa, 93
antacids, 8
antibiotic(s), 136, 139, 140, 141, 145, 150, 151

antibody, 3, 11, 67, 85, 89, 103, 105, 106, 118, 123, 184, 294
antidepressants, 4, 203
antigen, 3, 35, 53, 58, 64, 70, 76, 103, 123, 129, 183, 184, 185, 186, 195, 197, 222, 230
antigenicity, 116
antihistamines, 4, 35, 69, 74, 80, 97, 104, 144, 152, 176, 198, 224, 227, 229, 232, 235, 236, 244, 245, 281, 282, 287, 288
anti-inflammatory drugs, 125, 126, 137, 146, 163, 164, 166, 174, 175, 176, 230, 264
antipyretic, 174
anxiety, 31, 37, 61, 70, 71, 187, 201, 235, 239, 242, 243, 245
APC, 63
apoptosis, 263, 268
aqueous solutions, 147
Ara h 1, 89, 114
Ara h 2, 89, 113
Ara h 3, 89, 113
Ara h 8, 114
Ara h 9, 89, 114
arrest, 32, 187
arrhythmia(s), 65, 70, 74, 203, 264
artery, 40
ascites, 267
ascorbic acid, 197, 231
asphyxia, 58
aspirate, 264, 267, 278, 280, 287
aspiration, 35, 39, 170, 238
aspirin, 25, 43, 87, 118, 125, 126, 130, 131, 132, 163, 164, 167, 171, 172, 173, 174, 175, 176, 230
assessment, 4, 11, 22, 42, 43, 53, 58, 60, 61, 62, 70, 77, 80, 119, 121, 136, 170, 173, 175, 191, 261, 277, 278, 280
asthma, ix, 2, 20, 21, 22, 23, 24, 25, 27, 29, 33, 42, 43, 44, 45, 46, 67, 74, 79, 80, 111, 113, 115, 117, 118, 119, 120, 121, 122, 123, 131, 132, 133, 174, 175, 176, 217, 218, 219, 222, 246, 247, 248, 249, 252, 254, 255, 261
asthmatic airways, 64
asthmatic symptoms, 101
asymptomatic, 36, 37, 280, 287
atherosclerosis, 238
athletes, 128
atopic dermatitis, 64, 67, 103, 107, 118, 275
atopic eczema, 52, 55, 63, 156
atopy, 6, 8, 15, 22, 26, 107, 138, 192, 291
atracurium, 142

B

back pain, 61, 288
bacteria, 34, 277
basophil(s), 3, 52, 54, 55, 65, 71, 85, 106, 123, 145, 148, 149, 156, 170, 200, 222, 229, 231, 276, 277, 278
basophil activation, 56, 125, 127, 144, 148, 150, 157, 170, 176, 177, 197, 200, 224, 291
bee, 219, 222, 248
beneficial effect, 51, 105, 273
benign, 58
beta blocker(s), 33, 69, 75, 78, 80, 97, 193, 194, 208, 211, 213, 214, 239, 256, 257
beta-2 agonist, 74
bifodobacterium, 106
biological activity(ies), 183, 184
biological fluids, 265
biomarkers, 10, 49, 50, 55, 56, 59, 60, 61, 64, 210
biopsy, 41, 61, 144, 160, 232, 267, 275, 278, 280, 286, 288
biphasic anaphylaxis, 43, 44, 69, 80, 220, 270
bleeding, 32
blood, 42, 56, 58, 59, , 92, 129, 137, 146, 151, 222, 247, 267, 279, 280, 288
blood flow, 125, 127, 130
blood pressure, 3, 31, 70, 74, 76, 168, 187, 242, 244, 286
BMI, 73, 278
body weight, 235, 288
bone, 36, 142, 231, 232, 264, 266, 268, 272, 273, 274, 275, 278, 279, 280, 281, 283, 286, 287, 288, 289, 292, 295
bone marrow, 61, 231, 266, 267, 268, 269, 272, 273, 274, 275, 279, 287, 288, 289
bone marrow biopsy, 232, 264, 278, 280, 286
bone resorption, 273
bowel, 41
bradycardia, 32, 38, 46, 75
bradykinin, 9, 50, 51, 52, 53, 54, 63, 65, 184, 194
brain damage, 17, 137
breast cancer, 215
breathing, 38, 41, 70, 85, 242, 287
breathlessness, 35, 168, 169, 171, 213
bronchial asthma, 70
bronchiolitis, 35, 39
bronchoconstriction, 37, 53, 54, 74, 76, 167
bronchodilator, 255, 258
bronchospasm, 3, 31, 32, 34, 36, 37, 39, 50, 140, 155, 156, 168, 187, 233, 238

C

C1q, 231
C3, 35
C4, 35, 64, 126, 231, 268

Ca^{2+}, 54
CAD, 234, 239
calcium, 168, 264, 281, 282, 283, 288, 289, 294
caloric restriction, 240
cancer, 201, 215, 216, 284
candidates, 201
CAP, 196, 213, 214, 215, 222
carbohydrate(s), 89, 91, 149, 183, 184, 197, 222, 230, 248
carboxypeptidase A3, 51, 52
carcinoid syndrome, 35, 37, 41, 57, 58, 229, 230, 232
carcinoma, 35, 170
cardiac activity, 76
cardiac arrest, 70, 74
cardiac arrhythmia, 198
cardiac involvement, 37
cardiac output, 152
cardiac risk, 202
cardiogenic shock, 38
cardiologist, 199, 202, 213
cardiomyopathy, 38, 46
cardiovascular disease, 9, 33, 131, 138, 193, 194, 199, 201
cardiovascular system, 3, 30, 35, 41, 70, 79, 85, 108, 167, 168, 186
caregivers, 4, 69, 77, 99, 199, 217
catecholamines, 45, 184, 232
cathepsin, 51
cathepsin G, 50, 52, 63
CD25, 61, 231, 266, 275, 278, 280, 286, 287, 289, 293
cell culture, 131
cell differentiation, 59, 131
cell line(s), 264, 266, 267, 271, 277, 284, 288
cell signaling, 66
central nervous system (CNS), 4, 243
cephalosporin, 46, 140
cerebral hypoxia, 137
cerebrovascular disease, 239
chemical(s), 38, 147, 151, 163, 164, 165, 167, 171, 172, 173, 244
chemical reactivity, 147
chemokines, 52, 268
chemotaxis, 54, 265
chemotherapy, 215
chicken, 107, 111, 116, 244
childhood, 22, 24, 43, 46, 80, 91, 115, 131
chlorhexidine, 147
cholecalciferol, 294
choline, 140, 164
cholinergic urticaria, 125, 128
chopping, 99
chromatography, 277, 293
chronic diseases, 170, 284
chronic illness, 295
chronic obstructive pulmonary disease, 4
circulation, 35, 50, 54, 57, 59, 70
cisatracurium, 142, 153
cKit, 58
classification, 5, 30, 31, 67, 144, 164, 166, 167, 175, 187, 188, 191, 208, 233, 234, 238, 245, 265, 266, 267, 290, 294
clinical application, 50
clinical assessment, 50
clinical diagnosis, 56, 69, 147, 151, 173
clinical examination, 30, 242
clinical presentation, 12, 29, 30, 43, 49, 61, 113
clinical symptoms, 107, 149, 259, 265, 278
clinical syndrome, 128
clinical trials, 207
clonal, 175, 221, 292
clonality, 294
cloning, 113, 174
cluster, 206
coagulopathy, 35
codon, 231, 274, 280
cognition, 74
cognitive impairment, 293
colloids, 142
coma, 286
combination therapy, 258
comorbidity, 193
comparative analysis, 295
complement, 3, 50, 52, 55, 65, 186, 231, 265
complexity, 135, 157
compliance, 179, 194, 208, 216, 235, 236, 261
complications, 70, 234, 288
component resolved diagnosis, 216, 217
composition, 93, 167, 172, 183, 184, 185, 204
compounds, 137, 146, 150, 184
compression fracture, 288
conflict of interest, 79, 135
confounders, 67, 176
conjunctivitis, 192
consciousness, 70, 129, 131, 238, 244, 287
consensus, 1, 3, 20, 36, 45, 67, 74, 111, 126, 199, 201, 207, 290
consumption, 15, 24, 34, 78, 88, 104, 110, 116, 125, 164, 231, 269
contamination, 51, 57, 90, 98, 99, 100, 107, 109, 230, 277
contraindications, 201
control group, 59
controlled studies, 97, 130, 236
controlled trials, 74, 281

COPD, ix
coping strategies, 112
Cor a 8, 89
Cor a 9, 89
coronary arteries, 38
coronary artery disease, 40, 170, 234
coronary artery spasm, 46
coronary heart disease, 58
correlation(s), 55, 78, 89, 95, 149, 196, 200, 231, 293, 295
corticosteroid therapy, 229, 240
corticosteroids, 11, 34, 75, 79, 97, 137, 144, 151, 159, 198, 199, 201, 227, 229, 235, 240, 241, 245, 258, 287
cortisol, 288
cough, 32, 76, 130, 145, 168, 169, 171, 213, 242, 255
cough suppressant, 158
coughing, 107, 258
counseling, 69, 79, 126, 228
covering, 182
COX-1, 165, 166, 167, 168, 169, 172, 173
COX-2, 165, 166, 169, 172, 173, 174, 176
creatinine, 273, 278, 285, 287, 288
cromoglycate, 130, 133, 264, 265, 281
cross links, 85
cross-sectional study, 15, 85
croup, 35, 39
crystalline, 169
CSD, 233, 235, 240, 241, 245
cyanosis, 31, 35, 187
cyclooxygenase, 163, 164, 167, 174, 175, 176
cyst, 39
cytokines, 55, 66, 200, 268, 273
cytometry, 264, 278, 279, 289
cytoreductive, 264, 281, 294

D

death rate, 7, 19, 144
deaths, 6, 7, 19, 26, 44, 87, 96, 191, 192, 253, 257, 259
defecation, 288
degradation, 9, 52, 62, 63, 77, 90, 127, 132, 193, 277
demographic factors, 8
dendritic cell, 106, 114, 200
density values, 288
depression, 4, 39, 40, 242, 273, 284, 293
derivatives, 146, 164, 268
dermatologist, 275
dermatology, 293
dermis, 266
desensitization, 102, 103, 104, 121, 122, 140, 260
detectable, 50, 55, 59, 92, 95, 98, 101, 185, 196, 266, 274, 279, 286, 287
detection, 60, 150, 170, 188, 196, 197, 221, 274, 277, 286, 293
diabetes, 70, 132
diabetic patients, 70
Diagnostic and Statistical Manual of Mental Disorders, 36
diagnostic criteria, 3, 4, 30, 67, 231, 232, 249, 266, 280, 285
diagnostic markers, 116
diamine oxidase, 51
diaphoresis, 92, 232
diarrhea, 31, 85, 92, 105, 187, 233, 244, 255, 264, 265, 273, 286, 288
diclofenac, 164, 171
diet, 8, 85, 104, 105, 132, 277, 282, 283, 284, 293
dietary habits, 13
differential diagnosis, 39, 45, 146, 170, 277
digestibility, 133
digestion, 85, 94, 111
digestive enzymes, 89
diphenhydramine, 74, 75, 80, 234, 235, 244
dipyrone, 164, 169, 171, 177
diseases, 4, 8, 10, 17, 20, 23, 26, 67, 74, 77, 87, 94, 107, 127, 139, 165, 171, 193, 194, 201, 209, 211, 212, 215, 216, 219, 227, 245, 250, 259, 294
disinfection, 147
disorder, 2, 4, 14, 36, 58, 67, 77, 85, 94, 108, 231, 232, 233, 234, 241, 242, 245, 265, 266, 267, 268, 280, 285, 295
distress, 30, 34, 36, 44, 75, 132, 232
distribution, 137, 145, 188, 203, 247, 277
diversity, 5, 20, 89, 95
dizygotic twins, 85
dizziness, 31, 32, 34, 41, 60, 71, 147, 187, 202, 228, 232, 241, 270
DNA, 103
doctors, 33, 145, 179, 284
dolichovespula, 180, 182, 183, 185, 186, 203
dopamine, 76, 185, 207
dosage, 205, 209, 240, 243, 245
dosing, 73, 104, 202, 207, 208, 213, 214, 235, 253, 254, 256, 258, 259, 261, 294
double blind placebo controlled, 281
double blind study, 104
double positivity, 196, 216
drug allergy, 71, 140, 143, 166
drug interaction, 203
drug provocation tests, 149
drug reactions, 17, 25, 136, 164, 173, 174
drug treatment, 281

drugs, 4, 12, 17, 20, 32, 33, 37, 39, 66, 69, 78, 86, 87, 111, 112, 135, 136, 137, 139, 140, 142, 144, 145, 146, 148, 149, 150, 151, 152, 153, 154, 155, 156, 157, 160, 163, 164, 165, 166, 169, 170, 172, 173, 174, 175, 198, 230, 264, 270, 277, 282, 286
duodenitis, 269
dyes, 136, 137, 144, 151, 160, 162
dysarthria, 31, 187
dysphagia, 32, 170, 228
dysplasia, 267
dyspnea, 92, 168, 187, 232, 241, 257

E

eczema, 8, 12, 95, 105, 153, 252
edema, 32, 74, 76, 107, 152, 231, 232, 241, 242, 244, 255
egg, 15, 18, 26, 78, 83, 84, 85, 88, 90, 91, 98, 103, 104, 105, 110, 111, 115, 116, 118, 121, 122, 138, 244
elderly population, 239
embolism, 35, 44, 45
emergency management, 41, 61, 102, 216
emotional stimuli, 61
emphysema, 70
encephalopathy, 224, 243
endocrine, 41
endoscopy, 243, 244, 273
endothelial cells, 52
endotoxemia, 132
endotoxins, 125
endotracheal intubation, 76
environment(s), 12, 18, 55, 127, 128, 141, 142, 147, 151
environmental factors, 8, 20, 85, 135
enzymatic activity, 184
enzyme(s), 9, 10, 16, 23, 33, 43, 51, 52, 53, 54, 56, 63, 65, 69, 78, 126, 131, 138, 144, 183, 184, 193, 217, 248, 268, 277, 280
enzyme immunoassay, 131
enzyme inhibitors, 10, 16, 23, 43, 193, 217
eosinophilia, 59, 280
eosinophilic esophagitis, 85
eosinophils, 50, 52, 53, 64, 200, 229
epidemic, 17, 22, 109, 113
epidemiologic, 2, 20, 25, 146, 158, 160
epidemiology, 1, 2, 5, 6, 15, 17, 20, 21, 22, 23, 80, 112, 145, 158, 219, 292
epilepsy, 170
epinephrine, 70, 71, 72, 73, 75, 80, 96, 108, 117, 152, 158, 239, 281
epinephrine auto-injector, xii, 69, 73, 96, 120, 287, 288
epithelial cells, 106
epithelial transport, 127
epithelium, 126, 127
epitopes, 89, 91, 94, 114, 116, 196
esophagitis, 85, 111
ester, 146
ethanol, 4, 10, 294
ethnicity, 12
ethylene oxide, 160
etiology, 22, 111, 172, 220, 228, 250, 263
Etomidate, 141
examinations, 144, 241, 268, 272, 273, 274, 278, 279, 287, 288
excretion, 277, 278, 279, 283, 285, 288, 293
exercise, 4, 10, 15, 25, 33, 37, 38, 43, 46, 77, 87, 93, 94, 104, 108, 117, 118, 125, 126, 127, 128, 129, 130, 131, 132, 133, 175, 176, 230, 231, 240, 247, 248, 283, 288
exercise induced anaphylaxis, xii, 33, 43, 125
exertion, 15, 125, 130
exposure, 3, 4, 6, 8, 15, 16, 19, 24, 29, 30, 31, 32, 33, 34, 37, 58, 60, 78, 84, 85, 89, 92, 94, 100, 111, 121, 140, 143, 145, 147, 148, 149, 151, 152, 167, 168, 187, 188, 191, 192, 195, 199, 200, 201, 202, 216, 229, 231, 274, 282, 283
extracts, 55, 77, 149, 179, 185, 197, 203, 204, 206, 207, 209, 210, 212, 215, 216, 218, 223, 260, 261
extravasation, 92

F

failure to thrive, 85
false negative, 195
false positive, 150, 215, 276
families, 99, 235, 239, 245
family history, 138, 139, 195
family members, 77, 99, 192, 212, 219, 240, 242
fat, 22, 132
fatal, 5, 44, 67, 79, 87, 90, 109, 117, 188, 247, 249, 260
fatal anaphylaxis, 21, 23, 26, 45, 113, 220, 291
fear, 195, 214, 240, 287
feelings, 284
femur, 288
fentanyl, 146, 151, 156, 282
fetus, 243
fever, 9, 18, 37, 77, 273
fibrinogen, 52
FIP1L1-PDGFRA fusion gene, 59, 280
first aid, 199, 217
first generation, 4
fish, 24, 34, 35, 39, 40, 44, 56, 66, 83, 84, 88, 90, 93, 98, 99, 106, 108, 230, 277

fluid, 34, 35, 39, 44, 45, 74, 85, 92, 97, 137, 184, 287
flushing, 32, 36, 37, 269, 273
food additive, 117
food allergen avoidance, 83
food allergy, viii, 21, 42, 71, 79, 81, 83, 84, 85, 106, 109, 119, 123, 186, 219
Food and Drug Administration (FDA), 75, 254
food industry, 99
food intake, 130
food products, 44
food protein-induced enterocolitis syndrome, 85
formation, 65, 111, 117, 127, 274, 277
formula, 106, 123
fractures, 264, 267, 269, 273, 280, 281, 283, 287, 288, 289, 292
frequent, 167, 233
fruits, 78, 84, 128, 138, 182
fusion, 59, 280

G

Gal d 1, 91
Gal d 2, 91
Gal d 3, 91
Gal d 4, 91
galactose α-1,3 galactose, alpha-gal, 91, 230
gastroesophageal reflux, 243
gastrointestinal tract, 52, 85, 86, 167, 168
general anaesthesia, 46, 135, 142, 143, 148, 152, 157, 161, 282
general practitioner, 5, 11, 41, 164, 205, 268
genes, 12, 263, 268, 280
genetic alteration, 290
genetic engineering, 180, 212, 217
genetic factors, 168, 193
genetics, 45, 67
genome, 8
genus, 39, 180, 270
geography, 24, 191
GI tract, 125, 131
ginger, 244
gland, 182
glaucoma, 70, 240
globus, 230, 232, 235, 241, 242, 245, 250
glucagon, 69, 75, 80, 97
glucocorticoid(s), 74, 75, 249, 281, 282
glutamate, 35
glutamine, 126
Gly m 1, 91
Gly m 3, 91
Gly m 4, 91
glycerol, 138
glycoproteins, 222
granules, 50, 52, 276
grass(es), 171, 253, 254, 256, 258, 259, 261
growth, 58, 239, 265
growth factor, 67
guidance, 43, 49, 62, 99, 199, 234
guidelines, 2, 4, 21, 23, 32, 35, 47, 74, 80, 84, 87, 145, 147, 157, 161, 179, 191, 196, 201, 211, 214, 216, 218, 219, 222, 251, 257, 259

H

habitat, 197
hairless, 180
half-life, 51, 56, 57, 59, 76
hazards, 121
hazel nut, 89
HBV, 205, 209
headache, 32, 37, 40, 63, 70, 71, 129, 169, 255, 265
health, 4, 42, 80, 84, 99, 179, 180, 199, 222, 251
health care, 11, 17, 18, 23, 77, 79, 97, 217, 259
health care costs, 242
health care professionals, 79, 97, 259
health care system, 36
heart attack, 214
heart disease, 4, 23, 70, 213, 214, 286
heart rate, 71
hematopoietic stem cells, 268
hemisphere, 9
hemodialysis, 147
hemoglobin, 288
hepatomegaly, 267
herbal medicine, 103, 123
hereditary angioedema, 170, 231
heritability, 290
heteroaryl acetic acid, 166
heterogeneity, 30, 114
Hev b 1, 149
Hevea, 149
histamine, 42, 44, 46, 51, 56, 66, 93, 118, 119, 148, 248, 263, 268, 277, 293, 294
histamine N tau-methyltransferase, 277
histidine, 34, 51, 62, 277
histological examination, 41, 273, 289
HIV, 58
hives, 31, 32, 34, 74, 92, 167, 168, 191, 192, 228, 232, 233, 242, 244
HLA, 167, 175
honey bees, 19, 183
hormone(s), 231, 248
hospital death, 158
hospitalization, 11, 13, 85, 169
host, 39, 63, 127
house dust, 90

human, 42, 50, 52, 53, 54, 55, 63, 65, 67, 88, 103, 113, 117, 123, 127, 132, 164, 182, 222, 229, 247
human neutrophils, 66
human skin, 64
humidity, 128
hyaluronidase, 183, 184, 185
hydatid, 39
hydatid disease, 47
hydroxide, 206
hygiene, 8, 22
hymenoptera, v, 23, 67, 179, 181, 183, 184, 185, 188, 189, 197, 199, 218, 220, 221, 222, 223, 224, 228, 272, 290, 295
hymenoptera sting, 25, 43, 175, 180, 186, 191, 193, 198, 212, 216, 217, 219, 263, 264, 269, 270, 271, 273, 283, 289, 291, 292
hyperactivity, 4
hyperglycaemia, 70
hyperplasia, 275
hypersplenism, 267
hypertension, 37, 70, 71, 203, 232, 234, 269
hyperthyroidism, 70
hyperventilation, 170
hypnotics, 141, 145, 150
hypotension, 3, 30, 34, 35, 36, 38, 39, 50, 51, 53, 60, 74, 75, 76, 78, 92, 97, 142, 148, 154, 155, 156, 170, 199, 202, 213, 228, 231, 232, 233, 234, 238, 239, 241, 242, 254, 257, 264, 265, 270, 273, 286, 287
hypotensive, 75, 79, 85, 107, 202, 286, 287
hypothesis, 8, 22, 35, 126, 127, 137, 270
hypoxemia, 31, 168, 187
hypoxia, 35, 76, 92

I

ibuprofen, 61, 164, 166, 173
ICAM, 114
identification, 37, 50, 59, 79, 98, 102, 151, 152, 157, 177, 203, 279
identity, 88, 155, 156, 186, 203
idiopathic, 1, 6, 12, 14, 18, 19, 20, 35, 36, 37, 41, 45, 128, 227, 229, 231, 237, 246, 247, 248, 249, 265
IgE mediated, 15, 30, 39, 41, 50, 55, 58, 78, 84, 85, 90, 91, 108, 126, 148, 197, 214, 270
IgG4, 105, 114, 200, 210
IL-13, 55, 200
IL-8, 52, 63
immediate reaction, 167
immune reaction, 108, 151, 229
immune response, 84, 85, 94, 102, 106, 108, 127, 184, 200
immune system, 126, 151, 165
immunity, 29
immunization, 18, 26
ImmunoCAP, 78, 276
immunoglobulin, 116, 185
immunohistochemistry, 275, 286
immunologist, 148, 238, 239
immunomodulatory, 229
immunoreactivity, 275
improvements, 216
in vitro, 56, 114, 147, 148, 149, 170, 176, 177, 196, 197, 200, 203, 208, 210, 211, 222, 229, 247
in vivo, 53, 123, 149, 170, 247
incidence, 1, 2, 4, 5, 6, 8, 9, 11, 12, 13, 15, 17, 20, 22, 24, 30, 31, 33, 38, 44, 80, 85, 86, 87, 108, 109, 111, 113, 115, 119, 135, 136, 137, 143, 144, 145, 157, 158, 159, 191, 208, 209, 215, 220, 246, 256, 257, 258, 268
indications, 195, 200, 202, 279
individuals, 6, 7, 9, 11, 13, 16, 30, 34, 36, 37, 38, 39, 77, 78, 79, 84, 87, 89, 90, 91, 93, 96, 98, 99, 101, 107, 108, 109, 123, 142, 166, 183, 191, 193, 200, 203, 212, 222, 277
indolent, 57, 66, 193, 209, 221, 263, 264, 266, 268, 271, 275, 285, 289, 290, 292, 295
infancy, 110, 274
infants, 8, 15, 24, 31, 32, 74, 85, 91, 110, 115, 274
infarction, 202
infection, 22, 29, 37, 88, 123, 124
inflammation, 52, 53, 54, 64, 71, 85, 132, 169, 176, 292
inflammatory mediators, 37, 50, 52, 64, 127, 152, 165
infliximab, 58
influenza vaccine, 18
infrequent, 233, 259
ingest, 104, 234
ingestion, 4, 10, 13, 15, 39, 46, 57, 89, 92, 94, 97, 100, 105, 108, 117, 120, 126, 128, 129, 130, 170, 171, 175, 176, 230, 231, 242, 248
ingredients, 98, 99, 231
inhaler, 107
inhibition, 52, 64, 146, 165, 167, 168, 173, 176, 197, 200, 216
inhibitor, 33, 52, 53, 113, 169, 172, 185, 213, 231, 243, 248, 274
initiation, 126, 243
injections, 73, 121, 143, 150, 205, 206, 207, 208, 211, 212, 213, 215, 252, 253, 254, 260, 261, 287
injury, 125, 127
innate immunity, 63
insect venom, 14, 31, 32, 33, 43, 53, 56, 58, 62, 65, 77, 86, 92, 179, 183, 197, 201, 209, 218, 219, 221, 222, 223, 270, 279, 292, 295

insects, 16, 77, 90, 166, 180, 182, 183, 203
insomnia, 240
intensive care unit, 151, 169, 236, 257
interference, 58, 67, 276, 293
interferon, 282, 294
interstitial cystitis, 57
intervention, 76, 79, 130, 154, 155, 156
intestinal tract, 266, 269, 273, 289
intestine, 247
intradermal test, 154, 195, 214
intralymphatic, 212, 217
intramuscular injection, 73, 74
intravenous fluids, 79
intravenously, 60, 74, 142, 287
iodinated contrast, 160, 162
iodine, 144
ionic, 144
ionization, 144
ions, 127, 140
iron, 155
irradiation, 281
irritability, 32
ischaemic heart disease, 70, 213
isolation, 30, 50, 59
isotope, 293

K

kallikrein, 53
karyotyping, 280
kidney, 150, 277, 288, 293
kinetics, 51, 55
Kounis syndrome, 35, 37, 38, 40, 46

L

label reading, 98, 109
labeling, 98, 119, 120, 231
laboratory tests, 108, 196
Lactobacillus, 106
Langerhans cells, 103
laryngoscopy, 38, 242, 250
larynx, 255
lead, 8, 13, 50, 53, 59, 61, 70, 86, 102, 108, 127, 136, 182, 185, 239, 242, 243, 264, 270
lecithin, 138
legume, 13
lesions, 41, 66, 130, 235, 263, 264, 266, 267, 269, 274, 275, 279, 281, 284, 285, 286, 287, 288, 290, 292
lethargy, 85
leukemia, 170, 264, 266, 267, 277
leukocytosis, 279
leukotriene antagonists, 232
leukotrienes, 3, 50, 51, 52, 53, 61, 64, 139, 146, 150, 152, 165, 167, 168
LFA, 44
lifestyle changes, 8
ligand, 114, 247
lipids, 183, 185
lipooxygenase, 165
listeria monocytogenes, 122
liver, 41, 47, 264, 266, 267, 274, 280, 286, 287, 288, 289
liver cells, 247
liver disease, 150
living conditions, 197
local anaesthetics, 137, 141, 146, 151
local reaction, 202, 251
localization, 63
loss of appetite, 36
loss of consciousness, 16, 31, 187, 215, 228, 233, 238, 243, 255
low molecular weight heparins, 292
low risk, 199, 212
lubricants, 147
lumbar spine, 280, 281, 288
lung disease, 23
lupin, 24
luteinizing hormone, 231, 248
lymph, 267, 278
lymph node, 144, 145, 160, 264, 274, 280, 286, 287
lymphadenopathy, 267, 278
lymphoid tissue, 266, 289, 290
lymphoma, 267
lysis, 55, 185
lysozyme, 91

M

macromolecules, 127
macrophages, 54
magnesium, 164
Maillard reaction, 89
Mal d 1, 86
malabsorption, 288
malaise, 31, 147, 187
malignancy, 267
malignant, 233, 241, 249
mapping, 103, 144, 145
marrow, 61, 231, 232, 264, 266, 267, 269, 273, 278, 280, 286, 287, 288, 289
mass, 41, 270, 284, 289
mass spectrometry, 293
mast cell activation syndrome, 230, 249, 265

mast cell degranulation, 50, 52, 54, 57, 125, 126, 127, 131, 148, 232, 282, 288
mast cell stabilizer, 232
mast cells, 3, 30, 36, 50, 52, 53, 54, 55, 58, 63, 64, 65, 67, 71, 85, 103, 106, 126, 127, 131, 140, 145, 148, 168, 185, 186, 200, 228, 229, 231, 232, 247, 263, 265, 266, 267, 268, 270, 273, 274, 275, 276, 277, 278, 280, 282, 286, 287, 288, 289, 292, 293
mastocytoma, 269
mastocytosis, 32, 33, 35, 36, 43, 45, 58, 71, 79, 205, 208, 211, 223, 249, 265, 266, 268, 289, 290, 291, 292, 294, 295
meat, 92, 93, 116, 121, 230
medical, 9, 18, 34, 36, 53, 69, 77, 79, 80, 93, 95, 98, 102, 107, 109, 147, 148, 158, 159, 163, 165, 170, 199, 202, 205, 208, 238, 240, 241, 242, 243, 245, 246, 257, 258, 259, 268
medical alert bracelet, 69, 79
medical care, 9, 199, 242, 257
medical history, 163, 170, 243
medication, 11, 17, 19, 36, 70, 73, 85, 92, 99, 102, 146, 209, 214, 220, 224, 229, 230, 236, 238, 242, 244, 256, 284, 286, 292
medicine, 29, 42, 44, 246, 247, 249
Mediterranean, 114, 128, 180, 183, 193, 204
Mediterranean countries, 13, 203, 215
medulla, 37
medullary carcinoma, 35
melanoma, 160
meloxicam, 165, 166, 169
meningomyelocele, 26
menstrual, 94
menstruation, 15, 125, 126, 127, 131
mental disorder, 36
mental health, 4
meta-analysis, 84, 110, 122, 204, 223, 262, 283
metabisulfite, 93, 146, 230
Metaolic, 93
metabolism, 3, 126, 249, 273, 293
metabolites, 53, 66, 149, 264, 271, 273, 277, 278, 286, 288, 289, 292, 293, 294
metabolized, 165
Metacromatic, 278
methodology, 246
methylene blue, 142, 144, 151
methylprednisolone, 156
metrorrhagia, 155
mice, 116, 123, 124, 132, 212
microbiota, 132
micrograms, 74, 283
Middle East, 13
migraines, 93
migrants, 8
migration, 52
mild asthma, 107
military, 80
Milk, 90, 105
mobile phone, 41
models, 54, 65, 103, 105, 106, 107, 212
molds, 169, 171, 258
molecular weight, 14, 183, 184, 185, 218
molecules, 49, 50, 106, 126, 183, 204
monoamine oxidase inhibitors, 57, 78, 88
monoclonal mast, 193, 232, 263, 264, 265, 266, 279, 289
Monoclonal mast cell activation syndrome, 230
monomers, 143
monosodium glutamate, 170
monozygotic twins, 85
montelukast, 53, 130, 133
mood change, 240
morbidity, 2, 135, 136, 148, 157, 179, 180, 188, 199, 214, 236
morphine, 39, 140, 145, 146, 247
morphology, 231, 280, 286, 287
mortality, 2, 7, 17, 19, 20, 35, 54, 126, 135, 136, 137, 157, 158, 179, 191, 199, 214
mortality rate, 7, 17, 35, 126, 136, 137
mosquitoes, 16
MR, 46, 111, 176, 177, 261
MRI, 41
mucosa, 101, 116, 125, 127, 169, 171
mucous membrane, 32
mucous membranes, 32
mucus, 32, 92
mumps, 18
muscle relaxant, 139, 150, 160, 264, 282
music, 102
mussels, 40
mustard, 98, 244
mutagenesis, 105
mutation, 59, 61, 103, 231, 232, 263, 264, 265, 266, 268, 274, 278, 279, 284, 286, 287, 289, 290
mutational analysis, 278
mutations, 268, 280
myelomeningocele, 147
myeloproliferative disorders, 57, 277, 278
myocardial infarction, 30, 38, 39, 40, 46, 170, 202, 213, 239
myocardial ischemia, 152
myocardium, 38

N

N tau-methylhistamine (MH), 277
naproxen, 244

nasal polyp, 17, 167
natural course, 285
nausea, 31, 32, 34, 35, 37, 40, 92, 129, 187, 228, 264
nematode, 39
neoplasm, 267
nervous system, 32
neutrophils, 50, 52, 53, 54, 55
NHS, vii
nimesulide, 166
nitrogen, 293
nodules, 274
non-steroidal anti-inflammatory drugs (NSAIDs), 10, 14, 15, 17, 59, 61, 112, 126, 127, 130, 131, 137, 146, 149, 163, 164, 165, 166, 167, 168, 169, 170, 171, 172, 173, 174, 175, 176, 177, 230, 231, 244, 264, 265, 270, 281, 282
norepinephrine, 65
nursing, 45, 257
nutrient, 125

O

obesity, 132, 199, 277, 293
objective symptoms, 242
obstacles, 59
obstruction, 3, 40, 53, 63, 65, 129, 147, 198, 228, 233, 238, 241, 249
occult blood, 125
oedema, 11, 34, 35, 54, 76, 130, 152, 169, 202
oesophageal, 38
old age, 7, 211
omalizumab, 106, 123, 209, 224, 236, 241, 249, 283
opioids, 61, 136, 137, 141, 146, 264, 270, 282, 288
oral allergy syndrome, 85
oral food challenge, 13, 15, 84, 93, 95, 117, 118, 123
organ(s), 3, 30, 31, 36, 47, 65, 76, 84, 125, 167, 168, 187, 231, 232, 255, 266, 280, 292
organic disease, 170
orthostatic hypotension, 232
osmolality, 125, 126, 127, 144
osteoporosis, 240, 249, 264, 269, 273, 280, 281, 282, 283, 286, 287, 288, 289, 292
outpatient(s), 36, 78, 83, 86, 96, 119, 165, 190, 228
ovalbumin, 91, 116, 138
overlap, 30, 32, 34, 41, 54, 93, 232
overproduction, 286
ovomucoid, 85, 91, 111, 116
oxygen, 39, 69, 76, 97, 215, 242

P

pain, 31, 32, 36, 37, 39, 41, 85, 92, 166, 168, 169, 187, 198, 202, 215, 228, 231, 238, 244, 257, 287
palate, 32, 107
pallor, 37, 38, 71
palpation, 267
palpitations, 32, 37, 40, 71, 232, 286
panic attack, 30, 230, 243
panic disorder, 232, 235
parasites, 39
parents, 12, 69, 99, 102, 107, 155, 238, 239
parvalbumin, 90
pathogenesis, 50, 53, 54, 62, 91, 127, 228, 229, 245, 290
pathology, 294
pathophysiology, 30, 55, 62, 65, 83, 94, 117, 121, 127, 180, 227, 228
pathways, 9, 50, 52, 77, 165, 168, 186, 193
pattern recognition, 4
peanut allergy, 113
pediatric allergist, 120
penicillin, 6, 17, 46, 60, 140, 151, 171, 231
pepsin, 111
peptic ulcer disease, 281
peptide(s), 35, 126, 127, 183, 185, 207, 212, 218, 224
percentage of fat, 192
perforation, 286
perfusion, 74, 76
perinatal, 35
peripheral blood, 55, 229, 278, 279
permeability, 10, 53, 54, 71, 76, 94, 125, 126, 127, 130, 131, 132
persistent asthma, 236
PGD2, 53, 59
PGE2, 53, 167
PGF2, 53
pH, 87, 125, 126, 127, 250
phaeochromocytoma, 35, 37, 45
pharmaceutical, 258
pharmacogenomics, 294
pharmacokinetics, 209
pharmacology, 45
pharmacotherapy, 43, 239, 244
phenol, 138
phenotype, 172, 177, 232
phenylpiperidines, 151
pheochromocytoma, 45, 229, 232
phosphate, 146, 288
phospholipase, 183, 184, 185
phospholipids, 165
phosphorus, 293

physical activity, 94, 108, 125, 126, 128, 131
physical exercise, 127
physicians, 49, 61, 73, 77, 110, 199, 212, 217, 236, 238, 240, 241, 242, 243, 245, 253, 257, 259
physicochemical properties, 89
physiological factors, 29
piloerection, 32
placebo, 63, 89, 95, 97, 100, 104, 106, 122, 123, 124, 130, 166, 224, 236, 254, 256, 261, 281
plasma levels, 73, 273
plasma proteins, 58, 144
platelet activating factor, 55, 62, 65, 229, 247, 268
platelet aggregation, 52, 54
platelets, 54, 267
pneumothorax, 238
point mutation, 266, 280, 286
poison, 182
polistes, 180, 182, 183, 184, 186, 195, 197, 203, 213, 214, 215, 218, 222, 223
pollen, 15, 85, 89, 91, 94, 114, 149, 230, 248, 254, 256, 257, 258, 259, 261
pollination, 182
pollinators, 182
pollutants, 8
polyamines, 184
polymorphism(s), 12, 49, 52, 53, 55, 63, 65, 167, 268, 277
polyps, 269
portal hypertension, 267
positive correlation, 89
potassium, 115, 169
PR-10, 91
predictive accuracy, 95
prednisone, 75, 198, 199, 228, 233, 234, 235, 236, 238, 239, 240, 241, 242, 243, 244, 245, 246, 247
pregnancy, 62, 203, 243, 250, 277, 294
preoperative screening, 148
prevalence, 4, 5, 84, 110, 113, 115, 129, 189, 219, 271, 290, 291
prevalence rate, 18
prevention, 2, 4, 18, 21, 26, 34, 60, 62, 75, 78, 94, 98, 108, 130, 131, 144, 151, 152, 158, 179, 209, 216, 229, 249, 260, 282, 283, 294
primary prophylaxis, 26
primate, 42
probability, 5, 33, 87
probiotic(s), 106, 123
procurement, 69
prodromal symptoms, 129
progesterone, 155, 231
prognosis, 90, 179, 201, 227, 228, 239, 245, 246, 267, 284
pro-inflammatory, 8, 85
proliferation, 61, 263, 265, 268, 289
prophylactic, 61, 144, 249
prophylaxis, 136
propofol, 46, 138, 141, 153, 156
prostaglandins, 3, 50, 51, 52, 53, 61, 139, 165
prostration, 129
proteases, 52
protective mechanisms, 116, 222
protein kinases, 184
proteins, 35, 39, 85, 89, 90, 91, 94, 101, 102, 105, 108, 113, 123, 126, 129, 183, 184, 185, 200, 204, 218, 265
proton pump inhibitors, 8, 281
proto-oncogene, 264, 265
pruritus, 74, 86, 92, 97, 105, 128, 129, 130, 146, 147, 167, 168, 201, 228, 231, 238, 241, 242, 244, 252, 255, 256, 257, 259, 265, 279
psoriasis, 64, 275
psychiatric illness, 4, 38
psychiatry, 250
psychosomatic, 170, 194
puberty, 12, 263, 274, 284
public health, 2, 4, 80
pulmonary edema, 70
pyrazolones, 146, 165

Q

quality control, 58
quality of life, 102, 179, 180, 194, 199, 202, 212, 217, 222
quantification, 61, 64, 115, 149, 150, 170
questionable, 195, 233
questionnaire, 112, 116, 253

R

race, 70
rash, 3, 32, 34, 35, 41, 60, 171
RAST, 78, 216
reaction rate, 204, 253
reaction time, 167
reactivity, 85, 89, 90, 91, 104, 117, 132, 133, 141, 144, 148, 149, 150, 151, 159, 169, 183, 184, 185, 186, 195, 196, 197, 203, 212, 214, 215, 216, 229, 250, 259
reagents, 151
receptors, 53, 62, 70, 71, 75, 103, 106, 200
recognition, 4, 9, 21, 94, 99, 108, 120, 152, 173, 238, 256
recovery, 121, 130, 188, 222

recurrence, 50, 61, 77, 114, 192, 211, 212, 216, 236, 286
redistribution, 127
registry(ies), 115, 188
regression, 284
relevance, 52, 183, 267
remifentanil, 151, 154
remission, 215, 216, 227, 229, 234, 236, 238, 239, 240, 241, 243, 244, 245
renal cell carcinoma, 37
renal dysfunction, 293
renal failure, 58
renin, 50, 53, 65
research funding, 4
researchers, 13, 34, 228
resection, 41
residues, 126, 184
resolution, 33, 89, 91, 93, 122, 152, 263, 284
resource allocation, 4
respiratory arrest, 2, 35
respiratory failure, 169, 238, 257
respiratory rate, 32, 71, 76
rheumatic fever, 17
rheumatoid factor, 58
rhinitis, 11, 17, 53, 64, 93, 153, 169, 171, 257, 262
rhino, 192
rhinorrhea, 93, 146, 255
risk assessment, 43, 58, 77, 275, 291
risk factors, 1, 2, 8, 9, 12, 16, 19, 20, 23, 25, 34, 42, 43, 77, 83, 88, 97, 107, 108, 135, 140, 145, 152, 157, 159, 179, 180, 192, 193, 194, 200, 201, 202, 204, 205, 208, 209, 211, 216, 217, 218, 247, 259, 260, 291
risks, 99, 101, 109, 113, 119, 170, 174, 201, 235, 259
rocuronium, 142, 153
room temperature, 57, 278
rush, 205, 206, 259

S

salicylates, 94
saliva, 77, 121
salmon, 34, 40, 231
saturation, 76, 242
scleroderma, 229
scombroid poisoning, 34, 230
scope, 4, 13, 165, 182
seafood, 13, 47, 90, 94, 99, 108, 115, 126, 128, 131
secrete, 200
secretion, 169, 171, 200, 277
sedatives, 4, 33
sensation, 34, 35, 232, 235, 242, 244, 245, 250, 255
sensitivity, 17, 49, 51, 56, 58, 59, 60, 61, 66, 77, 89, 121, 126, 138, 148, 149, 150, 170, 172, 174, 175, 176, 186, 195, 196, 200, 208, 210, 214, 221, 222, 231, 258, 259
sensitization, 8, 13, 15, 18, 24, 26, 42, 69, 77, 78, 85, 89, 91, 92, 95, 103, 107, 114, 116, 127, 144, 145, 147, 149, 151, 152, 158, 160, 169, 180, 183, 185, 188, 192, 194, 195, 196, 197, 203, 212, 214, 216, 222, 248, 253, 260, 270, 283, 287
septic shock, 58
serine, 52, 184, 185, 186
serotonin, 37, 184, 207
sesame, 13, 24, 84, 98, 106, 110, 244
severe asthma, 9, 11, 35, 39, 231, 232
sex, 7, 34, 136
sex hormones, 23, 137, 249
shellfish, 10, 24, 44, 83, 84, 88, 90, 98, 106, 108, 128
shock, 32, 35, 38, 46, 54, 58, 65, 92, 117, 128, 146, 170, 187, 192, 238, 257, 261, 270
shortness of breath, 32, 40, 244, 255
shrimp, 13, 40, 90
side effects, 23, 105, 199, 205, 208, 209, 210, 211, 213, 214, 215, 217, 224, 235, 240, 241, 283
signs, 2, 3, 4, 16, 36, 50, 75, 78, 83, 92, 135, 147, 148, 152, 157, 167, 232, 235, 239, 253, 257, 265, 268, 276, 281, 282, 288
skeletal muscle, 126, 131
skeleton, 264, 283, 289
skin cancer, 281
skin prick test, 40, 95, 118, 130, 145, 149, 151, 154, 156, 213, 215
smoking, 283
smoldering, 267
smooth muscle, 52
social services, 240
social situations, 239
socioeconomic status, 9
sodium, 130, 133, 138, 164, 174, 230
somatic mutations, 263, 268
soy, 13, 15, 84, 88, 91, 108, 116
specialists, 3, 164, 170, 207, 209, 268
species, 63, 180, 182, 183, 185, 186, 193, 195, 196, 197, 203, 213, 214, 215, 221
specificity, 51, 116, 170
sphincter, 250
spina bifida, 18, 26
spinal cord, 170
spine, 280
spleen, 264, 266, 274, 280, 286, 287, 289
splenomegaly, 267
stable asthma, 257
starch, 142
stent, 46

sterile, 182
steroids, 34, 38, 69, 97, 213, 215, 227, 229, 232, 239, 242, 243, 244
stimulus, 265
stratification, 61, 89
stress, 4, 9, 41, 77, 242, 250
stridor, 31, 32, 38, 129, 168, 187, 228, 232, 241, 242, 244, 249, 255
stroke, 170
strontium, 282
structure, 151, 163, 164, 165, 167, 172, 174, 183, 185, 288
style, 284
subcutaneous injection, 73, 212, 252
sublingual immunotherapy (SLIT), 104, 209
substance abuse, 4
substance use, 157
substitution, 173
substrate, 125
success rate, 104, 204
sufentanil, 151
sulfites, 170
supplementation, 123, 264, 281, 282, 283, 288, 289, 294
suppression, 231, 247, 249
surgical intervention, 38, 155, 156
surveillance, 254, 261, 282
survival, 59, 265, 290
susceptibility, 8, 58, 87
suture, 147
suxamethonium, 142
swelling, 32, 40, 186, 191, 198, 241, 242, 244, 252, 257, 265, 274, 287
sympathoadrenal, 125
sympathomimetics, 198, 227
syndrome, 2, 10, 35, 37, 38, 40, 41, 45, 46, 61, 76, 79, 85, 89, 93, 103, 111, 128, 170, 177, 193, 230, 231, 232, 249, 263, 264, 265, 266, 267, 279, 285, 289
synthesis, 50, 51, 52, 165, 167, 168, 277
systemic mastocytosis, 57, 59, 61, 66, 193, 199, 209, 221, 228, 231, 232, 247, 264, 266, 267, 271, 272, 275, 279, 280, 285, 289, 290, 291, 292, 293, 294, 295
systemic reaction, xi, 16, 33, 78, 91, 100, 101, 103, 105, 108, 125, 141, 142, 148, 150, 152, 158, 163, 165, 166, 170, 172, 175, 179, 186, 187, 195, 202, 205, 208, 209, 212, 214, 216, 217, 218, 221, 251, 260, 261, 270, 273, 282, 292
systolic blood pressure, 31, 60, 168, 187

T

T cell, 55, 144, 165, 200, 224, 229
T lymphocytes, 229
T suis, 107
tachycardia, 38, 70, 71, 155, 156, 228, 264, 270, 286, 287
tachypnea, 71
task force, 120, 217
tau, 264, 277, 279, 285, 293
taxonomy, 180, 181
temperature, 51, 63, 89, 94, 128, 281
testing, 49, 56, 61, 69, 77, 78, 89, 95, 118, 139, 140, 141, 146, 148, 150, 157, 159, 161, 170, 171, 175, 176, 189, 194, 195, 196, 199, 211, 213, 215, 216, 229, 230, 244, 248, 253, 254, 260, 270
testosterone, 288
therapeutics, 45
therapy methods, 219
thermoregulation, 125
thorax, 180
threshold level, 201
thyroid, 35, 37, 170
tissue, 3, 31, 35, 64, 71, 73, 85, 132, 167, 168, 185, 187, 247, 266, 279
tissue transglutaminase, 126
TLR9, 106
TNF, 55, 273
tobacco, 295
tofu, 15
toll like receptor 9 (TLR9) agonists, 106
tonsillectomy, 153
toxicity, 34, 230
toxin, 66
trachea, 255
tracheostomy, 76
transfusion reactions, 3
translocation, 125
transport, 127, 132
transportation, 240
trauma, 281, 288
tremor, 70, 71
trial, 63, 104, 106, 123, 124, 212, 224, 241, 256, 261
tricyclic antidepressants, 70, 88
triggers, 1, 2, 4, 12, 13, 14, 17, 18, 20, 37, 38, 44, 54, 61, 69, 77, 88, 164, 220, 227, 229, 230, 231, 245
trypsin, 52, 63, 113, 185
tryptase, 45, 51, 56, 57, 58, 59, 60, 63, 66, 67, 76, 148, 276, 292
TSH, 288
tuberculosis, 17
tumor(s), 35, 37, 41, 45, 290
turnover, 292, 294